DATE DUE			

rists

T
RUST
ATION

Psychology for Psychiatrists

Edited by

DEEPA S. GUPTA, MB, ChB
Leeds Community and Mental Health Services

RAJINDER M. GUPTA, PhD
Dudley Psychology and Counselling Services

W

WHURR PUBLISHERS
LONDON AND PHILADELPHIA

British Library Cataloguing in Publication Data
A catalogue record for this book is available from the British
Library.

ISBN 1 86156 140 7

Printed and bound in the UK by Athenaeum Press Ltd,
Gateshead, Tyne & Wear

Contents

Contributors

Nick Banks, Social Sciences Department, University of Birmingham.

Mark Blagrove, Psychology Department, University of Swansea.

M.C. Chung, Lecturer in Social Sciences (Psychology) Applied to Medicine, University of Sheffield.

Guy Cumberbatch, Head of Psychology Department, University College Worcester.

Peter Davies, Department of Psychology, University of Leeds.

M. Eacott, Department of Psychology, Durham University.

Helen Graham, Psychology Department, Keele University.

Paul Humphreys, Senior Lecturer in Psychology, University College Worcester.

G. Kent, Department of Psychology, University of Sheffield.

G. Matthews, Department of Psychology, University of Cincinnati, Ohio.

John Pickering, Psychology Department, Warwick University, Coventry.

Helen Ross, Psychology Department, University of Stirling.

K. Sheehy, Head of Behavioural Science, Department of Special Education, St Patrick's College.

Richard Toogood, District Clinical Psychologist and Regional Clinical Advisor, Dudley Priority NHS Trust.

D. Trent, Consultant Clinical Psychologist, Walsall Community Health Trust and Director, Midland Psychological Services, Sutton Coldfield.

G. Turpin, Department of Psychology, University of Sheffield.

Janet R. Wheatley, Honorary Senior Lecturer, University of Birmingham, Deputy Director South Birmingham Psychology Service.

M. Williams, Department of Psychology, University of Reading.

Introduction

The major thrust of most psychiatrists' clinical work is the diagnosis, treatment and prevention of both mild and severe mental illnesses. In order to do this they require both medical training and a sound grasp of psychological knowledge. The latest MRCPsych Part 1 and 2 syllabi and the examination requirements reflect this. For example, primacy and latency effects may affect the point in the consultation at which information is given to the patient. Learning theory and behaviour or cognitive modification are used extensively in both child and adult psychiatry.

The genesis of this book lies in the first editor's first-hand knowledge and experience of MRCPsych Part 1 syllabus and examination. While preparing for the MRCPsych Part 1 examination she found that, although there were some excellent psychology textbooks on the market, none of them appeared to have been written specifically with these candidates' needs in mind. Many candidates who have to use these texts seem to feel that some have details that are superfluous to their needs and others may not be detailed enough or are not clinically relevant.

In planning and editing this book, we have tried to bear in mind the shortcomings of the psychology textbooks commonly used by psychiatrists in training and we have attempted to avoid these limitations in our book. In other words, this book has been written principally with 'psychiatrists in training' in mind. The book is also likely to be useful to other professionals, particularly school medical officers, pediatricians, community psychiatric nurses and social workers who, we believe, also require a good deal of knowledge of psychology in their day-to-day work.

The strength of this volume is twofold. First, it has contributions by some of the most prominent people in their field. They have tried to write their respective chapters in an accessible style (but retaining their individuality) while remaining very authoritative in their content. A few have been written by practising psychologists who have vast experience of working with psychiatrist colleagues, both trained and in training. We feel, therefore, that it is a positive feature that this book is multi-authored as opposed to written by just one or two people. Secondly, the book has been edited by the collaborative efforts of a psychiatrist and a psychologist. They have been able to oversee the contents of this book from two different perspectives, hopefully increasing its usefulness.

The book follows more-or-less the same format as the MRCPsych Part 1 syllabus except for a few minor changes. For instance, it has included neuropsychology and psychological assessment in the basic psychology section. The other change is that we have covered topics to do with methodology and measurement in the chapter entitled 'Some empirical approaches to individual differences', and this may be found in the first part of the book.

Psychology for Psychiatrists has two further features. First, each chapter provides a list of key concepts and the individuals they are associated with. For instance, in Chapter 1, the reader will notice that *structuralism* is associated with Wilhelm Wundt, Herman Ebbinghaus, Oswald Külpe and Edward Titchner. In Chapter 14, on human development, the concepts of *attachment and bonding* are associated with Bowlby. This inevitably means that there is some repetition in the book. For example, certain aspects of *attitude measurement* are covered in both Chapter 13 and Chapter 19. Our main rationale was that if a few concepts are repeated and presented in two different styles it would simply help the reader to consolidate them. Furthermore, we felt that too much editing might adversely affect the flow of the chapters.

Finally, it remains for us to thank the key people who have made this book possible. First of all our deepest gratitude goes to all our contributors, not only for making a contribution but also for their patience. The second editor would particularly like to thank Richard Toogood and Nicky Whitehead, his line managers, for their encouragement and for providing him with opportunities to continue working on the book. Our sincere thanks to both Graham Sherwood and Rahul Gupta who were always more than willing to help iron out all our computer related problems. Last, but not least, it is also a great pleasure to acknowledge the help we have received from 'the Publishers' who were always there to sort out any queries and deal with any technical aspects of producing a book.

Deepa S. Gupta
Rajinder M. Gupta

Part One:
Basic Psychology

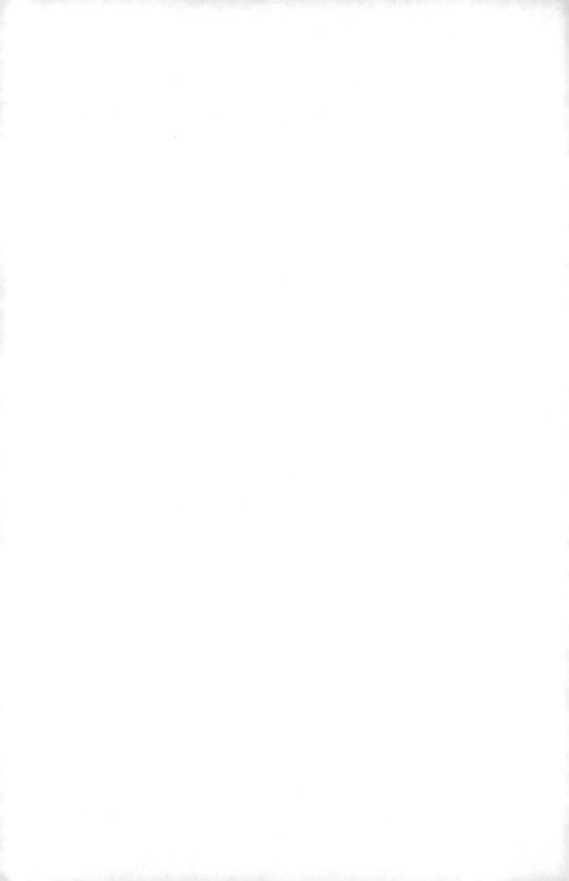

Chapter 1
Behaviourism and learning theory

DENNIS TRENT

Key concepts	Key names
Structuralism	Wilhelm Wundt, Hermann Ebbinghaus, Oswald Külpe, Edward Titchener
Functionalism	Charles Darwin, Sir Francis Galton, William James, G. Stanley Hall, James Cattell, John Dewey, James Angell, Harvey Carr, Robert Woodworth
Classical conditioning	Ivan Pavlov
Operant conditioning	B.F. Skinner, C.L. Hull
Systematic desensitization	J. Wolpe
Reciprocal inihibition	
Shaping	B.F. Skinner
Modelling	A. Bandura
Rational emotive therapy	Albert Ellis
Cognitive therapy	Aaron T. Beck
Habituation	
Reinforcement	
Escape	
Avoidance	
Punishment	
Behaviourism	
Cost response	
Chaining	

Introduction

Behaviourism, like all disciplines in psychology, began with the first people sitting around a campfire watching each other to discover whether or not it was safe to remain. Since then, the study of human behaviour has been one of constant understanding and misunderstanding.

Probably the most important event in the whole of psychology occurred in 1859 when the naturalist Charles Darwin published *On the Origin of Species by Natural Selection*. It was not really his idea, as his grandfather, Erasmus Darwin, had already written a treatise on the subject. Even he, though, did not have the idea. It can be traced back to the fifth century BC.

The importance of Darwin's work for psychology is that it formed the origin of the four major schools of psychology. Darwin's thesis argued that man had evolved from earlier forms, therefore if man was to be understood, we could look at animals to gain that understanding. After all, if one wants to understand the workings of a Ferrari, it is easier to start with an old Humber and work our way up because the basic functions remain the same.

Second, his theory stated that, since animals adapt to their environment, they must be learning – and the basis for learning theory and much of behaviourism came from this assumption. At the same time, the question of individual differences within any species arose and this in many ways formed the underlying structure for cognitive studies. Against this remained the creationists' view that man had been made separate and distinct from all other animals and was therefore unique in both origins and functions. This laid the groundwork for much humanistic/existentialist thinking.

It is easy, then, to see how Darwin became so integral to future work in the area of psychology. With so much discussion going on different ideas began to emerge and began to form into schools of thought. There was a rise in *structuralism* as an attempt was made to analyse consciousness into its component parts and discover the structure of consciousness. Early structuralists included Wilhelm Wundt (1832–1920), Hermann Ebbinghaus (1850–1909), Oswald Külpe (1862–1915), and Edward Titchener (1867–1927). It was the main aim of structuralism to turn psychology into a science that could be understood and tested in systematic and repeatable ways.

The structuralist study of the mind, while telling us how it worked, did not help people understand anything about the results or accomplishments of that activity. Not that it was supposed to, as science was not seen as describing at that time, but more as testing. As such, there began to grow a new school of psychology that focused on the functions rather than the structure of the mind. It was appropriately known as *functionalism*. These functionalists were far more interested in what the mind did and how it did it than in how it was structured. Again, we see the strong influence of Darwin as one of the driving influences in functionalism. The theory of evolution was, in its own right, an explanation in functionalist terms as it gave a mechanism as to how changes occurred.

Other functionalists included Sir Francis Galton (1822–1911) and his work on individual differences. In America we began to see the start of functionalism with people like William James (1842–1910), G. Stanley Hall (1844–1924), and James Cattell (1860–1944). These ideas continued with John Dewey (1859–1952), James Angell (1869–1949), Harvey Carr (1873–1954), and Robert Woodworth (1869–1962).

It was within this framework, with structuralism still holding on and functionalism beginning to stabilize as a mature school of thought, that behaviourism made its entrance as a major theoretical assumption. The introduction of behaviourism, unlike the slow transition from structuralism to functionalism, was abrupt, traumatic and total. This was not a realignment of past ideas, but was a total break with them which offered no compromise. The new leader was a man named John Broadus Watson (1878–1958). He argued for a totally independent and objective psychology that dealt only with observable behaviours that could be described in terms such as stimulus and response. His application of research techniques to human behaviour was a direct outgrowth of his work with animal behaviour, an area in which he had been active for some time.

Along with Watson, others were studying animals and their behaviours. Not only was Freud looking at animals to establish the structure of personality in the far more complex human, Edward Lee Thorndike (1874–1949) was using experimental investigations to develop an objective and mechanistic theory of learning. He again believed that psychology had to study only the behaviour of the animal and disregard the mental elements or conscious experience of the mind.

The early 1900s were pivotal in psychology. With individuals such as Freud, Watson, Thorndike and others, psychology was entering new areas and the study of man was no longer limited to the realms of physical illness. To paraphrase an old song, 'psychology was here to stay'.

As noted above, by the early twentieth century a great deal of work had already been started in the area of behaviourism and behavioural psychology within both Europe and North America. However, the first of two major impacts was not to come from within but – as is often the case – from an unrelated source, namely the work of Pavlov (1849–1936).

Behaviourism and conditioning

In his work, Pavlov used a method of tapping into the subject's (dog's) glands surgically so as to drain off the digestive secretions to a location outside the body in order to measure them. One aspect of his work dealt with the function of saliva, which would involuntarily be secreted when food was placed in the dog's mouth. His work went well until he began to obtain results that did not fit either with earlier results or expectations. What he discovered was that the dogs would begin to salivate when they heard the footsteps of the individual tasked with feeding them. The reflex had become attached to, or conditioned to, stimuli that previously would not have elicited the response but had been associated with feeding. These *psychic reflexes* as Pavlov originally called them, had developed by a phenomenon that was referred to as *association by frequency of occurrence*. This was later to be known as *classical conditioning*.

Classical conditioning

Classical conditioning refers to the process identified by Pavlov. It occurs when responses that naturally occur in relation to one stimulus are tied to an unrelated stimulus so that they occur in response to that stimulus. It can be demonstrated graphically quite easily (see Figure 1.1).

Unconditioned Stimulus ———————————————— Unconditioned Response

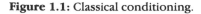

Conditioned Stimulus   ————————————   Conditioned Response

Figure 1.1: Classical conditioning.

The *unconditioned stimulus* is always the one that automatically causes the response. In Pavlov's case, the unconditioned stimulus was the food given to the dogs. It is a natural response for food to cause salivation in dogs and therefore no conditioning is required for the dog to salivate to food. The *unconditioned response* is the automatic response to a given stimulus. In Pavlov's experiment, the unconditioned response is the salivation. When food is given to a dog, the dog will salivate. It does not have to do or learn anything, it is automatic.

The *conditioned stimulus* is the new stimulus. It is the one that would not normally create the response that is occurring. The footsteps of the person feeding the dogs formed the conditioned stimulus in Pavlov's situation. The *conditioned response* is the same response as the unconditioned response. It becomes a conditioned response when it is tied to a new stimulus. Again, in Pavlov's work, the conditioned response is the dog's salivation; the same response as before, only now as a result of the new (conditioned) stimulus.

In this example, then, the food is the unconditional stimulus, the footsteps are the conditioned stimulus and the salivation is both the unconditioned and the conditioned response depending on whether it is tied to the unconditioned or conditioned stimulus. This tying together of a response to one stimulus with a new stimulus underlies the process of classical conditioning.

A simple experiment will show how classical conditioning works. Take a person and stand face to face. Draw in a breath so that it is audible and then blow a puff of air across the eyelash of the person who is acting as the subject. Blow hard enough so that it is clearly felt, but not so hard as to be uncomfortable. When the puff of air hits the person's eyelash, he or she will blink. The puff of air is the unconditioned stimulus and the blink is the unconditioned response. It is an automatic response to blink when a puff of air hits a person's eyelash. Audibly draw in another breath and do the same thing again. Do this five times and then, without telling the person acting as the subject, draw in a breath and hold it. Most people will blink in anticipation of the puff of air. In this case, the audible drawing in of breath becomes the conditioned stimulus and the blink becomes the conditioned response. It is conditioned because people do not naturally blink when someone draws in a breath.

Applications of classical conditioning

Classical conditioning is one of the first ways in which a child learns. As it is a pairing of two events, that pairing is unrelated to other skills or ability of the individual. Because of this, the person does not need to have an elaborate abstract symbolic representation of the event. In other words, it can occur before the individual becomes verbal. The individual does not need an in-depth understanding of what good and bad are in order to pair an event with displeasure. There is no need to even understand the idea of pleasure. As such, once something is experienced as either desirable or undesirable, and that feeling is paired with a conditioned stimulus, that stimulus will continue to elicit that response. This can be very powerful since if the conditioned pairing occurred before the individual had a mechanism for identifying and describing the stimulus, it will be difficult to identify and alter that pairing.

Classical conditioning is not all bad, however. Classical conditioning is extremely useful in trying to alter responses to events. As noted with 'Alex' in *A Clockwork Orange*, no thought or internal dialogue had to be entered into in order for him to respond in a different way. The original behaviours were also not unconditional. That is, it is not a natural response of humans to become violent or sexually aroused when meeting or seeing another human being. It is also not a natural response for an individual to become afraid of a stimulus or situation that would normally pose little or no threat. Classical conditioning, then, becomes one of the best ways of treating such irrational fears or phobias.

Wolpe (1958) used the term *reciprocal inhibition* to argue that, if anxiety could inhibit a normal response, a normal response could inhibit anxiety. This then became the prototype for a process he began called *systematic desensitization*. Systematic desensitization is a clear example of classical conditioning. In systematic desensitization, individuals are encouraged to make a *hierarchy* of their fears and to approach them in order while pairing them with positive responses. As the presentation of the stimulus creates fear or anxiety, the presentation of the stimulus under a systematic desentization regime is paired with a state of relaxation. There are, therefore, three definitive steps: teaching the individual deep relaxation techniques, helping the individual make a hierarchy of situations inducing anxiety, and the pairing of the two.

Deep relaxation is a skill that can be learned by anyone with the appropriate motivation. Relaxation is the natural state of the body and we have all been relaxed at periods of time throughout our lives. Either a *tense-release* or a *guided fantasy* can be used and once states of deep relaxation can be achieved comfortably with regularity, pairings can begin to take place. Even the process of achieving a state of relaxation can be paired. Russell and Sipich (1973) referred to pairing a word such as 'calm' or 'relax' with states of relaxation in order to function as a cue for deep relaxation.

While the individual is learning to achieve states of deep relaxation, the question of the hierarchy can be addressed. In order to build an effective hierarchy, it is imperative to remember that the hierarchy belongs to the individual and it is that person who must create it. The hierarchy is a listing of situations that produce sequentially higher degrees of anxiety when faced by the individual. For example, in the case of a fear of spiders, a five-step hierarchy where 'one' produces the least amount of anxiety and 'five' produces the most may look something like this:

5. Touching a spider or having it crawl on me.
4. Being in the same room with a spider, which is not contained.
3. Seeing a spider in a closed case (for example, in a zoo or one mounted in a display).
2. Seeing a picture of a spider.
1. Saying or hearing the word 'spider'.

Within such a hierarchy, the process is one of exposing the individual to events at the first level. As anxiety mounts, the individual attempts to relax until both the presentation of the stimulus and deep states of relaxation are achievable simultaneously. Once this is done, the individual moves up to the next higher level and repeats the process. This continues until stimuli that used to create high levels of anxiety are endurable in a relaxed manner. Again, however, it must be noted that if the items on the hierarchy are assigned arbitrarily or are chosen by someone other than the subject, the likelihood of success is going to be limited at best.

Stimulus–response and a new breed of theorists

Although much of behavioural research was focusing on classical conditioning, there were those who argued that any behaviour was nothing more than a response to a stimulus. This argument was put forth most cogently by a young experimental psychologist who believed that all behaviour could be broken down into discrete behaviour patterns. Burrhus Frederick Skinner (1904–90) began looking at the operations performed by the organism in relation to learning.

Operant conditioning

One of Skinner's main disagreements with Pavlov was in the area of the role of the subject. Pavlov saw classical conditioning as taking place respondently – that is, the organism (dog) did not have to interact with the world in any way to make the connection; all it had to do was to respond to the events around it. *Operant conditioning,* on the other hand, argues that the organism affects the world and vice versa. Skinner then argued that the organism is part of the process and has some control or effect in how that process takes place. It was his argument that, as the organism acted on its environment, the environment would react and thereby increase or decrease the likelihood of future actions by the organism.

In operant conditioning, the behaviour occurs without any observable external stimulus. It is the organism's actions that drive the learning rather than the actions of another. The organism's response appears spontaneous and independent of any known stimulus. Skinner believed that operant behaviour was much more representative of real-life human learning experiences and therefore the most effective approach to a science of learning behaviour was through the study of conditioning and the extinction of operant behaviours.

The underlying premise of operant conditioning is that behaviours that are reinforced are likely to continue and those that are not will become extinct or cease to occur. Conditioning, then, depends on the interplay between two functions; the *type of reinforcement* and the *timing of that reinforcement*. These again can best be represented in a figure. Figure 1.2 looks at the types of reinforcement.

	Increase	Decrease
Give	Positive Reinforcement	Punishment
Receive	Negative Reinforcement	Cost Response

Figure 1.2: Types of reinforcement.

Behaviour can be reinforced either by giving a person something or taking it away. Moreover, the intention of the reinforcement can either be to increase or decrease the likelihood of the target behaviour. If a person is given something in order to increase the likelihood that behaviour will reoccur; it is called *positive reinforcement*. In order for positive reinforcement to be effective, the reinforcer must be seen by the organism to be desirable. If the organism does not, it is highly unlikely that the reward would be seen as such and that the behaviour would be repeated. For this reason, it is advisable to allow the individual to be a participant in choosing the reward if possible.

If an organism is given something in order to reduce the likelihood of a given behaviour reoccurring, it is called *punishment*. As with positive reinforcement, punishment depends on the view of the organism. The organism must see the punishment as undesirable. If it is seen as desirable, then it is likely to be interpreted by the organism as positive reinforcement and the behaviour would increase. Clearly punishing children for bad behaviour by forcing them to eat ice cream is unlikely to have the desired effect.

If something is taken away from an organism in an attempt to increase the likelihood of a given behaviour, it is *negative reinforcement*. A negative reinforcer, like a punishment, must be seen as undesirable. It is the removal of the noxious stimulus that enhances the likelihood of a behaviour reoccurring. If the stimulus were to be seen by the organism as positive, its removal would be seen as a loss rather than as a gain and the behaviour would be likely to decrease. As an example, imagine a person with a headache. Let us assume that two behaviours were tried to make the headache go away. In the first effort an aspirin was taken and in the second, the person took a paracetamol. If the headache was not removed by the aspirin but was by the paracetamol, it is far more likely that the person will go directly to the paracetamol the next time a headache occurs. The noxious stimulus (the headache) was removed and the likelihood of the behaviour (taking paracetamol) is increased.

Finally, if something is taken away in order to decrease the likelihood of a behaviour reoccurring, it is called *cost response*. This is a common form of disciplining children. Taking away a child's freedom by 'grounding' the child is an example of cost response, as is not allowing them to watch a favourite television programme.

Clearly there can be some confusion. Cost response is often seen as punishment and is frequently included under that umbrella. The important difference is that punishment is given and cost response is taken away. That is, if I give you a slap it is punishment while if I take away your sweet it is cost response. A great deal of confusion is also likely to occur between negative reinforcement and punishment. Negative reinforcement is not applied, it is removed. It is frequently said that a little negative reinforcement needs to be applied to get someone to stop doing something; however, if it is applied to get someone to stop something, it is punishment, not negative reinforcement. Negative reinforcement is taken away and will increase, not decrease the likelihood of a behaviour.

Just to make things a bit more confusing, it will sometimes be the case that an individual will gain both positive reinforcement in the form of attention or advantages of some kind and negative reinforcement in the avoidance of some aversive consequences at the same time in regard to the same behaviour. This is referred to as a *secondary gain* in that the negative reinforcement is secondary to the primary reinforcer; that is, it comes along as a secondary rather than a primary reinforcer. A person who attempts to feign a mental disorder in order to avoid a severe penalty has a strong secondary gain underlying his behaviour. That is, while immediate attention and acceptance of his story may reinforce his behaviour, the secondary effect of avoiding a lengthy punishment will have a strong effect on his behaviour.

Remember that in order for a reward to be seen as a reward, the organism must see it as desirable. Because of this, the reinforcer for any given behaviour can change over time. Someone may see chocolate as a strong reward and respond accordingly. When pregnant, however, she may not be able to tolerate chocolate and its value as a reward is lost.

The other function of reinforcement is the schedule by which the reinforcement is applied. Figure 1.3 is a diagram of the possible schedule variations.

	Event	Time
Fixed	Fixed Ratio	Fixed Interval
Variable	Variable Ratio	Variable Interval

Figure 1.3: Schedules of reinforcement.

As with the types of reinforcement, the schedule, or the manner in which the reinforcement is applied, can also be displayed as a four-way matrix. In a schedule of reinforcement, items can either be based on a fixed schedule, that is one that does not change, or it can be based on a variable schedule, that is one that continually changes. Those changes can also be based either on each event or on a period of time.

Looking at Figure 1.3, it can be shown that the four options are a *fixed ratio*, a *variable ratio*, a *fixed interval* and a *variable interval*. Each of these has a different effect on the organism and its ability to learn a desired goal or behaviour.

A fixed ratio is one in which there is a constant ratio between the number of occurrences of the behaviour and the number of occurrences of the reward. The most common is a 1:1 ratio in which, each time the behaviour occurs, a reward is given. This is the fastest way to instil a new behaviour and is often used by persons trying to teach their pets new behaviours. In this pattern, each time my dog sits up, I give her a treat. The result is that my dog will begin to incorporate the behaviour in order to get the desired treat. Because the treat is something the dog wants and the intent is to increase the likelihood of the behaviour, the treat would be a positive reinforcement.

In a variable ratio, the frequency of the ratio is constantly changing. As such, I may give my dog a treat after the first occurrence and then after the second, the fifth, the third, and so forth. As the dog does not know when the treat is coming, she will continue to exhibit the behaviour in the hope that this might be the time a treat is given. This principle underlies the payout system on a gaming machine. Whether it is a fruit machine in a pub or a slot machine in Las Vegas or Monte Carlo, the coins go in on the chance that this may be the time this machine pays off. While a fixed ratio, especially a 1:1, is the fastest way to instil a new behaviour, a variable ratio is the best way to maintain behaviour.

A fixed interval schedule is one in which reinforcement is given based on the passage of a given amount of time regardless of the number of behaviours observed. An example of this would be to give my dog a treat every five minutes no matter how often she sat up. Since the giving of the reward is contingent on the passage of time rather than the exhibition of behaviours, it is time passage that will be learned, not the desired behaviour, and my dog is likely to learn how long five minutes is rather than how to sit up.

The fourth schedule is a variable interval schedule, in which a reward is given randomly without regard to either the passage of time or the exhibition of behaviours. In this case, the reward is not contingent on either and it is highly unlikely that the dog will learn anything.

It is clear, after looking at both types of reinforcers and the schedule by which they are given, that the primary necessity for a reward system to work is that the organism sees the reward as contingent on the behaviour. That is, the reward (or punishment) must be seen as occurring as a result of the production of the desired behaviours. Obviously, the closer the reward is given to the exhibition of the behaviour, the more likely the organism will see the two as related and learn from the experience. This can also be graphed as in Figure 1.4.

	Immediate	Delayed
Before	Ante-proximal	Ante-distal
After	Post-proximal	Post-distal

Figure 1.4: Proximity of reinforcement.

The farther the reward is separated from the behaviour, the less likely the organism is to make the connection between the two. As a result of this, rewards given either long before (*ante-distal*) or after a behaviour (*post-distal*) are likely not to function well as reinforcers. In each of these cases it is difficult for the organism to see the reward as contingent on the production of the desired behaviours. If the reward is given shortly before the behaviour (*ante-proximal*), a contingency may be seen by the organism, but is likely to be reversed such that the behaviour is seen as contingent on the giving of the reward and therefore will only occur once a reward is given. Clearly then, it can be seen that rewarding shortly after a behaviour (*post-proximal*) is the most effective and the closer the reward is given to the exhibition of the behaviour the more effective it will be as a reward.

Other forms of learning

Within the process of operant conditioning, it is necessary to break behaviours down so that each sub-behaviour can be seen as a compilation of other more finite behaviours. For example, for someone who is sitting watching TV to get a drink, the person must get out of the chair, move toward the kitchen, go to the sink, turn on the water, and so forth. If the behaviour desired is complex, it may be necessary to break it down into component parts. By doing this each component can be reinforced in sequence, thereby leading the organism to the desired behaviour. This process of *sequential reinforcement* or the reinforcement of closer approximations to a desired behaviour is referred to as *shaping*. Shaping is one of the ways we teach our children to walk, speak and act and is a very powerful method. A child may begin by producing an unclear 'th' sound and the parents will accept it. Over time, however, through reinforcing closer approximations to the desired sound, the child is able to redefine the sound so that it is produced appropriately. One very close to shaping is the technique called *cueing and fading*. Cueing essentially consists of introducing discriminative stimuli that have a very high probability of triggering the appropriate behaviours. This is a technical way of saying that a person can use something to trigger a response. An example is to use the word 'calm' in order to initiate or enhance a relaxation response. As the person continues to repeat the word, they become progressively more relaxed. Fading refers to the tendency for a response to fade or become weaker over time.

Fading occurs when a behaviour artificially reinforced on a contingent basis over time is slowly withdrawn. For example, in the case of my dog, I give her a treat each time she sits up. This would not happen in normal circumstances and is used by me to train her. Gradually the artificial reinforcement of giving her a treat will need to be faded out so that more natural reinforcers such as attention or approval can take over. The slow withdrawal of the artificial reinforcer (the treat) is called fading.

Another concept that must be understood in order to understand behaviour and learning theory is that of *extinction*. Extinction is the unlearning of a behaviour and occurs when behaviour is not reinforced over a period of time. In the example of trying to teach my dog to sit up, if no reward was given (that is, no artificial reward such as a treat or natural reward such as attention), after a period of time she would stop sitting up. This can occur either by my not giving my dog rewards, or her decision that the item I am giving her is no longer desirable. Since extinction is the process of unlearning, and since nothing can be totally unlearned, a behaviour will come back more quickly than when it was originally learned, however the speed with which a behaviour is recovered after extinction is determined by the type of behaviour, the reinforcer, the extent of extinction and the person. In other words, the speed of recovery of a behaviour cannot be predetermined.

Another form of classical conditioning involves a process called *aversion therapy*. Aversion therapy links a noxious result to a behaviour that previously had a positive one. One of the most powerful books dealing with classical conditioning was Anthony Burgess' *A Clockwork Orange* (1962). Burgess made a strong argument against classical conditioning when he wrote his book. In it, the main character, Alex, is extremely violent with little regard for the rights of others. After being sent to prison for a particularly violent offence, he is made to watch violent and pornographic films while being given a drug to make him nauseous. The two events, the violent or sexual thoughts and the nausea, are paired together through classical conditioning. The result is that whenever Alex thinks of either sex or violence, he becomes violently ill and cannot act out on his thoughts.

Burgess also points out one of the difficulties with classical conditioning. That is, one can never be certain of the pairing that is going on within the individual. While Alex is forced to watch the films, Mozart and Beethoven are being played as background music. Classical music is the only positive thing in his life. The result is that he is also inadvertently conditioned to become violently ill whenever he hears Mozart, Beethoven or other, 'music that was like for the emotions'. Those giving him the behavioural modification have thereby inadvertently removed the one positive source of enjoyment leaving him with only his negative, violent and sexual, sources of enjoyment. As with Alex, inadvertent pairings can occur with little or no recognition by the psychiatrist at the time.

One of the classic examples of this in real life was the use of electric shock, which was given to smokers who tried to quit. Every time the smoker would reach for a cigarette, a shock was given until the smoker paired the negative result of the shock with the action of reaching for a cigarette. This also underlies the use of substances like Antabuse with alcoholic patients. The nausea resulting from the interaction of the drug with the alcohol is paired with drinking and the drinker quits. If the aversive stimulus was no longer seen as aversive, it is likely that the behaviour would either continue or restart.

If a behaviour begins and is punished, the person may begin to recognize that it is about to be applied. The person may begin to anticipate the punishment and change behaviours before the punishment is applied, thereby avoiding the punishment. This is referred to as *avoidance training*. A simple example would be of a person who has been bitten by a dog. By avoiding all dogs, he avoids the punishment of being bitten by another one. If, on the other hand, the individual cannot avoid the punishment, but a rapid change of behaviours will terminate the punishment, the process is called *escape training* as the individual is escaping from the punishment rather than avoiding it. The case of applying electric shocks when a person lights a cigarette is an example. The shock continues until the person stops smoking or puts the cigarette out and then stops. It is clear within this example that escape training is a form of aversion therapy.

By now it is probably clear that there is a lot of overlap between classical and operant conditioning. For example, while aversion therapy may be seen as an operant process in which a punishment is administered in response to an undesired behaviour, it can also be seen as a classical pairing.

People also learn by observing or imitating others. *Observational learning* has also been called *modelling* as the person duplicates the actions of the model. This is the 'monkey see, monkey do' assumption where a person (or animal) watches another and performs in a similar way. We will find this when young people begin to dress or act like their heroes or idols. This was clearly pointed out in a no smoking campaign run a few years ago in which a father was seen washing his car and his son of two or three was washing the tyre with him. The father then went on to mow the lawn and the son followed along pushing a toy lawn mower. The third shot shows the father lighting a cigarette and the son reaching for the packet.

There is an old saying that children live what they learn and they learn a great deal by listening and watching others. Any parent who has had a child say something in public that they had said in private is aware of the process. Clearly the environment along with the relationship between the individual and the person whose behaviour is being imitated are the most important factors in determining the level and extent of learning within a modelling or observational learning paradigm. Bandura (1977) lists four processes inherent in modelling. They include attention to the modelled events, the retention of what is learned from that observation, the ability to reproduce a model's behaviour and the motivation to do so. The more important the model and/or the more to be gained by adopting the behaviours, the more likely that the behaviour will be incorporated into the person's repertoire.

General issues about behaviourism

If we accept that a stimulus elicits a response, it can be seen that, if the stimulus is repeated over time, the response will decrease. This is a process of *habituation* and is the result of the same basic process that requires more of a drug to be administered in order to obtain the same result. As the stimulus elicits the response, the response to the stimulus weakens. An example is the ticking of a clock. When a person enters a strange room in which there is a grandfather clock, the person is likely to turn to look at the clock when the ticking becomes known. After a while, however, the ticking fades into the background and the person no longer responds to it. The response has been habituated since the ticking has not changed. Spontaneous recovery occurs if the stimulus is withheld. The response will tend to recover over time. If a behaviour is habituated and spontaneously recovered repeatedly over time, habituation becomes more rapid. Other things being equal, the more rapid the frequency of stimulation, the more rapid and/or more pronounced is the habituation. By the same token, the weaker the stimulus, the more rapid and/or more pronounced the habituation. Strong stimulation may yield no habituation. *Dishabituation* is the opposite of habituation, which is the process of becoming more rather than less responsive to a stimulus. An example may be the sensitivity a soldier develops to gunfire. Even after a behaviour is fully habituated, repeated exposures will make it more resistant to dishabituation.

Hull (1943) argued that the power of any reinforcer may be transferred to another stimulus situation by constant and repeated association. This is very close to the same process that Pavlov set out as classical conditioning. After the reinforcement power has been transmitted to one previously neutral stimulus, it can be transferred to any number of other stimuli in a chain or series whose length is limited only by the conditions which bring about the consistent and repeated associations set up by the primary reinforcement.

Cognitive behavioural techniques

Albert Ellis, among others, was dissatisfied with the idea that people were behaving only as responses to stimuli. First of all it called the idea of free will into question and, secondly, it did not explain why two people who experienced the same event responded in different ways. It, to some degree, explained the 'how' but not the 'why'. He began what he called *rational emotive therapy* (RET) which is the forerunner of *cognitive behavioural therapy* (CBT). Aaron T. Beck has done a lot of work in this area, especially with depression, and refers to the entire area as *cognitive therapy*. The idea is that it is not the stimulus that elicits the response, but the person's perception of the stimulus. It can best be explained as the A-B-C theory of behaviour.

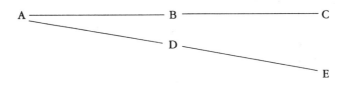

Figure 1.5: A-B-C behaviour theory.

Cognitive behavioural therapy argues that, because it is the perception of an event or situation that determines the response, if one changes that perception the response must change. An example is to become terrified of the book you are holding. Do not pretend you are terrified or act as you would if you were, but actually become terrified of it. You probably cannot because the book does not present a threat to you. If you were to perceive the book as dangerous in some way, however, it would create fear. The reality is that you cannot feel fear without the sense of threat and if a threatening object or situation loses that threat, you cannot retain the fear. It is the perception of threat that drives the feeling or response, not the stimulus.

How behaviourism works

So how does behaviourism work in the real world? Let us create a person named Sam. As a child, Sam is very interested in sports and decides to emulate his hero, who is a noted football player. Sam begins to walk like his hero and to act in the way that he has seen his hero act while on television. Sam is now engaging in *modelling* or *observational learning*. As Sam grows older, he gets a dog and wants to train his dog how to retrieve the ball for him. Clearly he cannot tell the dog directly because the dog cannot understand him. Rather he begins to *reinforce* the dog's behaviours. He reinforces behaviours closer and closer to the desired behaviour and continues to reinforce them each time they occur. He is now *shaping* the dog's behaviour with a 1:1 ratio reinforcement schedule.

While training the dog, he was bitten by a spider and became ill. This occurred while he was in the back garden and Sam paired being in the back garden with the illness so that whenever he went into his back garden he became ill. We now have a case of *classical conditioning*. He then generalized this to all back gardens and now will not enter into any rear garden. As his girlfriend enjoys siting in the back garden and Sam wants to be with her, he goes to see a therapist who has him set out a hierarchy tied to a relaxation process which ultimately results in his relaxed presence in rear gardens. Sam has now begun a *systematic desensitization* process. He also decides that he would like to stop smoking in order to play better. His therapist applies mild electric shocks to his fingertips each time he reaches for a cigarette. Sam has now experienced aversive therapy.

Finally, Tolman (1948) noted what he termed *sign learning*, in which rats gained an idea about what to expect within a maze. He called these expectations *cognitive maps* and hypothesized that they represented a perceptual map of the maze. Restle (1957) tested this theory by training rats to run a maze. He then flooded the maze and the rats were able to swim the maze without error even though they did not have the same set of stimuli.

It now can be seen that behaviourism has far-reaching applications and can effect wide and enduring changes in people's behaviour.

Summary

Clearly it is not the intention of this chapter to give a full, in-depth review of all behavioural theory. The works of Watson, Thorndike and others have been glossed over and their contribution to the understanding of behaviour has been woefully underrepresented. As with any overview, however, it is not possible to do justice to everything. A recognition, however, of both classical and operant conditioning along with an understanding of the different types and schedules of reinforcement is essential if one is to understand the concept of behaviourism or learning theory.

Knowing the principles and mechanics, however, is not enough. As with any concept or process, the more powerful it is the more good, or harm, it can do. Behavioural techniques are one of the most powerful interventions that can be made and as such, if poorly understood or inappropriately applied, they can be markedly harmful. Over the past years programmes such as the 'pin-down' programme used in Staffordshire have been in the news, not for the good that might have come from them if they had been appropriately designed and applied, but for the harm they caused from their inappropriate design and application. Pin-down was an attempt to apply behavioural techniques to the management of the behaviour of children in care, however it was not well designed and was inappropriately applied. It brought out the worst in behavioural modification because the people using it were not appropriately trained.

References

Bandura A (1977) Social Learning Theory. Englewood Cliffs: Prentice-Hall.

Burgess A (1962) A Clockwork Orange. New York: Buccaneer Books.

Hull CL (1943) Essentials of Behaviour. New Haven: Yale University Press.

Restle F (1957) Cited in Gross RD (1988) Psychology: The Science of Mind and Behaviour. London: Edward Arnold.

Russell R, Sipich J (1973) Cue-controlled relaxation in the treatment of test anxiety. Journal of Behavioural Therapy and Experimental Psychiatry 4: 47–9.

Tolman EC (1948) Cognitive maps in rats and men. Psychological Review 55: 189–208.

Wolpe J (1958) Psychotherapy by Reciprocal Inhibition. Stanford: Stanford University Press.

Suggestions for further reading

I would suggest that the starting point for further reading is a good basic textbook in behaviour therapy. A good one is:

Rim DC, Masters JC (1979) Behavior Therapy Techniques and Empirical Findings. London, New York: Academic Press.

There are a number of others available. You may also want to check out the following:

Dryden W (ed.) (1995) Rational Emotive Behaviour Therapy: A Reader. London: Sage.

This is a good source of general information. It brings together some of the most important writings of the past decade on rational emotive behavioural therapy (REBT).

Dryden W (ed.) (1995) Brief Rational Emotive Behaviour Therapy (Wiley Series in Brief Therapy and Counselling). Chichester: John Wiley & Sons.

This book looks at a brief form of therapy consisting of a fixed number of sessions within an REBT process. This is an easily read book with a lot of good information.

Gilbert P (1997) Overcoming Depression: A Self-Help Guide using Cognitive Behavioural Techniques. London: Robinson Publishing.

This is one of a series looking at cognitive behavioural therapy (CBT) techniques targeted at specific disorders. They are again written in plain English with little or no jargon. Other titles focus on anxiety and panic, with anorexia and low self-esteem planned along with others.

Chapter 2
Sensation and perception

HELEN E. ROSS

Key concepts	Key names
Nativists	Gestalt psychologists, Kant
Empiricists	Helmholtz
Tabula rasa	Locke
Proprioception	
Exteroception	
Kinaesthesis	
Extrasensory perception (ESP)	
Telepathy	
Clairvoyance	
Precognition	
Psychokinesis	
Psychophysics	Weber, Fechner, Stevens
Outer	
Inner (neurophysiology)	
Weber's law	
Signal detection theory	Swets
Theories of colour vision	Young, Helmholtz, Hering
Phi phenomenon	
Gestalt theory	Wertheimer, Koffka, Köhler
Isomorphism	
Constancy	Gestalt psychologists
Figural aftereffects	
Contingent aftereffects	McCullough
or McCullough effects	
'Carpentered world' hypothesis	
Synaesthesia	
Hypnagogic (or hypnogogic) imagery	
Hypnopompic imagery	
Eidetic imagery	

Definition of perception

Perception covers a range of topics, from basic sensory processes to complex perceptual analyses. Basic processes include the mechanisms of neural coding for individual sensations and the laws of psychophysics. Complex processes include the interaction of the senses, the perception of objects and events, and the relationship between perception and action.

It is difficult to make a sharp distinction between sensation and perception. Most authors treat sensory processes as innate, but argue about the extent to which perception is learned. Traditionally, the *nativists* (such as the Gestalt psychologists in the early 1900s) believed that perception was innate, while *empiricists* or *constructivists* (for example Hermann von Helmholtz, 1821–94) believed that it was learned. The nativists followed the philosopher Immanuel Kant (1724–1804) who proposed that humans are born with knowledge of causality, space and time. The empiricists followed the philosopher John Locke (1632–1704), who likened the mind to a *tabula rasa* (blank writing slate) on which sensory experience leaves its mark. Most authors now accept a compromise and try to identify which components are innate or learned. The modern emphasis is on the difference between *bottom-up processes,* which depend on automatic mechanisms, and *top-down processes,* which depend on higher mental processes.

Individual sensations

How many senses are there?

Traditionally, following Aristotle (384–322 BC), it was argued that there were five senses (vision, hearing, taste, smell and touch) and a 'common sense' to unite them. A more recent division was the *special senses* – referring to four of the head senses (vision, hearing, taste and smell) – and some other more general senses. These divisions are no longer in use: the vestibular system is recognized as another head sense; the skin and muscle senses are further subdivided; and it can be argued that vision should be divided into two or more systems. There are also various internal sensations such as hunger, thirst, sex, and a sense of time. *Proprioception* (self-perception) is a general term for internal sensations, as opposed to *exteroception* (the perception of the outside world). *Kinaesthesis* is a branch of proprioception, and is the perception of one's own body movement and joint position. There are thus a variable number of senses, depending on the classification system.

It is sometimes claimed that humans (all or some) possess a 'sixth sense', which does not require the stimulation of a sense organ. This is known as *extrasensory perception* (ESP), and can be divided into three main categories: *telepathy* (the transfer of thoughts between people); *clairvoyance* (the awareness of objects or events without the use of any known sensory channels); *precognition* (knowledge of future events). It is also claimed that some people possess *psychokinesis* – the ability to manipulate or influence objects without touching them. Few academic psychologists accept these claims. Most would argue that much of the evidence is fraudulent and depends on the tricks used by magicians; the rest of the evidence is poorly controlled, or improperly analysed statistically. Nevertheless, many lay people are fascinated by the occult, and have strong beliefs in some form of ESP.

Neural coding

The sense organs are normally stimulated by their own specific energies; photochemical for light in the eye, auditory vibrations for the ear, and so on. *Intensity* is usually coded by the rate of firing, and by the number of different fibres firing. *Quality* is usually coded according to which particular fibres are firing, and by the pattern of firing over different fibres. Coding strategies differ for different sense organs (or *modalities*).

Psychophysics

Psychophysics is concerned with the measurement of basic sensations, such as the relation between a physical stimulus and the subsequent sensation. The subject was developed by Ernst Heinrich Weber (1795–1878), Gustav Fechner (1801–87), and more recently by S.S. Stevens (1906–73). Fechner made a distinction between *outer* and *inner* psychophysics. Outer psychophysics is concerned with the relationship between the physical stimulus and the observer's sensation or response, whereas inner psychophysics is concerned with the internal neural coding between the stimulus and the response. (Most textbooks equate psychophysics only with the outer variety, and call the inner variety *neurophysiology*.) There are two main areas of psychophysics: *sensory discrimination* (or thresholds) and *sensory magnitude*. There is also the question of whether there is a relation between the two.

Discrimination

This topic can be subdivided into *absolute* thresholds and *differential* thresholds.

The absolute threshold is the smallest amount of energy that can be detected by a sensory system. This varies in different systems. The human visual system is very sensitive (equivalent to a candle flame seen at 30 miles on a dark, clear night), whereas the sense of smell is poor compared with that of a dog.

The differential threshold is the smallest difference in a stimulus that can be discriminated. According to *Weber's law*, it is a constant fraction of the stimulus intensity. The fraction varies in different modalities from around 2/100 to 10/100.

Modern psychophysical methods are often based on *signal detection theory*, which was developed by John Swets in 1964. The mathematical theory can be applied to all senses, but it is based on an acoustical model in which the observer has to discriminate an auditory signal from a noisy background. The observer's performance is determined partly by his sensory ability and partly by his *criterion* or *response bias*. The criterion is the cut-off point for the sound level, above which the observer says that a signal is present and below which that no signal is present. The criterion can be manipulated by offering different costs and rewards for different kinds of errors and correct judgements. Errors can occur for saying 'yes' when there was no signal (a false positive), and for saying 'no' when there was a signal (a missed positive). If it is very important not to miss a signal, while false positives do not matter much, the observer will set a low criterion for his threshold and may appear to be very sensitive. However, if the proportions of true and false positives are measured, the underlying sensitivity can be calculated. This gives a better measure of sensitivity than those methods in which false positives are not taken into account. The criterion can also be manipulated by different payoffs: a plot of true versus false positives then gives a family of data known as a *receiver operating characteristic* (or ROC) curve.

Sensory magnitude

This topic is concerned with the apparent intensity of a stimulus, and how it varies with the physical magnitude. Several mathematical formulae have been proposed. The matter is complicated, partly because the nervous system adapts rapidly and stimuli become reduced in apparent intensity. There is continuing argument about whether there is any relation between the discriminatory ability of a sensory system and the scaling of intensity.

Perceptual systems

Visual system

Vision is possible because patterned light is focused on the retina, and the neural messages are analysed in the brain.

The retina and brain

The *retina* is the layer of receptor and other cells at the back of the eye, which generate the neural messages down the optic nerve. The retina contains two types of receptor cells: rods and cones. The central part of the retina is the *fovea,* and it contains only cones; the outer part is the *periphery,* and it contains rods and some cones. The fovea is concerned with detailed pattern vision and colour vision. The periphery is concerned with detecting low levels of light and with movement. The fovea occupies only about 5 degrees of the visual field (equivalent to about three thumbnails held at arm's length). The fovea is good at resolving detail because the cones there each link on to one ganglion cell and have a near one-to-one connection with cells in the brain. Further from the fovea, a few cones may link on to one ganglion cell, providing less detail. The rods link in larger clusters on to one ganglion cell: detail is lost, but the advantage is increased sensitivity to the presence of any light, and to movement. The sensitivity of the periphery can be noticed when searching for stars in a dark sky: a star may be seen out of the corner of the eye, but it disappears when fixated. Similarly, a fluorescent tube may be seen to flicker in peripheral vision but it becomes steady when fixated.

Inside the eyeball is a fairly clear fluid, which may contain tiny particles of debris. These cast a shadow on the retina and may be seen as *floaters* (dark patches, blobs and squiggles), which follow the gaze of the eye. They are particularly visible when looking at the sky, and may give rise to impressions of flying saucers or other unreal celestial objects.

The nerve fibres from the retinal cells form the optic nerve. The point where they leave the retina is known as the *blind spot,* because there are no receptors there. The blind spot lies to the nasal side of the fovea, and is not normally noticed as the other eye sees the corresponding part of the visual field.

It is an interesting fact that the spatial arrangement for visual processing in the brain is 'reversed' with respect to the outside world – both left/right and up/down. This is not a problem for perception: the brain happens to be wired up that way, but could in principle process the information if it were wired up in some other systematic manner.

Light and dark adaptation

The eye responds to a very wide range of light intensities. It achieves this by adapting to the ambient light level. Dark adaptation is slow and depends on the regeneration of the photopigments. Light adaptation is relatively rapid, and is the result of neural reorganization. Rapid neural adaptation also occurs to changes in light level as a cloud goes over the sun. Adaptation enables the nervous system to make maximum use of the available rates of neural firing: the system can respond over a wide range of intensities and nevertheless be sensitive to small changes in intensity.

Sensitivity after dark adaptation increases about 100 000 fold, though pattern discrimination remains poor. As a result, people may make visual errors in dim light and think they see objects that are not there. (This is not the same thing as hypnagogic imagery that occurs before sleep with the eyes closed.)

Pattern vision

Sensitivity to light is not enough for good vision. To have visual acuity we need to discriminate pattern. Neural coding enhances contrast. Each neuron in the visual pathway has a *receptive field*, corresponding to the area of the retina to which it responds when stimulated. The neurons closest to the photoreceptors respond by increasing their rate of firing when the light intensity in their receptive field increases. At the level of the ganglion cells, the response becomes more complicated. Some cells are *on-centre, off-surround* and others are *off-centre, on-surround*. The first type of cell gives a burst of firing when the light is in the centre of the receptive field, and returns to its normal rate when the light is switched off; and it slows its rate of firing when the light is in the surrounds, increasing to normal when the light is switched off. The opposite is true of the other type of cell. If the light covers both centre and surround there is no response. This receptive field organization helps to enhance contrast. Further processing occurs in the *lateral geniculate nucleus* (LGN) and *cortex*. The cortex contains *feature-detecting cells*, whose response is more specific. David Hubel and Torsten Wiesel first investigated these in the 1960s. It is now known that there are several types of cells: *simple cells*, whose 'on' and 'off' areas are arranged side by side, and which respond best to bars of a particular orientation; *complex cells*, which respond best to the latter moving in a particular direction; and *hypercomplex (or end-stopped) cells*, which respond best to corners or short bars moving in a particular direction. Further processing in other areas of the brain leads to very specific feature detectors, such as cells in the temporal lobe that respond to faces.

It is now thought that there are two main visual pathways or streams flowing from the primary visual cortex. One system serves *conscious visual perception* and *object identification*, and follows the ventral stream to the inferior temporal lobe; while the other serves *motor action* (eye, limb and head position) and follows the dorsal stream to the posterior parietal lobe. Some brain-damaged patients may have one system intact but not the other.

Colour vision

Theories of colour vision are of two main types, the *trichromatic theory*, and the *opponent process theory*. Both of these apply, but at different levels of processing. The trichromatic theory is sometimes known as the Young–Helmholtz theory, because it was proposed by Thomas Young in 1802 and was modified by Hermann von Helmholtz in 1852. The theory was based on the perceptual phenomenon that most colours can be produced by suitable proportions of only three coloured lights, provided the lights have widely separated wavelengths. As three primary colours were sufficient, it was assumed that there were three types of cones. It was later shown by *microspectrophotometry* and by electrical recordings that single cones respond to short, medium or long wavelengths. The trichromatic theory was therefore established at the level of the cones. However, the cones are connected to the retinal ganglion cells in a manner that operates according to the opponent process theory. Ewald Hering proposed this theory in 1878. It was based on the perceptual phenomenon of *complementary colours*, shown as contrast colours and colour aftereffects (*negative afterimages*). Complementary pairs of colours are so called not because they are pleasing ('complimentary'), but because they complement or complete each other to form white light when combined. Red/green and blue/yellow form such pairs. After staring at a red light a green afterimage is seen, and after blue a yellow afterimage, and vice versa. The contrast colours can also be induced in a neutral grey patch adjacent to the primary colour. The *opponent process theory* explains these phenomena by supposing that individual cells can code information about two complementary colours by firing fast for one colour and slow for the other.

Colour constancy refers to the fact that objects appear approximately constant in colour despite quite wide variation in the overall illumination. Perceived colour depends on the ratios of wavelengths reflected by adjacent objects. Constancy breaks down if the illumination is strongly monochromatic.

Colour blindness is an inherited condition that affects mostly males. The most common condition is red–green confusion, which usually results from the malfunction of the green cones. Such people are known as *dichromats* as they have only two types of cones and can match any pure colour with a mixture of only two colours. People with normal vision are *trichromats* as they have three types of cones and have three colours to make a match. *Albinos* lack pigment in their skin, hair and cones, giving them their distinctive fair skin, white hair and bloodshot eyes: they are dazzled by bright light, and function mainly with rod vision.

Depth perception

We use various types of information to enable us to see distance or depth. Bishop George Berkeley called these sources *cues* in 1709, because he believed that we learn to see depth. However, both empiricists and nativists often use the term. Depth cues can be subdivided in various ways, such as *monocular* (one eye) versus *binocular* (two eyes), or visual versus proprioceptive.

The *monocular cues are all visual,* and are mainly those that can be seen in a picture. The following make objects appear further away: relatively small image size; texture gradients; converging lines; interposition (partial covering by nearer objects); height in the visual field; aerial perspective (objects appearing bluer and having lower contrast). Shading also produces relief, on the implicit assumption that the light comes from above rather than below. A further monocular cue that cannot be seen in a picture is *movement parallax*: when the head is moved the foreground appears to move in the opposite direction, and to move more than objects further back. The brain partially compensates for this effect, and its absence in pictures can produce the opposite direction of effect: the eyes and head of the Mona Lisa appear to follow one as one walks around the picture.

Binocular cues provide further depth information. Some of this is *muscular*, and depends on the degree of convergence of the eyes required to bring the images of the two eyes into register: more convergence is required for nearer images. Linked to this is the degree of *accommodation* of the lens, which also increases at near distances. However, this does not provide much distance information on its own. *Binocular stereopsis (binocular parallax, binocular disparity)* is more effective. This depends on the slight difference in the shape of the images received by the two eyes due to their *interocular separation* (about 6 cm). Provided the disparity is not too great, the brain fuses these images to produce an impression of solidity and depth. Most cells in the visual cortex are monocular, responding to one eye or the other, but some are binocular and respond only when both eyes receive a stimulus simultaneously. Stereoscopic displays can be produced artificially by presenting slightly different (laterally displaced) images to each eye. The views of the two eyes can be separated by means of prisms or a mirror stereoscope; or through the use of red and green filters, or oppositely oriented Polaroid filters. *Anaglyphs* can also be produced as pictures with plastic grids over them, which act as prisms allowing the two eyes to see different pictures. Random dot paired stereograms were developed by Bela Julesz in 1971, in which some of the dots were systematically shifted to the left or right in relation to the surrounding dots. More recently, single patterns of this type have been produced by computer, which can be fused by *free fusion* (diverging or converging the eyes voluntarily) to reveal marvellous figures and patterns in depth. Free fusion can also occur accidentally when looking at repeating wallpaper patterns or at the coils on ropes. The false fusion disturbs the apparent depth and size of the object.

Some environments give an almost uniform visual field with little pattern or depth information. Examples can be seen when walking or skiing in a snow 'whiteout', driving in a fog, diving in low-visibility or empty water, and flying through cloud. These conditions can lead to *empty-field myopia*, when the eyes are focused to a near point instead of the distance, with a loss of acuity for any distant objects that may be present. The lack of a visual scene also produces a feeling of isolation or 'break-off', similar to that caused by other types of sensory deprivation.

Movement perception

The movement of an image across the retina is easily detected by the visual system, because of the overlapping receptive fields of cells. A moving spot of light enters and leaves the centre and surrounding areas of many retinal cells, causing sudden changes in firing rates. These changes are picked up by movement-detecting neurons in the brain. True movement is not necessary, as lights flickering on and off at the right time interval and spatial separation mimic the same effects; this is known as the *phi phenomenon*, and it enables us to see movement at the cinema, in 'flip picture books', and in various advertisements.

However, the perception of visual movement is complicated, because movement is always relative to some other stationary or moving reference. An image can move across a stationary eye, or a moving eye can track it; and the observer's head and body may also be moving. The brain has to calculate whether movement of a retinal image represents movement in the outside world or not. There are two main theories to explain how this is done. The empiricist explanation maintains that we take into account our own eye, head and body movements, and cancel them out against retinal movement. The nativist explanation maintains that it is unnecessary to do this: instead, we assume that if the whole visual scene moves then our own bodies are moving, whereas if part of the visual scene moves then only that part is moving. Evidence in favour of the latter explanation is the *moving train illusion*: when our own train is standing at a station and another train moves by, we feel our own train moving in the opposite direction. This happens because the moving train fills the whole of the visual scene visible through the window.

Movement aftereffects also create illusions. The *waterfall illusion* is a familiar example. After staring at descending water, and then turning one's gaze to the side, the stationary landscape appears to drift upwards for a while. The effect is not due to any eye movements, but is probably caused by adaptation of cells that are specialized to detect motion in a particular direction. These cells are paired with opponent cells, which detect the opposite direction of motion. Fatigued cells fire at less than the resting rate, and the brain takes the difference between the firing rates of the opposed cells to indicate the direction of motion.

Auditory system

Sound waves are produced by objects vibrating in a medium such as air or water. The waves consist of alternate compressions and rarefactions of the molecules, and the effects can be transmitted a long way through the medium. Wavelength and wave frequency are inversely related, so that long wavelengths have low frequency and short wavelengths high frequency. Audible sound is that part of the energy spectrum that the ear is capable of transforming into neural messages. For humans, this lies in the frequency range of approximately 30 to 20 000 Hertz (Hz) or cycles per second. Human speech is around 1000 Hz, and musical sounds (distinguished by their regular wave patterns) range from about 30 to 3000 Hz. Below the audible range is infrasound and above it ultrasound. Some animals can hear frequencies that humans cannot: for example, bats can hear up to 150 000 Hz.

Coding for pitch and intensity

The neural coding systems for pitch (frequency) and intensity are complicated as they vary with the frequency. There are two mechanisms, known as the *place theory* ('pitch-is-which') and the *frequency theory*. The details of the place mechanism were worked out by Georg von Békésy in 1949. He found that high frequency sounds produced most stimulation of the basilar membrane near the stirrup, and low frequency sounds at the far end (the apex of the cochlea): the *tonotonic map* continues to the auditory cortex, although localization is poor for low frequency sounds. On the place theory, pitch is coded by which hair cells are firing most, and intensity is coded by the rate and number of cells firing. Rutherford suggested the frequency theory in 1886, and proposed that the auditory nerve fired at the rate of the various frequencies, like a telephone wire. On this theory pitch is given by the rate of firing, and intensity by the number of cells firing. The maximum firing rate of a nerve fibre is about 1000 Hz because of the refractory period between nervous impulses. However, up to four groups of fibres can work in relay, producing a combined firing rate (or *volley*) of up to 4000 Hz. The volley theory was proposed by E.G. Wever in 1949, and evidence for such *phase locking* was later produced. However, at the cortical level, neurons do not phase lock to frequencies much above 1000 Hz. *The frequency system works best for frequencies below 1000 Hz, and the place system above 5000 Hz, although both systems overlap in the intermediate range.* However, the frequency system clearly includes the range for human speech, and most musical tones.

Auditory localization

We can localize the angular direction of a sound source quite well, and its distance rather poorly. Direction is determined mainly by two sets of binaural cues: the difference in the time of arrival at the two ears and the difference in intensity. If the sound source is straight ahead it affects the two ears similarly, but if it is to one side it reaches the nearer ear first and is also louder. The importance of these cues varies with the frequency. The time difference is difficult to detect with high frequency sounds, because the difference is too short. The loudness difference is difficult to detect with low frequency sounds because long wavelengths flow around the head leaving no sound shadow whereas short wavelengths are reflected off the head, giving a reduced intensity at the further ear. Stereophonic sound can be reproduced with a headset delivering different sounds to the two ears, or with two or more speakers arranged around a room. There are thought to be binaural cells in the brain that respond to interaural time and intensity differences.

The distance of a sound source is more difficult to determine. Sound waves lose energy with distance, so distant sounds are quieter. There is also a selective loss of high frequencies, changing the quality of distant sounds. Distance can also be detected from the ratio of reflected sounds (echoes) to unreflected sounds, further sources having more reflected sound. We show some degree of *loudness constancy,* in that sounds seem to lose intensity less rapidly with distance than is physically the case. Sometimes we make mistakes: for example, when half asleep, a small creak in the room can be mistaken for an explosion outside.

Sounds can also be used to detect the presence of objects, on the sonar principle. This is known as *echodetection* or *echolocation.* High-frequency sounds are bounced off objects and the echoes provide information about the nature and distance of the objects. Blind people use this technique; and bats are especially adept at it, having excellent hearing in the high frequencies. We do not normally hear short echoes as such, but they affect the qualities of sounds. The acoustic properties of concert halls vary with the proportions of reflected sound (echoes or reverberation) and direct sound.

Other sensory systems

The other sensory systems cannot be described in detail here, but they follow similar principles of coding and perception to the visual and auditory systems.

The *vestibular system* lies next to the cochlea in the inner ear. It has three semicircular canals oriented at right angles to each other, each containing a *cupula.* The relative changes in firing rates of the nerves from the different canals determine the perception of rotary motion. Illusory self-motion (or *vertigo*) occurs when the cupula is moved in an abnormal manner: for example by changes in air pressure (*alternobaric* vertigo in divers), by changes in temperature (*caloric* vertigo), or by changes in membrane density through alcohol intake (*alcoholic* vertigo). The vestibular system also contains the *otolithic* organs in the utricle and saccule, which are responsive to linear acceleration such as the constant force of gravity, and the linear component of acceleration while travelling. The otoliths respond to constant head tilt, because the effect of gravity is always present. Unusual combinations of head orientation, accelerative forces, and of visual movement information, can cause illusory movement perception and motion sickness. This is known as the *sensory conflict* account: it can explain travel sickness on land, sea sickness, space sickness (in astronauts), and also the sickness brought on by cinerama and other visual displays when there is no physical movement.

Taste (*gustation*) and smell (*olfaction*) are closely related chemical senses. The sense of taste actually depends to a large extent on smell, as becomes evident when the latter is impaired with a head cold. Tastes are generally subdivided into four basic categories: salty, sweet, bitter and sour. Odours are less easy to classify.

The skin contains several types of receptors: the *Pacinian corpuscles* respond to mechanical pressure or touch, and there are also *thermoreceptors* (temperature) and *nociceptors* (pain), and some others. However, the receptors do not map very neatly on to specific sensations as some respond to more than one type of stimulus. The resulting sensation depends on the overall pattern of stimulation. The locus of the stimulation is analysed in the parietal lobes of the brain. The accuracy of localization depends on the receptive fields of the neurons, which is particularly fine in the fingertips.

Kinaesthetic information from the joint and muscle receptors goes to the parietal lobe. The various sensory and motor systems are coordinated in many reflex and learned responses. Perception and action are interlinked – a point stressed by J.J. Gibson and his followers.

Complex processes

Many aspects of perception seem complex and seem to demand high level processing by the brain. It may be that learning or higher cognitive processes are involved, as was argued by Helmholtz. Alternatively, innate brain structures may provide sufficient processing, as was argued by the Gestalt psychologists and more recently by the Gibsonians.

Gestalt theory

Gestalt theory developed in opposition to orthodox empiricist theory, which took the view that we learn to combine simple sensory events into the perception of the objective world. The *Gestalt* ('configuration' or 'form') psychologists were most notably represented by Max Wertheimer (1880–1943), Kurt Koffka (1886–1941) and Wolfgang Köhler (1887–1967). They believed that the perception of form was more than the sum of its parts (or elementary sensations). They stressed the innate nature of much perceptual organization, and speculated on the neurophysiological mechanisms involved. They believed in *isomorphism* (the idea that brain processes were similar in form to the object of perception). The neurophysiological ideas have been discarded, but the basic phenomena of perceptual organization remain interesting. The main principles for organizing complex visual patterns into figures or groups are: *similarity* (similar images are grouped together even when separated physically); *proximity* (nearer images are grouped); *closure* (gaps are filled in to complete a shape); *good continuation* (images that appear to continue in the same direction are grouped); and *common fate* (images that move together in a scene are grouped). Other Gestalt phenomena are figure–ground differentiation and reversible figures (such as the Necker cube), object constancy despite variation in the proximal stimulus, and perceptual set (expectations).

Many of the Gestalt principles apply to auditory phenomena. For example, the ability to pick out speech or music from a noisy background is similar to figure–ground differentiation in vision. Sounds that are similar in pitch are generally perceived as coming from a single source. This accounts for musical streaming, in which alternating high and low tones sound like separate high and low streams coming from two different instruments or voices. However, if the pitch changes gradually between high and low, only one source is heard. The former effect follows the principle of similarity, and the latter of good continuation. Tunes are also recognized as the same when played in different keys, provided the main relations between the notes are maintained. However, if the timing is changed too much the tune is perceived as different: rhythm is perhaps the most basic element of music. Speech recognition is also remarkably good, despite wide variation in accents. Listeners are adept at picking up a shift in vowel sounds or consonants, and interpreting ambiguous sounds within that speaker's context.

The constancies

Objects in the real world appear fairly constant in size, shape, brightness, colour, location and other qualities despite considerable variation in the retinal image. There is thus some compensation or scaling for distance, tilt, illumination and so forth, although the compensation is not usually complete. In vision there is size constancy despite a reduction in image size with viewing distance; shape constancy despite a change in image shape with slant; colour constancy despite changes in the predominant wavelength of the illumination; brightness constancy despite changes in the intensity of illumination; position constancy despite changes in the retinal location of objects with eye movements; and speed constancy despite a reduction in the velocity of an image movement across the eye with viewing distance. Constancies also occur in other sense modalities. In audition there is loudness constancy despite a reduction in the intensity of the proximal stimulus with the distance of the sound source; direction constancy despite turning the head; melody constancy despite a change in key; and so on.

The Gestalt psychologists invented the name *constancy*, and stressed its automatic nature, whereas the empiricists stressed the role of experience. Colour and brightness constancy are generally thought to be largely innate, and to depend on the ratios of wavelengths and intensities in the visual scene. Size and shape constancy are more complex: the empiricists argue that we 'take account of distance' (often called *size–distance invariance*), although nativists argue that we perceive size in relation to that of surrounding objects or texture gradients (see Figure 2.1).

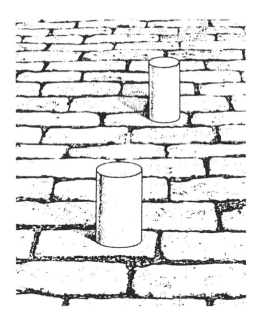

Figure 2.1: Gradient as a size cue.

Adaptation and aftereffects

Many illusory effects are caused by simple sensory adaptation. For example, staring at a bright light bleaches the photopigment in part of the retina: this produces an afterimage, which appears to move with the eyes. Temperature adaptation is also easy to demonstrate: if one hand is immersed in cold water and the other in hot water, and the two hands are then placed in lukewarm water, the same water will feel hot to the cooled hand and cool to the warmed hand.

Figural aftereffects (FAEs) are rather like simple sensory aftereffects. Some FAEs are called Gibsonian and others Köhlerian. Gibsonian normalization occurs after staring at an 'off-normal' shape such as a curved line or slanting line. A straight line (or vertical line) will then appear curved (or slanted) in the opposite direction. Köhlerian displacement occurs after staring at some pattern, and then looking at a test figure that has contours adjacent to the original figure: the adjacent contours are then displaced. FAEs are thought to be due to the adaptation of various types of feature-detecting cells in the brain.

Contingent aftereffects (or *McCullough* effects – reported by Celeste McCullough in 1965) are more complex, and result from linking two different sensory aspects. For example, an observer may stare at a pattern consisting of red horizontal stripes and green vertical stripes: when the pattern is replaced by similar black and white stripes, the opponent colour is seen faintly (green horizontal stripes and red vertical stripes). The effect is not a local afterimage, as it occurs when the eyes are moved around, and it may reoccur days later. The sensory mechanism remains controversial.

Perceptual modification is even more complex, and its neurophysiological basis more uncertain. The name refers to such phenomena as adaptation to optical distortion. For example, in 1896 George Stratton wore inverting prisms and after several days learned to carry out normal activities. On removing the prisms he had aftereffects when the normal world seemed inverted. Most distortions are not as extreme as this. For example, sub-aqua divers experience distortions of size, curvature and distance when looking through a facemask in water. They partially adapt to these distortions, and experience a short aftereffect on leaving the water. Experienced divers adapt more rapidly than novices, as they build up a contingent expectation about appearances in water.

Geometrical optical illusions

Some geometrical illusions are similar in form to the combined inspection and test components of FAEs. For example, in the *Zöllner illusion* (Figure 2.2) the oblique cross ties cause the vertical lines to appear to converge and diverge. This is thought to be due to the strong stimulation of oblique feature detectors in one direction, which makes vertical lines appear slightly tilted in the opposite direction.

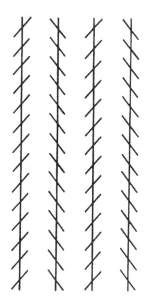

Figure 2.2: Zöllner illusion.

Many illusions can be described as examples of contrast effects. Another example is the *Ponzo illusion* (converging railway lines – Figure 2.3) in which size contrast is shown: the upper bar appears larger than the lower bar, perhaps in contrast to the smaller space between the enclosing lines. However, some authors have sought to explain such size illusions as examples of inappropriate size constancy: they argue that the upper bar appears enlarged because it appears 'as if' further away, and is scaled accordingly. The explanation runs into difficulties, because the figures normally appear flat on the paper.

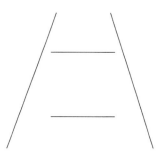

Figure 2.3: Ponzo illusion.

An interesting and much-discussed illusion is the *moon illusion* – the phenomenon that the moon (and sun) appear larger on the horizon than higher up in the sky. It is not an optical effect caused by refraction, but is the result of various factors that contribute to size constancy. It is often argued that the moon appears to lie on the apparently flattened bowl of the sky: it appears further away on the horizon, and is then enlarged by size–distance invariance (see Figure 2.4). However, observers claim that the moon appears both nearer and larger on the horizon. It is therefore likely that factors other than apparent distance make it appear larger – factors such as the relative size of other horizon objects, an orange colour in misty conditions, the orientation of the observer's head and body and the state of convergence and accommodation of the eyes.

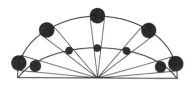

Figure 2.4: Moon illusion.

The development of visual perception

Perception develops in infants partly through maturation of the visual system, and partly through experience. Infant perception can be investigated behaviourally through preferential looking techniques, habituation procedures and reaching behaviour. It can also be investigated physiologically by measuring the visual scanning of the eyes, and visual evoked potentials in the brain.

Studies show that full colour vision develops by the age of about 2 to 3 months. Visual acuity and contrast sensitivity is poor at 1 or 2 months, due to undeveloped cones and cortical connections, but develops rapidly in the first 6 months; it does not reach adult level until over the age of 1 year. Accommodation and binocular convergence develop by about 3 months. *Stereoacuity* (based on binocular disparity) develops rapidly after about 3.5 months; however, there is a critical learning period for binocular development over the first 2 years or more, and children who have an early squint (*strabismus*) often fail to develop true binocular stereovision when the squint is later corrected. The use of pictorial depth cues develops between 5 and 7 months. Some degree of size constancy is shown by 3 months. 'Visual cliff' experiments were reported by Eleanor Gibson and Richard Walk in 1960. They found that crawling infants were reluctant to venture out on a glass shelf over a drop, showing that good depth perception had developed by 6 months. Animals born on the hoof, such as sheep and goats, show depth perception at birth.

Studies of perceptual development in later life are rather less informative. Several cases of recovery from blindness (usually through removal of cataracts) have been investigated, and they show that adults are slow to recover normal vision, or never do so. However, such cases are not typical of normal development: it is often hard to know how much vision was present before blindness set in, or how much damage was done to the visual system through lack of stimulation.

Environmental effects on perception have also been studied in normal children and adults. In particular, various authors have investigated the 'carpentered world' hypothesis – the idea that life in a built-up environment sensitizes the visual system to vertical and horizontal lines, and makes us more susceptible to certain geometrical illusions. For example, the *Müller-Lyer* illusion may be interpreted as representing buildings or books, in which case city dwellers should be more susceptible to it than people living in empty countryside. On the other hand, the *horizontal–vertical* illusion can be interpreted as representing a road receding into the distance, in which case people living in flat open country should be more susceptible to it than those living in a dense forest or a cluttered city (Figure 2.5). While the evidence gives some support to this idea, it is also possible that the differences between groups are due to differences in education, age, test conditions and so on. Moreover, developmental studies of the illusions generally show a reduction with age – a surprising finding if the illusions are supposed to be caused by environmental experience.

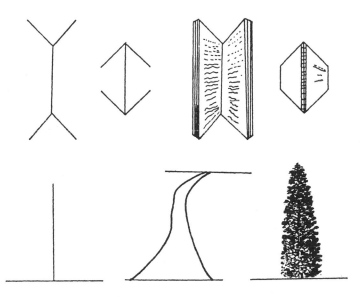

Figure 2.5: Müller-Lyer and horizontal–vertical illusions.

Illusions, hallucinations and other psychopathology

Many illusions caused by normal perceptual processes have been described in earlier sections. Almost everyone is subject to these. The other effects described here are mainly concerned with imagery, and not everyone experiences them. Many of the effects are common enough not to be considered abnormal. For example, *synaesthesia* is a normal association between different sensory systems, where letters of the alphabet may seem coloured, or strange diagrammatic forms may be used as schemes for ordering numbers and calendars. Synaesthesia is more common in children than adults.

Other illusions are associated with various states of consciousness (some normal and some abnormal); and some with drugs, brain damage or psychopathology. Sir Francis Galton (1904) studied many types of imagery and argued that they formed a continuum rather than distinct categories: there are waking and dream images; imagery between sleeping and waking; eidetic imagery; quasi-hallucinations; and gross hallucinations.

Waking imagery

Mistaken perceptions can include faces in the fire, or dark shadows interpreted as wild beasts or murderers. *Pseudohallucinations* occur when hallucinatory imagery is known to be false.

Sleep and near-sleep imagery

Hypnagogic (or *hypnogogic*) imagery is vivid imagery occurring just before falling asleep, and sometimes on waking. It is rather like viewing random picture slides. It is common to see faces, sometimes horrible ones. A person's body image may also be distorted, with limbs that change size (as with Lewis Carroll's Alice). There may be an experience of falling. Such experiences may cause nightmares in children. Imagery may occur in other senses: for example voices, music, odours, and occasionally kinaesthetic activities. *Hypnopompic* imagery occurs while waking from sleep, and is like a continuation of the dream state. Auditory imagery is quite common, such as hearing an alarm before it goes off. There may also be wishful imagery of getting up and dressing, when the person is still drowsing in bed. There may be tactile experiences, such as being shaken awake; or sexual imagery, giving rise to the religious idea of involuntary intercourse with the devil. *Eidetic* imagery is a vivid and detailed image of a scene corresponding exactly to the original perception. It is usually visual, but may be proprioceptive or auditory. It tends to occur at night after learning a new skill, such as skiing or a musical instrument.

Unusual states of consciousness

Imagery can be brought on by meditation, isolation or sensory deprivation. Extreme emotion, such as grief at the death or desertion of a loved one, may make one hear or see that person. *Out-of-the-body* experiences may also occur under times of stress.

Derealization is a feeling that the world is unreal. It may be accompanied by a distortion of depth perception. It may occur in psychiatric patients, and in epileptic episodes; but also in normal people after experiencing intense excitement or danger – such as wartime aircraft sorties. Memory of the action has a dreamlike quality.

Mental illness

A common symptom of schizophrenia is that patients feel that their mental processes are controlled by others. They may hear voices telling them what to do, talking about them in a derogatory manner, or threatening them. They may hear their thoughts spoken aloud (*echo de pensée*), or have other hallucinations and delusions. These may take a religious form for religious people, or a pseudoscientific form for others (such as belief in UFOs, capture by aliens and so forth). Patients may also have tactile hallucinations, and feel that they are being sexually assaulted by the devil. Some patients may have olfactory hallucinations, believing that they are giving off foul odours, causing people to avoid them.

Effects of drugs and neural damage

Drugs that cause hallucinations are known as *hallucinogenic* drugs. They include LSD, PCP (Angel Dust), mescaline, psilocybin, marijuana (cannabis, hashish, THC) and some others. Strongly coloured patterns are commonly seen, and there may be distortions of depth and size perception.

Alcohol damage can cause delirium tremens, in which the patient sees frightening images, and may feel that lice are creeping over the skin.

Shortage of oxygen can cause pleasurable hallucinations, and is sometimes used to heighten sexual pleasure (with occasionally fatal results). Shortage of oxygen also occurs near death, and may be responsible for visions of angels.

Further reading

Consult the chapters on sensation and perception in a detailed first year psychology text such as:

Atkinson RL, Atkinson RC, Smith EE, Hilgard RC (1996) Hilgard's Introduction to Psychology (12 edn). Fort Worth: Harcourt Brace.
Gleitman H (1994) Psychology (4 edn). New York: WW Norton.

For more specialized information consult an advanced text, such as:

Goldstein EB (1996) Sensation and Perception (4 edn). Pacific Grove, London: Brooks/Cole Publishing Co.
Sekuler R, Blake R (1994) Perception (3 edn). New York: McGraw-Hill.
Bruce V, Green PR, Georgeson MA (1996) Visual Perception: Physiology, Psychology, and Ecology (3 edn). Hove: Psychology Press.

For two visual systems see:

Jeannerod M (1997) The Cognitive Neuroscience of Action. Oxford: Blackwell.

For geometrical illusions:

Gregory RL (1970) The Intelligent Eye. London: Weidenfeld & Nicolson.
Coren S, Girgus JS (1978) Seeing is Deceiving: the Psychology of Visual Illusions. Hillsdale NJ: Erlbaum.
Frisby JP (1979) Seeing: Illusion, Brain and Mind. Oxford: Oxford University Press.

For outdoor perceptual phenomena, and the moon illusion:

Ross HE (1974) Behaviour and Perception in Strange Environments. London: Allen & Unwin.
Hershenson M (ed.) (1989) The Moon Illusion. Hillsdale NJ: Erlbaum.
Plug C, Ross HE (1994) The natural moon illusion: a multi-factor angular account. Perception 23: 321–33.

For the constancies:

Walsh V, Kulikowski JJ (eds) (1998) Perceptual Constancy: Why Things Look as They Do. Cambridge: Cambridge University Press.

For synaesthesia:

Baron-Cohen S, Harrison JE (eds) (1997) Synaesthesia: Classic and Contemporary Readings. Oxford: Blackwell.

For hallucinations and parapsychology:

Siegel RK, West JL (eds) (1975) Hallucinations: Behaviour, Experience and Theory. London: Wiley.
Blackmore SJ (1995) Parapsychology. In Colman AM (ed.) Controversies in Psychology. London: Longman.

Chapter 3
Attention and information processing: applications to schizophrenia

GERRY KENT, GRAHAM TURPIN

Key concepts	Key names
Theories of attention	
Filter theory	Broadbent
Processing theory	Deutsch and Deutsch
Controlled and automatic processing	Shiffrin and Schneider
Supervisory attentional system	Norman
Assessing attentional biases	
Spatial attention	Posner
Thresholds	
Shadowing	
Stroop task	
Visual probes	Mathews and MacLeod
Clinical assessment	
Schizophrenia	
Filtering dysfunction	Hemsley, McGhie and Chapman
Stress–vulnerability model	Nuechterlein and Dawson
Continuous performance test	
Cognitive theories	Cowan, Frith
Attributional styles	Bentall

Introduction and overview

We imagine that you are reading this chapter while sitting, perhaps in a room where there is some extraneous noise around you. There are certainly many objects to look at besides this book yet you are able to read these words without being unduly distracted by any irrelevant sounds or visual input. Although we usually take it for granted, this ability to concentrate on the present task of understanding these words involves a complex process of attending to some stimuli while ignoring others. Without being able to do this, you would be overwhelmed by stimuli that are unrelated to your current aims and purposes. At the same time, you are also able to shift your attention when necessary. If the telephone rings or someone calls your name you can alter the focus of your attention away from this book and deal with this additional auditory input.

These are very sophisticated abilities, and also very important ones, as we can see when people have attentional difficulties. Someone with a phobia may find that their attention is 'captured' by the feared object whenever it is encountered and, indeed, may be hypervigilant to its presence. Individuals with a cat phobia, for example, may be constantly on the look out for cats, to the extent that they are unable to concentrate on other stimuli. Someone else who ruminates excessively may not be able to focus their attention on anything other than their thoughts and worries (Wells and Morrison, 1994). Another good example of this is hypochondriasis, where undue attention to bodily sensations can lead to severe disability (Warwick and Salkovskis, 1989). In other words, an ability to select appropriate stimuli and deal with them effectively is critical for our sense of self and wellbeing.

As we will see later in this chapter, an inability to focus attention and to filter out extraneous stimuli has been frequently suggested as a core psychological deficit underlying the experience of schizophrenia. An understanding of psychological models of attentional dysfunction in schizophrenia may assist the clinician in two important ways. First, consideration of these models prompts the clinician to attempt to understand the inner subjective world of the person with schizophrenia. What if, when reading this chapter, you were continually being distracted by external stimuli (such as traffic noise, distant conversations, flickering strip lights, inner thoughts and sensations)? What if you could not prioritize these stimuli and you were overwhelmed with irrelevant environmental events? What effect would this have on your ability to concentrate and process the information written within the chapter? Would you feel frustrated or at ease? Would you feel in control of the task or aimless? What effect would these feelings have on your own sense of self-identity and wellbeing? It is likely that many people with schizophrenia continuously experience sensory overload and an inability to remain focused on the task at hand. Accordingly, this may result in other behaviours such as an inability to concentrate, to engage in and follow conversations, to understand and process emotions, to attend to social interactions in a meaningful way, to withdraw from intense or distracting social situations and so forth. Such an understanding may assist in developing therapeutic relationships between clinician and patient. Moreover, it may also be beneficial to educate relatives and carers in attempts to understand the inner world of the person with schizophrenia.

Second, by identifying the cognitive processes underlying these attentional deficits and handicaps, it may be possible to develop therapeutic methods that may assist the person with schizophrenia to deal more effectively with the experience of psychotic symptoms and the disruptive effects that they frequently have on their everyday functioning. Recently, a range of psychological treatment methods have been proposed that deal effectively with hallucinations and delusions in some patients, even those who have been resistant to pharmacological treatment methods. The application of these psychological interventions will be briefly described in the final section of this chapter.

The purposes of this chapter, therefore, are (a) to outline the ways that psychologists and psychiatrists have understood the processes involved in how we manage to attend to only some features of our environment to the exclusion of others and (b) how we can direct the focus of our attention to accomplish the tasks we need to function effectively. The third purpose of this chapter is (c) to illustrate how these psychological approaches to attention can be used to understand the attentional difficulties that schizophrenic patients can experience.

Models of attention

It is useful to provide a brief historical review of the ways in which psychologists have studied and understood attentional processes. William James noted the importance of attention in 1890, but experimental studies of attention did not begin in earnest until the 1950s. Initially, Broadbent (1958) was concerned with the ways in which some stimuli are attended to while others are filtered out. Subsequently, Deutsch and Deutsch (1963) advocated the idea that some stimuli are processed more fully than others: unattended messages are not so much filtered out as not consciously perceived. More recently, Schneider et al. (1984) have made an important distinction between automatic and controlled attentional processes.

These models have some commonalities. They have in common the notion that people have only a limited capacity to process information. If a task requires considerable cognitive effort there may be little capacity left over for other activities. You will have noticed this on many occasions, such as when learning to drive. On the first occasion behind the wheel of a car all your cognitive effort was given to remembering the correct sequence to start the car, get it into gear and move off. Another situation may have been when you give a public presentation of some kind. When feeling nervous much attention is given to how you present your message, perhaps leaving less capacity to attend to how the audience is receiving what you have to say. A second similarity between models is that memory processes (see Chapter 4) are involved in attention, because they determine to some extent which messages are attended to and which are discarded. Memory needs to be involved at some level so that we can attend to stimuli that have previously been experienced as relevant, or else our attention would be focused randomly without influence from wider strategic aims.

Filter theories

Much of the early research in this area was inspired by Cherry's (1953) 'cocktail party problem'. We have all been in a noisy room at a party where many people are chatting loudly, yet we are able to attend selectively to our own conversation, ignoring others'. Cherry began to study this ability using the *dichotic listening task*. In this task, people wear a set of headphones, with different messages coming into each ear. They are asked to attend to only one message – usually by repeating the words out loud, termed *shadowing*. Cherry and others found that the second, unattended message is not processed consciously. People are unable to say what the nature of the message was afterwards. Broadbent (1958) proposed a filter model that could account for this phenomenon. He argued that information received by the senses first entered a short-term store but then entered a *selective filter*, which let only one message through to be processed more centrally. This filter was needed because attentional capacity was limited to only one message at once.

However, later research showed that some messages from the unattended ear were processed, as long as they were important enough. For example, the person's name was often heard and could be remembered later. Treisman (1964) modified Broadbent's model slightly to take such findings into account, arguing that there are really a set of sequential filters that examine the message for a variety of characteristics. If an unattended message is of sufficient importance for individuals – such as their name or a telephone ringing – it will pass through a filter. Such preferences for selected stimuli or *attentional biases*, as they are called, are particularly important when understanding attentional dysfunction in psychopathology. It has been shown that, for many psychological disorders, a pathological bias towards symptom-related stimuli such as those associated with anxiety are selectively attended to, even within an unattended channel or unconsciously (Williams et al., 1997).

Extent of processing theories

Broadbent and Treisman argued that only selected messages go beyond the initial stages of processing, Deutsch and Deutsch (1963) and Norman (1968) took quite a different view. They contended that all messages undergo processing, but vary in the extent of this processing. Their model implied that all information is perceived, even if we may not be able to recall all of it. One of the more important studies supporting their model was conducted by MacKay (1973). In this study, participants were asked to shadow sentences such as 'They threw stones at the bank yesterday' in one ear. This is an ambiguous sentence, because the word 'bank' could refer to a building or the side of a river. MacKay played related words on the unshadowed ear, either 'river' or 'money'. Participants were then asked to choose which of the following sentences was similar in meaning to the original message:

(a) They threw stones toward the side of the river yesterday

or

(b) They threw stones toward the saving and loan association yesterday.

According to the Broadbent and Treisman models, the choice should not be influenced by the words from the unattended ear, but MacKay found that the results supported Deutsch and Deutsch (1963). Even though the participants could not recall the word from the unattended ear, their choice of meaning was affected by whether they heard 'river' or 'money': they were more likely to choose the meaning consistent with the unshadowed message. This is an important finding because it suggests that we attend to much material that we do not use or are not aware of.

Controlled and automatic processing models

Most recently, there has been much interest in the ways that people, despite having limited attentional capacity, are often able to do two things at once. It is difficult to realize how often we do this. For example, it is easy for most people to walk and talk, or to eat and listen to music, at the same time. In light of the idea presented above that people have limited attentional capacity and can often attend to only one aspect of the environment at a time, how are these dual activities possible?

Studies of practice and skill acquisition provide much information in this respect. To return to some examples used earlier, you will recall how learning to drive a car required full use of your attentional capacity. You had to concentrate on the mechanics of driving, leaving little room for any extraneous noise or demands. You might have preferred to turn the radio off or not converse with your instructor, for example. However, as you became more practised, your ability to engage in other tasks increased. By the time you passed your driving test you felt able to talk to others and listen to the radio.

This process of gaining additional attentional capacity with practice illustrates a distinction between controlled processing and automatic processing as outlined by Shriffrin and Schneider (Schneider et al., 1984). Learning to drive involves a great deal of slow and effortful processing. Learners need to run through the tasks of driving sequentially (for example, check the mirror, turn on the ignition, put the car into gear and so forth), all of which require considerable attention. Once the skill is acquired, however, the tasks can be done quickly and with little effort. They can also be done in parallel and require little conscious attention. Well-learned tasks are also rather difficult to modify, so experienced drivers may have become set in unsafe routines that are difficult to change. Also, once drivers are well practised, they can find it difficult to describe what they are doing to others, such is the level of automaticity involved.

Similarly, as public speakers become more practised in giving presentations, they become more fluent and more able to interact with their audience.

These types of observation have led to the most recent theories of attention. According to these approaches, information can be processed in two ways – one automatic and non-conscious, the other conscious and controlled (Brewin, 1988). The former process is responsible for dealing with many of our perceptions of the external environment and internal bodily states. Much of what we do and much of our environment is familiar, so most everyday tasks require little conscious effort and our brains can deal with a considerable amount of information without using much attentional capacity. This process usually operates outside of conscious awareness. This is the system we use when we are well-practised and accomplished car drivers.

The controlled system of processing, on the other hand, operates within our conscious awareness, and is the process that we use to describe attention in everyday terms. Its capacity is severely limited, it requires conscious effort and is sequential – we attend to one aspect of the environment after another rather than all at once. A person's controlled processing can be disrupted by stress or by having many competing demands at the same time. For example, students may find it difficult to concentrate on academic work if there are many interpersonal demands at the time or if they find that there are too many tasks to accomplish in a short period of time.

We become aware of its importance only when there is an unusual task to accomplish. The *Stroop task*, where people are asked to name the colour in which words are written, is an example. If the words are unrelated to colours – such as 'desk', 'car' or 'table' – the colour of the print is compatible with meaning, and the task can be accomplished easily and quickly. If the words refer to colours, however – such as 'yellow', 'red' or 'blue' – and the words are themselves written in a different colour – such as the word 'yellow' written in red ink – the colour-naming task takes much longer. Thus in the Stroop task there is a competition between the automatic and controlled processing systems.

The relationship between automatic and controlled processing has led to the notion of some higher order mechanism responsible for supervising and shifting the level of task engagement from automatic to controlled, or non-conscious to conscious. This has been termed the *supervisory attentional system*. The control of either non-conscious or conscious processing by some central executive function has also become a focus for research in psychopathology, particularly in schizophrenia. Researchers such as Frith (1979) have argued that when non-conscious material inappropriately accesses consciousness, patients become aware of anomalous experiences, which might form the bases of psychotic phenomena such as hallucinations and delusions.

Measuring attention

Clinically, psychologists and psychiatrists can gain much information about clients' attentional difficulties by simply asking them about the focus of their attention. For example, hypochondriacal clients would be asked about how often they reflected on bodily sensations, and phobic ones about their vigilance for the feared object. We have already discussed some methods for measuring the direction of someone's attention in laboratory settings. In the dichotic listening task, people were asked about the content of the unattended channel. When they could not recall its content, Broadbent and others concluded that no attention was given to it. However, as the study by MacKay (1973) showed, attentional processes are more complex than this. There can be some attentional processing occurring of which the person is not conscious. Simply because a person cannot recall something does not mean that it was never attended to. In order to study unconscious automatic processes, other more sophisticated methods are needed. This section of the chapter outlines some approaches to these issues by providing a description of some techniques which have been used by laboratory-based psychologists when attempting to understand attentional biases in anxiety disorders.

Attentional biases

As described elsewhere, one of the defining characteristics of anxiety is the tendency for attention to be 'captured' or biased towards the feared object. There are many methods that can be used to study the ways people shift their attention towards some aspects of the environment rather than others. Investigators have examined this bias through the examination of eye-movements and measures of visual attention, auditory thresholds and the use of the shadowing technique, the emotional Stroop task and the visual probe technique.

One method is to record eye movements: as people look at an object or picture they scan it in an orderly way, depending on the shape of the object (for example, whether it is regular or irregular in shape), the points of interest in the object (people look at the eyes of faces more than any other characteristic), and their purposes (people will scan different parts of a picture depending on the aspect of interest). Reaction times to targets presented at different spatial locations in the visual field may also be used to study visual attention. Indeed, an influential theory of visual attention proposed by Posner and Peterson (1990) seeks to establish the neuropsychological basis for different components underlying attention. Posner's model was developed by studying patients with different focal lesions such as the parietal lobe and the mid-brain, and assessing the extent to which these lesions disrupted performance on *spatial attention tasks*. He argued that different brain areas are responsible for the separate processes of disengaging current attention, switching or shifting attention, and reengaging attention to a new stimulus.

Parkinson and Rachman (1981) examined the possibility that people who were anxious about an upcoming event would have a lower *detection threshold* for words associated with that event. They played a tape of music to mothers whose children were about to have a tonsillectomy. Embedded within this tape were words associated with physical danger (injection, operation, bleeding) at varying volumes. The mothers were asked to repeat the words when they heard them. The mothers were able to report hearing the words at significantly lower volumes compared with a control group of mothers whose children were of the same age but who were not being admitted to hospital. This lowered threshold was not found for similar neutral words (such as inflection, operatic, breeding) or dissimilar words (such as bird, uniform, newspapers).

Mathews and MacLeod (1986) used the *shadowing* technique with anxious clients and matched controls. While the participants shadowed one message, threatening or neutral words were played on the unattended channel. At the same time they were asked to respond quickly to a visual stimulus on a computer screen. Although the anxious participants were consciously unaware of the threatening words when asked about them, their reaction time to the visual task deteriorated when the threatening words (but not the neutral ones) had been played to the unattended ear. It seemed that that the threatening words had been attended to at some unconscious level.

As described above, the Stoop task involves testing for the interference between the semantic meaning of a word and its colour. Watts et al. (1986) asked a group of spider phobics to read words related to their feared object (such as 'hairy', 'crawl') and other words that had an emotional content but that were unrelated to the phobia. They showed that words directly related to their phobia produced greater interference than the unrelated emotional words. Furthermore, this interference decreased after desensitization treatment for their phobia, suggesting that this technique might be one way of assessing the efficacy of treatment.

The *visual probe technique* is somewhat more complicated. To simplify somewhat, participants are asked to watch a computer screen, where words are presented for a short period of time (0.5 seconds). Their task is to press a button as soon as possible whenever a dot appears. MacLeod, Mathews and Tata (1986) showed that anxious participants' reaction times after the appearance of the dot were greater when one of the words involved a threat than when both were neutral, a finding that did not hold for the matched controls. This and other studies (Williams et al., 1997) have indicated that that the anxious participants' attention had been drawn away from the reaction time task and, instead, towards the threatening word. Non-anxious individuals, on the other hand, demonstrate an opposite attentional bias whereby they tend to *avoid* threatening material.

The above examples of laboratory paradigms illustrate the range of methods that psychologists have employed to study attentional dysfunction within psychopathology. They also illustrate the important contribution that cognitive models of attention and memory have recently made to the understanding of neurotic disorders such as anxiety and depression. In the next section of this chapter we will illustrate some further attentional paradigms that have been used specifically to study psychosis and schizophrenia.

Attention and schizophrenia

The remainder of this chapter will focus on the application of models of attention to an understanding of schizophrenia. We will describe, from both the clinician's and patient's perspectives, the experiences that have led to the proposal that a dysfunction in attention underlies schizophrenia. We will then briefly review the empirical evidence regarding attentional deficits and the methodological limitations surrounding some of these studies. In particular, the utility of the *stress–vulnerability model* as providing a framework for understanding such deficits is emphasized. Several theories that seek to explain these deficits will be appraised and their relationship to the experience of schizophrenic symptoms outlined. Finally, the relevance of these theories to the clinical management of schizophrenia and the development of psychological treatments will be discussed.

Clinical observation and subjective experience

Ever since Kraepelin's description of dementia praecox, dysfunctional attention has been implicated within schizophrenia. Kraepelin, himself, distinguished between passive or automatic attention and active or voluntary attention (Nuechterlein and Asarnow, 1989), and suggested that the disorder was primarily characterized by dysfunction of active attention, although passive attention might also be disrupted either during the acute or chronic stages of the disorder. Similarly, other psychiatrists and psychologists in attempting to understand the subjective experience of people with schizophrenia have frequently emphasized disruption of attention. Hemsley (1993) when reviewing different attentional models of schizophrenia placed particular emphasis on early accounts of attentional dysfunction and identified some specific quotations which captured the essential nature of the dysfunction: 'A lack of continuity of his perceptions both in space and over time. He saw the environment only in fragments' and 'A schizophrenic can't see the wood for the trees . . . and examines each tree with meticulous care'. These accounts would seem to emphasize a disruption of selective attention whereby shifts in voluntary attention have become fixed or stilted, patients losing flexibility in their ability to direct attention over a range of stimuli and situations. Other researchers have also stressed an inability to concentrate and an experience of 'sensory overload' whereby the individual is continuously overwhelmed by environmental stimuli, being unable to selectively attend to those stimuli of specific interest or relevance to the task at hand. In particular, McGhie and Chapman (1961) on the basis of detailed studies of individual patients with schizophrenia proposed a defective attentional filtering mechanism as the primary deficit in schizophrenia. More recently, Anscombe (1987) has also stressed the patient's inability to focus attention in a purposeful manner. On the basis of these clinical observations and first person accounts of the schizophrenic experience alone, it can be argued strongly that the major dysfunction within schizophrenia is a fundamental disruption of cognitive processing resultant in various attentional deficits.

Empirical studies of attention within schizophrenia

It is not surprising, therefore, that studies of attention and information processing have become a major focus for research in schizophrenia (Braff, 1993; Nuechterlein and Subotnik, 1998). Several different goals may be identified as underlying this research. First, many researchers have attempted to empirically locate the nature of the attentional deficit using a variety of standardized experimental and neuropsychological assessments (Green, 1992). Second, on the basis of such findings, theoretical models of the aetiology of schizophrenia and its associated symptoms might be formulated with respect to identifying specific cognitive processes that are thought to underlie the attentional deficits, together with an understanding of the neurophysiological and anatomical substrates underlying these processes (for example, Braff, 1993; Hemsley, 1993). Third, the development of cognitive models of these attentional deficits might give rise to accounts of the origins and maintenance of schizophrenic symptoms such as delusions and hallucinations (for example, Frith, 1979; Hemsley, 1993). It may then be possible to identify psychological interventions based on theory that might be used to ameliorate the presence of these symptoms. Indeed, the past decade has seen the emergence of a variety of psychological treatments for schizophrenia ranging from those directed at enhancing attentional and cognitive abilities through to cognitive therapy that seeks to challenge the meaning and attributions associated with the presence of hallucinations and delusions (see Wykes, Tarrier and Lewis, 1998).

Methodological issues

Before summarizing the research evidence surrounding attentional and cognitive deficits within schizophrenia, it is important to identify several important methodological obstacles that have hindered progress in this area considerably. We will only identify some of the problems and the interested reader should consult reviews by Braff (1993) and Green (1992) for a more detailed discussion of these issues. First, it has to be recognized that schizophrenia represents a heterogeneous collection of symptoms and may well arise from several distinct underlying aetiologies and pathologies. Indeed, such diversity has caused many psychologists to challenge the overall validity of schizophrenia as either a useful diagnostic (Bentall, Jackson and Pilgrim, 1988) or scientific concept (Boyle, 1990). People diagnosed as schizophrenic, therefore, frequently differ amongst themselves and across time, presumably reflecting different presentations, types and stages within the disorder. Such marked variations can themselves give rise to heterogeneous and often inconsistent patterns of findings on a single standardized test. Neuroleptic treatments for schizophrenia are also undoubtedly associated with cognitive side effects either directly as a result of their therapeutic action or as a consequence of anticholinergic medications prescribed in order to control side effects (for example, Goldberger and Weinberger, 1996). It is also difficult to identify unequivocally a specific pattern of performance that can be argued to represent an underlying and primary schizophrenic deficit. Generally, people with schizophrenia are said to exhibit high levels of distractibility and poor motivation. Even if these deficits are specific to the disorder, they will result in poor performance on nearly any given task that requires concentration and voluntary cognitive effort. Accordingly, a performance deficit on a task performed by people with schizophrenia compared with other control groups (both patient and non-patient) might reflect general difficulties related to engagement with the task rather than a specific underlying attentional deficit.

Taken together, the above methodological barriers have until recently obscured the identification of specific cognitive deficits associated with the disorder. However, the recognition of these limitations to research in this area and the emergence of theoretical frameworks that incorporate these factors have recently given rise to a clarification of the empirical findings within this area. The most influential conceptual advance has been the adoption of the *stress–vulnerability model* (Nuechterlein and Dawson, 1984). Essentially, this model identifies a number of vulnerability factors (for example, genetic, familial, cognitive) that predispose individuals to developing schizophrenia sometime in their lifetime. The emergence of symptoms of schizophrenia, however, relies on an interaction between these vulnerability factors and environmental stressors (such as social adversity, expressed emotion, life events, substance misuse) that precipitate the disorder. Hence, individuals who are vulnerable to schizophrenia will display episodes of symptoms throughout their lives, which reflect variations across time in their ability to withstand environmental stressors and the moderating effects of other environmental factors (such as medication, social networks, enhanced coping strategies).

This stress–vulnerability model has important implications for the interpretation of experimental findings relating to cognitive deficits and how they might be identified. According to the model, if a deficit or cognitive marker is observed within a person who is acutely ill, several distinct interpretations may be entertained. Traditionally, the difference may be taken as an actual vulnerability marker reflecting a primary cognitive deficit underlying schizophrenia. However, given the vulnerability model, an illness episode may also reflect the influence of some precipitating environmental event. Hence, the deficit might represent an episode marker that reflects the manifestation of the psychotic illness state that the individual is experiencing. An example would be the general distracting effects of hearing voices on the performance of some cognitive task. The deficit arises, therefore, due to the episode of the illness and may not be specific to the underlying disorder. Moreover, a performance deficit could also arise more generally due to the non-specific effects of environmental stressors on performance, which may have precipitated the episode.

Research paradigms

In order to tease out these alternative explanations and to identify specific vulnerability markers underlying the disorder, several different study paradigms have been evolved. Essentially, there are two basic methods: the comparison of patients who are acutely ill with those in remission, and the conduct of high-risk or familial studies. If vulnerability is a stable trait-like factor that predisposes people to schizophrenia, vulnerability markers should be evident even when the individual is in remission. The study of remitted patients allows the identification of such vulnerability markers and may also be achieved in some circumstances in the absence of medication effects or the non-specific effects of experiencing an acute episode of the illness. Similarly, if it is assumed that vulnerability is associated with either genetic or familial causes, studies of relatives should also identify underlying vulnerability markers. Hence, in recent years there have been many (a) cross-sectional studies of cognitive functioning within the relatives of people with schizophrenia and (b) longitudinal studies (high risk) of the offspring of people with schizophrenia. In summary, the demonstration of specific cognitive deficits during an episode of schizophrenia, together with the presence of the same deficits both in remitted patients and relatives, provides good evidence of a specific deficit underlying cognitive vulnerability within schizophrenia.

Recent reviews of studies (such as Braff, 1993; Green, 1992; Nuechterlein and Subotnik, 1998), which have adopted the above paradigmatic approach are revealing a promising degree of consistency. First, there appears to be a deficit in the early perceptual processing of stimuli, especially when presented in difficult discrimination tasks. One particular paradigm that has demonstrated consistent deficits across patients who have been acutely ill, who were in remission and also in relatives and offspring of people with schizophrenia, has been the *continuous performance test* (CPT) (Green, 1992; Neuchterlein and Subotnik, 1998). This is essentially a vigilance-type task whereby a series of letters or digits are rapidly presented and certain infrequent targets (such as the letter 'x'), usually of brief duration (200 ms), require identification by a motor response. Measures derived from the CPT include: missed targets, false alarms when non-targets are identified, and hit rates for targets. The degree of task difficulty can be altered by varying the discriminability between the series and the targets. Using a high-load CPT that employs degraded letters (fuzzy indistinct lettering), a specific performance deficit has been shown in both remitted patients and relatives. A particularly interesting finding is that performance appears to be affected most by patients displaying negative symptoms rather than in individuals with active psychotic symptoms. Similar deficits have been observed on other tasks that also rely on early perceptual discrimination. These include backward masking tasks and the forced-choice span of apprehension (Neuchterlein and Subotnik, 1998).

A second type of deficit has also been suggested recently, which involves a disturbance of working memory used to cue the relevance of current stimuli. This deficit has been shown within a different type of CPT (3–7 CPT) whereby clearly focused digits are randomly presented at a rate of one per second. The target is the digit '7' but only when it is immediately preceded by the digit '3'. Hence, a preceding stimulus is used to cue whether the current stimulus is a target or not. This involves the operation of a working memory component in order to either release or inhibit the response to the current target (digit '7') depending upon the identity of the previous cue (digit '3' or other number). Again, patients in remission perform poorly on this version of the CPT but not as poorly as acutely ill patients.

Theories of attention and cognitive deficits in schizophrenia

The above findings give rise to two questions: how can these deficits be explained given contemporary models of attention, and do such explanations account for the experience of psychotic symptoms? Neuchterlein and Subotnik (1998) have related these deficits to a current influential model of attention advocated by Cowan (1988). Essentially, Cowan's model describes several different functional modules involved in the cognitive processing of incoming stimuli. Rather than representing a serial model whereby stimuli are processed sequentially through the information processing system (cf. Norman, 1968), these modules interact extensively during stimulus processing. Stimuli at first enter a brief sensory store which has unlimited capacity. Features of these stimuli then activate codes in a long-term store. Activated units representing a limited capacity short-term store are also located within this long-term store. If these activated units then enter consciousness, this represents a shift in the focus of attention. Cowan suggests that such shifts occur either because stimuli are intentionally selected by a *central executive* or stimuli are novel and capture attention accordingly. Finally, automatic and controlled actions are identified depending on whether the central executive module was required for their execution.

Neuchterlein and Subotnik (1998) employ Cowan's model to account for early perceptual processing deficits underlying the degraded stimulus CPT. Performance on the task involves the passive registration of stimuli in the sensory store, activation of corresponding stimulus features within the long-term store, and the active search for additional features necessary for target/non-target discrimination. The latter is said to be the responsibility of the central executive, which facilitates the entry of specific target codes into the focus of attention and their subsequent detection. They claim that these processes underlying early perceptual identification are compromised in schizophrenia. Poor performance on the CPT (3–7) task is also accounted for by the model. This task involves the activation in long-term memory of incoming stimuli, identification of stimuli as cues ('3's), differential attention to stimuli following these cues, and either voluntary initiation of a response ('7's) or withholding a response when the stored cue is absent. These processes all involve the central executive interacting with activated short-term memory, which has frequently been termed *working memory*. In summary, from Cowan's perspective these deficits imply a deficit in the initial passive phase of perception whereby incoming stimuli activate long-term codes, together with a further deficit in the second phase of perception involving the active search for specific stimulus features taking into account the stimulus context.

Other models to account for these deficits have also been suggested. In particular, Hemsley (1987, 1993) has been influential in applying information-processing models to account for schizophrenia and its associated symptoms. As with Neuchterlein and Subotnik's emphasis on a working-memory-based deficit in the use of cue-relevant stimuli, Hemsley (1987) has stated that 'it is a weakening of the influence of stored memories of regularities of previous input on current perception which is basic to the schizophrenic condition'. One demonstration of this was a choice reaction time task, which required differential responses to the letters 'A' and 'B'. These targets were regularly flanked by accompanying letters 'X' and 'Y' (thus 'XAX' and 'YBY') but occasionally the flanking would be reversed ('YAY' and 'XBX') while the correct response was still to be cued by the target 'A' or 'B'. Non-patients show a slowing in reaction time when the flanking letters are unexpectedly changed and the context shifted. However, if patients are influenced less by such past regularities such as context, they should be less affected by the shifts. This was found to be the case for acutely ill but not chronic patients. Hemsley and colleagues have extended this model, applying the latent-inhibition and blocking paradigms from animal learning theory and have modelled their theory both in animals and man (Gray et al., 1991; Hemsley, 1993).

Perhaps one of the distinctive features of the above model is that, although it is firmly grounded in a neurobiological substrate, it also attempts to account for the origins and maintenance of individual psychotic symptoms and experiences. Essentially, Hemsley argues that the reduced influence of previously stored memories on current stimulus processing leads to a number of clinically relevant consequences. Firstly, people with schizophrenia have a reduced ability to make use of redundancy and the patterning of input, which may give rise to states of sensory overload. A consequence of this may be that patients adopt adaptive strategies in order to contain or reduce such overload. Hemsley (1993) suggests that negative symptoms, such as social withdrawal and poverty of speech, might represent these coping strategies, together with a preference for highly structured and predictable environments. A second consequence of the reduced utilization of past regularities is a heightened awareness of irrelevant stimuli and the experience of unstructured and ambiguous sensory input. The ongoing experience of unrelated and ambiguous stimuli, together with the intrusion of unintended material from long-term memory, may give rise to the development of both hallucinations and delusions. Hence, hallucinations may arise from the perception of uninhibited material released from long-term memory being experienced as real and apparently deriving from external stimulation. Delusions, on the other hand, would arise due to faulty inferences linking irrelevant features and unexpected intrusions from long-term memory. Again, Hemsley (1993) links his theoretical model of symptom formation with first-hand accounts of psychotic experiences. He stresses previous descriptions by others: 'patients seeing non-fortuitous coincidences everywhere' and a patient stating: 'out of these perceptions came the absolute awareness that my ability to see connections had been multiplied many times over'. However, Hemsley also suggests that in addition to anomalous perceptual experiences, delusions can arise from abnormal reasoning styles, which may result in patients making abnormal causal inferences surrounding extraneous and unrelated events.

Another cognitive model that locates the primary dysfunction later on in the information processing system is that proposed by Frith (1992). His latest theory is a detailed neuropsychological model that extends his earlier theorizing concerning the role of consciousness in schizophrenia. Essentially, he posits a disorder affecting a self-monitoring system that results in the patient experiencing his perceptions, thoughts, and actions as if they originated from a source external to the self. He suggests that whereas a self-monitoring system or central executive usually provides feedback on our willed intentions and plans, the monitoring system for a person with schizophrenia becomes disconnected from intentional acts and results in the patient attributing self-generated actions and thoughts as if they originated externally. Such a dysfunction might account for hallucinations and passivity delusions, together with other positive symptoms. Negative symptoms, on the other hand, are said to arise from a disconnection between goals/plans and the generation of willed actions.

Finally, some mention should be made of Bentall's (1994) social cognition model of delusions, particularly those involving paranoia. The origins of Bentall's model require us to return to the Stroop task, which was discussed in relation to anxiety-related biases in a previous section of this chapter. Bentall and Kaney (1989) required paranoid, depressed and normal individuals to colour name threat-related, depression-related and neutral words. The paranoid individuals demonstrated a slowing to threat-related material. Further studies by these authors also confirmed biases in recall and autobiographical memories for threatening material within paranoid patients. In addition to specific cognitive biases, Bentall also examined *attributional styles* using various self-report questionnaires. Essentially, he demonstrated that paranoid patients, in comparison with either depressed or normal individuals, tended to make abnormally internal attributions for positive events and abnormally external attributions for negative events. Taken together, Bentall argues that these cognitive biases are responsible for the paranoid patient preventing any thoughts related to threats to the self becoming conscious, thereby maintaining a sense of positive self-esteem despite the presence of threatening information. Threats, on the other hand, are externally attributed to others. Such a mechanism is similar to psychodynamic formulations for paranoia being a defence against depression and low self-esteem.

Implications of cognitive models for management and therapy

As has already been discussed within the introduction, the study of attentional dysfunction in schizophrenia has two important implications for the management of schizophrenia. First, it should assist patients, clinicians and carers to gain greater insights into the phenomenology of the schizophrenic experience and hence be beneficial by developing a good understanding of the inner world of a person with schizophrenia. Clearly, this is limited by our rather impoverished third-person accounts of the experience. Moreover, it also requires consideration of the emotional impact and consequences of psychotic symptoms such as hallucinations and delusions. Nevertheless, such an approach is directed at attempting to understand the often *superficially* chaotic nature of a person's schizophrenic experience rather than the mere identification and labelling of individual psychotic symptoms.

Second, in addition to facilitating an understanding of the subjective experience underlying psychosis, cognitive models may also suggest new treatments aimed at ameliorating the impact of psychotic symptoms. Recently, several different types of psychological intervention have been developed for schizophrenia. These range from cognitive retraining programmes targeted at reversing or improving the basic cognitive deficits underlying the disorder (for example, Brenner et al., 1992), coping strategies aimed at more effective methods for dealing with distracting stimuli such as hallucinations (for example, Haddock, Bentall and Slade, 1996; Barrowclough and Tarrier, 1992), through to cognitive therapy techniques that challenge the meanings and attributions underlying hallucinations and delusions (Chadwick, Birchwood and Trower, 1996; Fowler, Garety and Kuipers, 1995). Indeed, recent randomized control trials have demonstrated that such therapeutic approaches can give rise to significant benefits in people diagnosed with schizophrenia and with histories of treatment resistance to medication (for example, Kuipers et al., 1997).

Summary

Psychological models of information processing and attention are constantly being updated and revised. Accordingly, we have been able to provide within this brief chapter only an introduction to the development of attentional models and a flavour of some of the major theories and concepts. Nevertheless, the importance of these models for understanding psychological disorders is becoming more and more influential for both psychiatrists and clinical psychologists. On the one hand, recent advances in neuroscience and brain imaging, in particular, purport to identify different brain areas and neurotransmitter systems implicated in psychiatric disorders. However, such advances in knowledge will only benefit psychiatrists if anatomical differences and anomalies can be related to cognitive models of information processing and ultimately to the expression and experience of psychiatric states and symptoms. At the other pole of the treatment dimension, there is an increasing demonstration of the clinical effectiveness of psychological methods of managing psychotic symptoms. Many of these approaches are based upon cognitive therapy models and in particular contemporary cognitive theories of information processing dysfunctions within psychosis. In conclusion, we would argue that an understanding of cognitive processing in schizophrenia is a fundamental area of knowledge for the inquisitive and innovative clinician.

References

Anscombe R (1987) The disorder of consciousness in schizophrenia. Schizophrenia Bulletin 11: 241–60.

Barrowclough C, Tarrier N (1992) Families of Schizophrenic Patients: Cognitive Behavioural Interventions. London: Chapman & Hall.

Bentall RP (1994) Cognitive biases and abnormal beliefs: towards a model of persecutory delusions. In AS David, J Cutting (eds) The Neuropsychology of Schizophrenia. London: Erlbaum, pp. 337–60.

Bentall RP, Kaney S (1989) Content-specific information processing and persecutory delusions: an investigation using the emotional Stroop task. British Journal of Medical Psychology 62: 355–64.

Bentall R, Jackson H, Pilgrim D (1988) Abandoning the concept of schizophrenia. Some implications of validity arguments for psychological research into psychotic phenomena. British Journal of Clinical Psychology 27: 303–324.

Boyle M (1990) Schizophrenia: a Scientific Delusion. London: Routledge.

Braff DL (1993) Information processing and attention dysfunctions in schizophrenia. Schizophrenia Bulletin 19: 233–59.

Brenner HD, Hodel B, Roder V, Corrigan P (1992) Treatment of cognitive dysfunctions and behavioral deficits in schizophrenia. Schizophrenia Bulletin 18: 21–6.

Brewin C (1988) Cognitive Foundations of Clinical Psychology. London: Lawrence Erlbaum.

Broadbent D (1958) Perception and Communication. Oxford: Pergamon Press.

Chadwick P, Birchwood M, Trower P (1996) Cognitive Therapy for Delusions, Voices and Paranoia. Chichester: Wiley.

Cherry E (1953) Some experiments on the recognition of speech, with one and two ears. Journal of the Acoustical Society of America 23: 915–19.

Cowan N (1988) Evolving conceptions of memory storage, selective attention, and their mutual constraints within the human information-processing system. Psychological Bulletin 104: 163–91.

Deutsch J, Deutsch D (1963) Attention: some theoretical considerations. Psychological Review 70: 80–90.

Fowler D, Garety P, Kuipers E (1995) Cognitive Behaviour Therapy for Psychosis. Theory and Practice. Chichester: Wiley.

Frith C (1979) Consciousness, information processing and schizophrenia. British Journal of Psychiatry 134: 225–35.

Frith CD (1992) The Cognitive Neuropsychology of Schizophrenia. Hove: Lawrence Erlbaum.

Goldberger TE, Weinberger DR (1996) Effects of neuroleptic medications on the cognition of patients with schizophrenia: a review of recent studies. Journal of Clinical Psychiatry 57 (suppl 9): 62–5.

Gray JA, Feldon J, Rawlins JNP, Hemsley DR, Smith AD (1991) The neuropsychology of schizophrenia. Behavioral and Brain Sciences 14: 1–20.

Green MF (1992) Information processing in schizophrenia. In DJ Kavanagh (ed.) Schizophrenia: An Overview and Practical Handbook. London: Chapman & Hall, pp. 59–78.

Haddock G, Bentall RP, Slade P (1996) Psychological treatment of auditory hallucination: focusing or distraction. In G Haddock, PD Slade (eds) Cognitive-Behavioural Interventions with Psychotic Disorders. London: Routledge.

Hemsley DR (1987) An experimental psychological model for schizophrenia. In H Hafner, WF Gattaz, W Janzarik (eds) Search for the Causes of Schizophrenia. Berlin: Springer Verlag, pp. 179–188.

Hemsley DR (1993) A simple (or simplistic?) cognitive model for schizophrenia. Behaviour Research and Therapy 31: 633–45.

Kuipers E, Garety P, Fowler D, Dunn G, Bebbington P, Freeman D, Hadley C (1997) London East Anglia randomised controlled trial of cognitive behavioural therapy for psychosis 1: effects of the treatment phase. British Journal of Psychiatry 171: 319–27.

McGhie A, Chapman J (1961) Disorders of attention and perception in early schizophrenia. British Journal of Medical Psychology 34: 103–16.

MacKay D (1973) Aspects of the theory of comprehension, memory and attention. Quarterly Journal of Experimental Psychology 25: 22–40.

MacLeod C, Mathews A, Tata P (1986) Attentional bias in emotional disorders. Journal of Abnormal Psychology 95: 15–20.

Mathews A, MacLeod C (1986) Discrimination of threat cues without awareness of anxiety states. Journal of Abnormal Psychology 95: 131–8.

Norman D (1968) Toward a theory of memory and attention. Psychological Review 75: 522–36.

Nuechterlein KH, Asarnow RF (1989) Cognition and perception. In HI Kaplan, BJ Sadcock (eds) Comprehensive Textbook of Psychiatry, Vol 5. Baltimore: Williams & Wilkins, pp. 241–56.

Nuechterlein K, Dawson M (1984) A heuristic vulnerability/stress model of schizophrenic relapse. Schizophrenia Bulletin 10: 300–12.

Nuechterlein KH, Subotnik KL (1998) The cognitive origins of schizophrenia and prospects for intervention. In T Wykes, N Tarrier, S Lewis (eds) Outcome and Innovation in Psychological Treatment of Schizophrenia. Chichester: Wiley, pp. 17–41.

Parkinson L, Rachman S (1981) Intrusive thoughts: the effects of uncontrived stress. Advances in Behavior Research and Therapy 3: 11–118.

Posner MI, Peterson L (1990) The attention system of the human brain. Annual Review of Neuroscience 13: 25–42.

Schneider W, Dumais S, Shiffrin R (1984) Automatic and controlled processing. In R Parasuraman, D Davies (eds) Varieties of Attention. London, Orlando: Academic Press.

Treisman A (1964) Selective attention in man. British Medical Bulletin 20: 12–16.

Warwick H, Salkovskis P (1989) Hypochondriasis. In J Scott, J Williams, A Beck (eds) Cognitive Therapy in Clinical Practice. London: Routledge.

Watts F, McKenna F, Sharrock R, Trezise L (1986) Colour naming of phobia related words. British Journal of Psychology 77: 97–108.

Wells A, Morrison A (1994) Qualitative dimensions of normal worry and intrusive thoughts: a comparative study. Behaviour Research and Therapy 32: 867–70.

Williams JM, Watts F, MacLeod C, Mathews A (1997) Cognitive Psychology and Emotional Disorders (2 edn). Chichester: Wiley.

Wykes T, Tarrier N, Lewis S (1998) Outcome and Innovation in Psychological Treatment of Schizophrenia. Chichester: Wiley.

Chapter 4
Remembering and forgetting

M. EACOTT

Key concepts	Key names
Primary/secondary memory	James
Short-term store	
Long-term store	
Rehearsal	
Recency effect	
Primacy effect	
Memory span	
Digit span	
Chunking	
Working memory	Baddeley
Declarative memory	
Semantic	Tulving
Autobiographical/episodic	
Procedural memory	
Explicit/implicit tests	Schachter
Free recall	
Recognition	
Cued recall	
Decay	
Interference	
Law of disuse	Thorndike
Retrieval failure	
Context-dependent memory	
Incidental learning	
Intentional learning	
Maintenance rehearsal	
Elaborative rehearsal	
Levels of processing approach	Craik and Lockhart
Deep encoding	
Shallow encoding	
Encoding-specificity principle	
Schema	
Amnesia	
Korsakoff's amnesia	
Hysterical amnesia/fugue	

We rely on memory for much of our everyday functioning, yet we often take our prodigious memory ability for granted. All the words in our vocabulary, the names and faces of all our friends, family and acquaintances and the results of our formal education are stored in memory, as well as a great deal of gossip and other incidental information. Still, we may be annoyed or embarrassed when we fail to place a familiar person we pass in the street, or fail to attend a scheduled meeting. These are clear examples of memory failures, but psychologists have long been aware that there are several different types of memory, each with its own characteristics, and which may fail us in characteristic ways.

Primary and secondary memory

The idea that there are distinct types of memory is an old one within psychology. As long ago as 1890, the psychologist William James suggested that there are two types of memory experience, which he called *primary* and *secondary memory*. By primary memory, James meant the information that you are holding in mind at this very moment, your current thoughts. By secondary memory, he meant those things that you have known or experienced in the past but about which you are not consciously thinking at the moment. This idea that there are two distinct forms of memory has become central to psychological views of memory. However, as we have come to understand the properties of these two types of memory more fully, the terms *short-term store* (STS, or sometimes STM for *short-term memory*) and long-term store (LTS or sometimes LTM) have replaced James's original terms (Atkinson and Shiffrin, 1968).

Primary memory or STS refers to what you are currently focusing upon, for example remembering a telephone number between looking it up in the telephone book and dialling. The important aspect of STS is its fleeting or temporary nature. The telephone number, for example, is unlikely to remain stored in memory for long – once you have dialled, the memory of the number will quickly fade from your consciousness. In fact, perhaps surprisingly, you will have almost no memory of the number as little as 20–30 seconds after you dial (Peterson and Peterson, 1959). However, if the number is engaged and you wish to redial in a minute or two, you will want to keep the number in memory for rather longer than this. Fortunately, you can prevent the telephone number being lost from STS by *rehearsal* – that is, by mentally reviewing the number to be dialled. Rehearsal may involve saying the number out loud, but subvocal repetition ('the inner voice') is more common and equally effective. However, if another telephone call interrupts the mental rehearsal of the number, the number will quickly be lost from memory. Thus the important characteristics of STS are its short duration (up to 30 seconds) and the need to mentally rehearse information held within it if we wish to keep it in STS for longer than this period.

Of course, the telephone numbers of our family and friends need to be stored in memory for longer than a few seconds if we don't want to look them up every time we telephone them. These numbers will have to be retained in secondary memory or long-term store (LTS). Long-term store can retain information over periods of up to 80 years or more without any active rehearsal (Bahrick, 1984). This means that you may easily be able to remember events that took place 10 or more years ago and about which you rarely think. Short-term store and LTS are linked so that information in STS may be transferred into LTS for long-term storage. Equally, information from LTS may be transferred into STS for active use. Telephoning a member of your family, for example, may involve retrieving the number from LTS and bringing it into the active consciousness of STS so that you may dial.

The operation of LTS and STS can be seen in a very simple demonstration, which is similar to an experiment carried out by Postman and Phillips (1965). Imagine that you read a list of 20 unrelated words. After reading the list, you try to recall as many of those words as possible. Given such a task, you would probably start by writing down the last few words you heard, those that are still in STS. Next, you try to recall all the other words you heard. People trying this task are often most successful in remembering the last few words on the list, those they wrote down immediately. They also remember the first few words on the list relatively well. Those words that formed the middle portion of the list are least well remembered. The superior recall of the last few words is called the *recency effect.* The recency effect shows recall of words that were in STS. If you delay recalling the words for a few minutes, for example by writing your name and address before attempting to recall the words, the recency effect will no longer be seen. We can understand this by realizing that, when writing your name and address, you are unable to actively rehearse the words. The time spent writing is long enough for the words to be lost from STS. Any words that you then recall are retrieved from LTS and therefore there will be no recency effect. Remember that recall of the first few words on a list is also relatively good. This is true regardless of whether you write your name and address before attempting to recall the words or not. This tendency to recall the first few items better than subsequent items is known as the *primacy effect,* and reflects the operation of LTS. Items at the beginning of a list or sequence of events have preferential access to LTS, causing the observed primacy effect. The primacy effect is also seen in real-life settings as well as in bizarre laboratory examples. For example, Ley (1979) looked at what patients remembered following a visit to their doctor. The patients remembered the first few things they had been told better than subsequent information. Perhaps one can draw the conclusion that the really important information should come early in a consultation if it is to be well remembered by the patient.

One important difference, therefore, between STS and LTS is the time span over which each operates. Without rehearsal, memories in STS last only a matter of seconds whereas those in LTS can extend over many years and decades. However, there are also other important differences between LTS and STS. In STS, information is often held in a phonological form – that is, according to how it sounds (Conrad, 1964). For example, when we hold a telephone number in STS while waiting to dial, we hold the numbers in the form 'won-too-three-for'. When we rehearse the number we also rehearse this phonological form so that we have 'an inner voice' that we may hear rehearsing. One result of this phonological coding of the information in STS is that mistakes may occur between phonologically similar items in memory. For example, if I wish to remember my postcode between looking it up and writing it on a form, I hold the information as the sounds of the letters and numbers. Should I make an error in STS I am likely to mistake a letter that sounds similar to the one I meant. Thus I may accidentally write CH1, as it sounds similar to DH1. In contrast, the sound of the items does not play an important role in LTS (Baddeley, 1966). Instead, LTS primarily stores the meaning of the item – it is semantically based. To demonstrate this, stop now to try to remember what is the difference in time span between LTS and STS. You will probably find that you can recall the meaning of what was said earlier in this chapter, but you will almost certainly not be able to recall the exact words that were written. You read that sentence too long ago for it still to be stored in STS and so have lost the phonological form of the words. You will have recalled the information from LTS. LTS is good at retaining the meaning, or gist, of information, but is poor at retaining the sequence of words that were used. We can therefore distinguish between the phonologically based coding in STS and semantic (or meaning based) coding in LTS.

Short-term store and LTS differ in one other important aspect. LTS is very unlikely to ever become full. As a result, you can always learn something new however old you are, or however much you already know. To some extent, therefore, you can teach an old dog new tricks. In contrast, STS has a very limited storage capacity. The amount that STS can retain at any one time is about seven numbers. So, you might reasonably hope to keep a telephone number in STS, but you would be unwise to attempt to remember two telephone numbers simultaneously. The amount of information that can be held in STS is called the *memory span,* but, because it is often tested using numbers, it is also sometimes known as the *digit span.* A digit span of seven numbers is entirely normal. There is, of course, some variation in the digit span of normal people but most people can recall between five and nine digits, that is seven plus-or-minus two (which is usually written as '7 ± 2'). George Miller (Miller, 1956), in a now classic and much quoted paper, called seven *the magic number.* To demonstrate this, try reading the following and then reproducing it on a scrap of paper after several seconds.

101007747765

There were a total of 11 numbers, more than you can hold in STS, and so you may have found it difficult to recall more than about seven successfully. However, if you succeeded, you may have helped yourself by noticing some patterns in the numbers. For example, there were two zeros followed by two sevens. This is an example of chunking – the principle of combining separate pieces of information into one meaningful chunk. Had you noticed that the number actually consisted of just four chunks of information, you may have found this task even easier (101, 007, 747 and 765). So, when we describe the capacity of the STS system as being just seven items, we should note that this might be much more than just seven numbers, letters or words. By combining the information into meaningful combinations, we can remember about seven chunks (plus or minus two). Using this principle, you will probably be able to recall more than seven of the following letters:

BBCUFOFBITSBGPO.

In summary, the differences between STS and LTS can be seen in three major ways. The first is the time span over which each retains information (30 seconds versus decades or more). The second major difference is the form in which they hold the information (phonological versus semantic coding). Finally, they differ in the amount of information that can be held at any one time (seven chunks versus an unlimited amount).

Working memory

Short-term store, however, is important for more than just temporarily remembering telephone numbers or strings of letters. It also has a more active role to play. For example, try to add the following numbers:

47, 31, 25.

When you attempted this, you probably found that you had to keep the result of 47+31 temporarily held in STS while you set about adding 25. But where was the mental activity of adding 25 taking place? Alan Baddeley suggested that STS not only held the numbers, but was also the place where the mental operation of addition took place. Thus Baddeley suggested that STS served as a 'workbench of mental operations', rather than just a passive holding area (Baddeley and Hitch, 1974; Baddeley, 1992). To emphasize this new active view of STS, Baddeley renamed it *working memory*. Working memory is another name for what is also known as STS, but takes the view that it is an active workbench for carrying out mental operations. These mental operations include simple mathematical operations such as addition and subtraction as well as other cognitive operations. For example, working memory will play a part in searching through LTS to answer the question 'when was the last time it rained' or even in understanding this sentence.

In addition, Baddeley realized that while most items in working memory are coded phonologically, it is possible to retain information that does not contain any sound. For example, imagine a question mark on a piece of paper. Now imagine turning the question mark through 180 degrees so that it is upside down and then picking up the paper and turning it face down on the desk. Does the opening in the curve of the question mark now lie to the left or the right of the page? This is just the sort of mental operation that Baddeley believes is carried out in working memory. However, if you have attempted this, you will have found that it would be impossible to get to an answer while dealing with this problem phonologically (i.e. on the basis of the speech sounds involved in the question). You will almost certainly have had to conjure up an image of how a question mark might appear on a page, and then manipulate that image. This implies that working memory may use visual, as well as phonological, information. In fact, because working memory in Baddeley's view is more than just a passive store of phonological information, he suggested that it consists of several smaller subcomponents. There is a component that can passively hold phonological material, a separate area that may passively hold visual images (such as the question mark), and an area that serves as the workbench for working on and manipulating the information that may be held in the other components. Together, these three components make up working memory.

Divisions within long-term memory

Long-term store is a system that retains the meaning of information over long periods of time. Unlike information in working memory, information in LTS does not need constant rehearsal to prevent it being lost. In fact, you may be able to remember the name of your primary school teacher despite the fact that you may well not have thought about your school days for many years. It is often said that you will never forget how to ride a bike, despite the fact that one rarely thinks about cycling. However, in one sense these two memory abilities are different. Many people can recall the name of their primary school teacher, but if asked how to ride a bike, would probably find it quite difficult to give a good answer. However, one would not necessarily conclude from this failure that they do not know how to ride a bike. Instead, the failure highlights the fact that not all information in LTS is in a declarative form – one that can easily be stated. *Declarative memory* is any memory that you can bring to mind and is often, although not necessarily, capable of being spoken. Knowledge of a teacher's name is declarative as it can be brought to mind and, if necessary, spoken. Equally, the answers to the questions 'What did you eat yesterday?' or 'What is the capital of Germany?' would demonstrate declarative memories. However, not all memories are of this type. Knowledge of how to ride a bike, how to drive, swim or write is unlikely to be declarative. These non-declarative memories are called *procedural memories*. By their very nature, procedural memories are very hard to pass on to others because the information cannot be brought to mind and verbalized. Complex procedural skills, such as how to do surgical operations, cannot therefore be taught in a classroom by passing on verbal information, but are usually taught using observation or supervised practice. However, the distinction between declarative and procedural memories is not always so clear-cut. Often one event may give rise to information, some of which is stored in a declarative form and some in procedural form. For example, if you were to do the same jigsaw puzzle each day for a week, you would gradually improve your ability to do the jigsaw, completing it progressively more quickly. At the end of the week you would have some declarative memories about your experience with the jigsaw – for example you would be able to report the picture depicted on the jigsaw. However, you are unlikely to be able to report how you were able to complete it more quickly at the end of the week than the beginning. This information is of a procedural nature and cannot be reported or consciously inspected. As you will have noticed, procedural memory often involves skills and for this reason is also sometimes known as *skills memory*.

In contrast to procedural memory, declarative memory often involves events and facts. Psychologists have further divided declarative memory into memory for events and memory for facts. Fact memory is called *semantic memory* and includes all general knowledge, including the meaning of words. For example you can draw on semantic memory to answer the following questions: Is a robin a bird? What is the Dead Sea? What shape is the Earth? Semantic memories are usually common to all members of a culture, although in the case of a flat earthist, may not be. Semantic memory can be contrasted with *episodic memory*, which contains memory for specific episodes in your life. For this reason, episodic memory is also sometimes known as *autobiographical memory*. You can draw on episodic memory to answer the following questions: When was the last time you saw a robin? Have you ever been to the Dead Sea? What did you do yesterday? While most readers of this chapter will have given identical answers to the first set of questions, drawing on a semantic memory which is shared by most members of a culture, episodic memory is specific to the person and will have been answered differently by each reader. However, note that there is, of course, an important interaction between semantic and episodic memory. In order to answer the question 'When did you last see a robin?' you must first extract the meaning of the words present from semantic memory and useful associated information (what is a robin and where might a robin be seen?)

before attempting to extract an answer about the last sighting from episodic memory. The second way in which the episodic and semantic information interact can be seen from the following example: suppose you are asked for a definition of the concept of declarative memory. At first glance the question appears to be asking for the meaning of words and therefore to require accessing semantic memory. However, if this word is new to you, you may instead remember that declarative memory was defined earlier in this chapter, so you may try to recall what you read there. This involves recalling a specific incident in your recent life – what you read a few minutes ago. Recalling what you read is a clear example of using *episodic* memory. Thus it is important to realize that the nature of the information stored is the important difference between semantic and episodic memories, not the question that elicits the information. Semantic memory contains memory about facts and concepts that are not linked to a specific time or place – you do not know how you know that a robin is a bird or when you learned it. In contrast, episodic memory is specific to a time or place, as each episode occurred at a specific time and place and is tied to that time and place.

The above distinction between the types of memories in LTS was proposed by Tulving (1985). However, an alternative way of describing the different stores in LTS was proposed by Schachter (1987). He distin-guished between explicit and implicit tests of memory. For example, if a subject has been shown a list of words including the word aardvark, he noted that there are several ways in which you can test for memory of the words. First, one could ask 'Can you remember the words on the list you saw?' This is a *free recall* test of memory. Alternatively one could test memory by presenting a choice of words and asking the subject to indicate which words were on the list ('Which of these words was on the list: anteater or aardvark?'). This is called a *recognition test of memory.* An intermediate condition is to provide hints or clues to aid recall, without giving the actual words to recognize. For example, one could give the initial letters or a word associated to words on the list ('Can you think of a word on the list which was an animal beginning with A?') This is called a *cued recall test.* All these are examples that ask the person to recall the event, and therefore test *explicit memory* for the words. However, it is possible to test the contents of LTS without overtly asking the person to attempt to remember at all. This is called an *implicit test* of memory – a test of memory that does not actually ask the subject to attempt to recall. For example, one could ask the subject to think of any word beginning with the initial letters of words which were on the list ('Can you think of an animal which begins with A?'). There is no need to refer to the memory of the list at all, although many people will produce words that were on the list. Schachter (1987) noted that declarative memories are often explicit in nature and procedural memories are usually implicit. However, the above examples show that there is not a one-to-one correspondence between the two ways of viewing types of memory. An alternative way of subdividing LTS therefore is into those memories that are explicitly available and those that are only implicitly available.

Forgetting from long-term memory

Decay and interference

As we have discussed, LTS has a vast, probably limitless, capacity for storing information. Despite this, we cannot always recall information when we need it. Indeed, we are most aware of our memory when it lets us down and we have forgotten something. But what does it mean when we say we have forgotten? What we tend to mean is that we have attempted to get some information from memory and have failed, despite a feeling that we once knew this information. However, we may ask why we failed. Perhaps because we have the impression of emptiness when we fail to remember, one view is that the information has been lost from memory. In particular, we tend to find that we forget relatively old memories, things that we have not remembered for a while. This may suggest that memories that are not reviewed once in a while will decay, leaving no trace. Indeed, in 1914 Thorndike proposed the *law of disuse*, which suggested that unused memories will gradually fade away. This might appear to be an efficient strategy to adopt, like a library disposing of books that have not been borrowed for some years. However, although information may decay quickly in STS, the fact that we will occasionally recall something that we have not thought of for many years suggests that memories may not decay in LTS. Instead, it has been suggested that new memories may interfere with memories already in store and make the older memories harder to recall. Given time, a memory will appear to fade away, not through decay itself, but because other, newer memories interfere with it so we can no longer access it. To assess whether new information might interfere with memories already in store, one can vary the level of interference caused by new memories and measure the amount of forgetting. If interference is the cause of forgetting, we will forget more when there is more interference. However, if forgetting is simply due to decay of memories caused by the passage of time, the amount of interference should be irrelevant to the rate of forgetting. To test this, McGeoch and McDonald (1931) taught a list of words to a group of subjects. Once they had learned the list of words well, they were given varying amounts of interference from new information. For example, one group of subjects now learned a different list of words, which had similar meanings to the first list. For this group, the similarity between the lists would be expected to be a cause of interference between the two lists in memory. Another group of subjects learned a list of unrelated words that should interfere much less with the first list. A third group just rested, an activity that should cause very little interference at all. Finally, all three groups were tested on their recall of the original list of words. It was found that those who had learned interfering lists of words recalled more poorly than those who had just rested. Moreover, the greater the similarity between the two lists learned, the poorer the recall of the original list. This study suggests that interference between the information in memory and subsequent similar information is the cause of at least some forgetting. This is supported by our own intuition that unusual events are well remembered, perhaps because there are few similar events to interfere.

Failures of retrieval

Sometimes we try to recall something without success, only to find that the required information pops into our mind at some later moment. This is a particularly common experience with people's names, when we search in vain for the name of an acquaintance or political figure, only to remember it quite clearly when the moment has passed. The fact that the name can be remembered at a later moment clearly indicates that the name was present in memory. Why then was it not recalled at the critical moment? This common and infuriating experience suggests that forgetting does not always mean that the information is not stored in memory, simply that you failed to locate and retrieve the memory at that particular moment. Thus forgetting may not only result from interference from other memories, but also from a *retrieval failure*. This is particularly apparent when you fail to recall something but can instantly recognize the correct answer should someone else suggest it. (Perhaps this is why a multiple-choice examination, a test of recognition memory, is preferred by many to forms of examination that test free recall of information.) Sometimes we have the experience of feeling that we know the answer we are seeking, but cannot quite find it. This feeling is known as the *tip-of-the-tongue* phenomenon (also abbreviated to *TOT phenomenon*). Often providing extra cues to memory can help a retrieval failure. So, for example, should you fail to retrieve the answer to the question 'What is the name shared by a German Chancellor and a famous ship?' you may be helped by the clue that it begins with B. However, sometimes one can provide oneself with additional cues to help resolve a retrieval failure in memory. For example, if you fail to remember something, it can help to return to the place in which you learned it. Being in the same place, with the same surroundings, sounds and smells, may be sufficient to trigger the elusive memory. If the situation is very evocative, memories may even be triggered without a conscious search through memory at all, as Proust famously found. Many people have reported returning to a childhood home town or old school only to find long-forgotten memories flooding back. It is not even necessary to actually visit a place to evoke the memories. Simply imagining the place or situation may be sufficient to retrieve a flood of memories (Smith, 1979). This is an example of *context-dependent memory* where the situation or context in which you find yourself is a determinant of the ability to retrieve memories (Godden and Baddeley, 1975). In general, the greater the similarity between the context in which you are attempting to retrieve a memory and the context in which the memory was stored, the better the recall will be. This can have important practical implications as skills will be recalled much better if taught in the setting in which they will be used, rather than in a classroom setting. For example, it may be more appropriate to teach resuscitation techniques in a ward rather than in a classroom, if the techniques are to be well remembered when the need arises on a ward.

However the context in which you attempt to recall does not just include the physical environment. The current mood or the drug state of a person can be considered as an internal environment in which the learning or remembering is taking place. It is a common observation that, when sober, one cannot recall what occurred when drunk, only to remember again next time we drink too much. Goodwin and his colleagues showed a very similar effect in an unusual laboratory study which involved subjects drinking high-strength vodka (Goodwin et al., 1969)! This is an example of the internal context (alcohol intoxication) aiding retrieval of memories of events that occurred in a similar context. In a different internal context (sober), the memories are less easily retrieved. Marijuana causes similar effects. Of course, our internal environment may also include our mood (Bower, 1981). This would imply that, when depressed, one may best recall events which occurred when one was depressed and one will recall less well events that occurred in happier times. It has been suggested that this phenomenon may serve to maintain clinical depression. A depressed patient will tend to focus on events that happened during periods of depression and will have difficulty recalling more positive moments. Of course, the converse effect may also be seen. Most people are fortunate enough to have relatively happy lives and therefore find it easier to recall examples of cheerful rather than unhappy events (Linton, 1975).

Using your memory efficiently

We remember quite a lot of information that we did not aim to memorize. For example, I can recall what I ate last evening, despite the fact that I did not set out to learn this information. This is an example of *incidental learning* – learning or memory that occurs without conscious effort to commit to memory. However, there are circumstances in which we want to deliberately commit something to memory and we want to be able to recall it on demand. This is called *intentional learning*. The revision process is an example of intentional learning, where we attempt to commit information to memory in the hope of being able to retrieve it during the examination. Can we use our understanding of the processes of memory to gain a better memory, or at least better examination results? Fortunately the answer to this question is 'yes'.

We have already discussed how information may be kept in STS by the process of rehearsal. However, this is not useful when attempting to learn the material as the information will disappear only seconds after we cease actively rehearsing it. Moreover, the limited capacity of STS means that we could keep very little information in store this way anyway. This may explain why rote learning is not an efficient way of learning (Craik and Watkins, 1973). This sort of rote repetition of material is known as *maintainance rehearsal*. It serves only to maintain the information in STS and does not succeed in transferring it into LTS for longer term storage. To succeed in a revision process we need to efficiently transfer information from STS into LTS. How can we achieve this? Remember that LTS is based on the meaning of the information, and so considering the meaning of the material to be learned helps the learning process (Craik and Tulving, 1975). This is sometimes called *elaborative rehearsal*. Elaborative rehearsal is any process that involves active consideration of the meaning of the material to be learned. If you attempt to learn a list of unrelated words, for example, elaborative rehearsal may include trying to think of a sentence involving each word. Elaborative rehearsal of a telephone number may involve looking for patterns or associations (your age, followed by your old house number, for example). Elaborative rehearsal of lists of unrelated words or telephone numbers may require some imagination on your part, but elaborative rehearsal of meaningful material, such as most examination material, should be easier. It will involve any active attempt to organize and understand the meaning of the material and it is often useful to relate it to other things you know. For example, in discussion of context dependent memory above, it would be helpful to attempt to think of a personal example of a context-dependent memory. Why does elaborative rehearsal aid memory? One way of answering this question is to consider the *levels of processing approach* (Craik and Lockhart, 1972). The 'levels of processing' approach suggests that encoding of material can occur at different levels, with deeper encoding associated with better recall. *Deep encoding* means processing the material according to deep properties, such as its meanings or associations. Deep encoding can be contrasted with *shallow encoding,* which is processing the surface properties, such as the sound of the word or the appearance of the letters of a word on a page. Elaborative rehearsal results in deep encoding of material and will therefore result in better recall. However, we can also consider why deep encoding should aid recall. We have already suggested that many memory failures are actually failures to find and retrieve the memory at the appropriate moment. Deep encoding of material means that the information is stored in LTS with all the results of the elaborative processes that you engaged in during elaborative rehearsal. This provides many associations or links to the material, all of which are stored in memory. These links can be seen as paths by which the material can be approached when we try to remember. The deeper we encode the material or the greater the number of elaborative associations we make to the material, the greater the number of potential retrieval paths there is. This will improve the likelihood of successfully retrieving the information when we need it. This thought may remind you that we have earlier suggested that the physical environment and the internal state may also serve as retrieval cues. In fact, anything that you encoded at the time of learning can provide a link that can serve as a cue to remembering. This idea is called the *encoding-specificity principle* (Tulving and Thompson 1973). Perhaps you should pause now and engage in some elaborative rehearsal and deep encoding of the ideas in this section in order to ensure good recall of its contents later.

Inaccurate remembering

Discussion so far has implied that once information is stored in memory, it is either successfully retrieved or not. We have not raised the possibility that one may recall inaccurate or even false information. However, by comparing the memories of two people who are describing the same event we will often find inconsistencies in their accounts that suggest that memory cannot always be entirely accurate. This may be crucial if one is to rely on one person's account of his or her medical history without considering that it may contain significant errors. Psychologists have investigated these inaccuracies, both to understand in what circumstances memories may be inaccurate but also to further our understanding of the normal memory processes that result in these inaccuracies.

One of the sources of inaccuracy that has been identified is something we have already considered – interference from related information in memory. We previously discussed the idea that interference from similar memories may make a particular memory unavailable, so that it is forgotten. However, the effect of interference may be to give someone the impression that they remember something, although their memory may be inaccurate. For example, Elizabeth Loftus and her colleagues have carried out a series of experiments in which she asked people to watch videos of staged car crashes or other similar events. In one of these studies she showed a video of an accident that included a car stopping at a stop sign (Loftus, Miller and Burns, 1978). In subsequent questioning the experimenter referred to the sign as a give-way sign. This interfering information was enough to change the memories of a significant proportion of the subjects. When later asked about the sign, these subjects recalled it as a give-way sign. They did not simply forget all about the sign, but their memory of it had changed in a major detail. We can conclude that the misleading information from the experimenter (that it was a give-way sign) interfered with the memory that it was a stop sign.

Sometimes the interfering information comes not from an experimenter but from our own expectations. Our expectations are themselves derived from our memory of what normally happens or what might be expected to happen. Psychologists suggest that people have a range of ideas and expectations about the likely course of events for a great many situations. These may be helpful in understanding what happens. For example, if I told you that I went to a new restaurant in town last night you may assume a great many things about my evening based on your knowledge about evenings in restaurants. Thus on hearing about my visit to the new restaurant, it would be natural to ask me 'how was the food?' despite the fact that I had not said that I ate anything there. However, your knowledge about restaurants and visits by academics to them allows you to assume that I ate (however, would you make the same assumption if you knew that my job was, in fact, a food hygiene inspector?). Bartlett (1932) introduced the term *schema* (the plural of which is *schemata*) for this sort of stored knowledge. It is schemata that allow you to make useful assumptions about known situations. Schemata consist of knowledge about people and events stored in semantic LTS and can be thought of as scripts for the typical events that allow us to explain events that happen around us. Thus you retrieved your restaurant schema to allow you to ask about the food. If I tell you more about my restaurant visit you may need your restaurant schema again to understand it 'I went to the new restaurant in town last night. The service was slow and the coffee was cold so I didn't leave a tip'. Your schema allows you to make certain assumptions. You assume I sat down at the restaurant, I ordered food as well as coffee, and that I was annoyed about the slow service and cold coffee and this is why I didn't leave a tip. You might reasonably be able to assume that I shall not be returning to this particular restaurant in the future. However, if asked tomorrow to recall exactly what I had told you about my evening, you may find it difficult to distinguish between what I told you and those things that you assumed. In this case, there is interference between what I told you and your schema such that you may mistakenly recall things that you were not told. You may believe that I told you that I shall not return to the restaurant, when this was only your entirely reasonable assumption. In the restaurant example, this effect may be trivial; indeed the advantage of schemata is that you don't need to be told things that are standard items in a particular situation. However, schemata may sometimes lead to more serious assumptions being made, which one can believe are based on memory for real events. For example, one may mistakenly believe that the barman said he smoked, because one's schema for barmen includes smoking, while this barman's wheezing may not be due to heavy smoking.

In some circumstances, schemata may also serve to distort information stored in memory rather than simply add to it. Carmichael, Hogan and Walter (1932) showed this most forcefully when they showed subjects a series of ambiguous drawings that had one of two labels. For example, two circles connected by a horizontal line were labelled either as dumbbells or as spectacles. Later the subjects were asked to draw from memory what they had seen. The drawings produced were clearly influenced by the labels that had been used. Those who had heard the label spectacles drew figures that resembled spectacles more closely than the original. Equally, the drawings of those who had heard the label dumbbell drew recognizable dumbbells. However, both sets of subjects drew objects that were clearly based on the original drawing, so it is not the case that they simply remembered the word 'spectacles' and drew a pair of spectacles. This suggests that the memory of the object seen has interacted in memory with a schema of the concept 'spectacles' and that the original memory has become distorted so that it resembles more closely the label used.

Memory disorders

The above discussion has concerned only normal memory, but these processes can be disrupted. The simplest and most widely known case is organic amnesia. *Amnesia* means a loss of memory and *organic amnesias* are those losses of memory that occur as a result of brain dysfunction. This dysfunction may, of course, have many different causes. One much studied form of organic amnesia is *Korsakoff's amnesia,* a form of organic amnesia that follows prolonged alcohol abuse, causing brain damage. In fact, the definition of a loss of memory is not precise enough because patients with organic amnesia have not lost all memory. A simple bedside test of memory, such as testing the digit span, will reveal that the operation of STS is entirely normal. Equally, asking the patient to add, subtract, or make simple judgements will reveal that there is no impairment in working memory. However, after brain damage, a devastating loss of episodic memories may be apparent. This can take two forms, although they often co-occur. First, the patient may have lost memory for episodic events which were once stored in LTS. For example, the famous patient, 'HM', became amnesic following surgical damage to his brain in an attempt to control intractable epilepsy (Scoville and Milner, 1957). As a result he no longer recalled events that had occurred in the period before his brain damage, including the fact that his much-loved uncle had died three years prior to his operation. More generally this can be demonstrated by asking patients about salient experiences that are known to have occurred in the weeks, months or even years before brain injury. This loss of episodic memories that were stored before brain damage occurred is known as *retrograde amnesia.* The amount of time lost from memory can vary from a few months to years or even decades. However, the lost memories always start at the time of brain injury and extend back in time.

Many patients have also lost the ability to form or retain new episodic memories, a condition called *anterograde amnesia.* A severe anterograde amnesia may mean that a patient is unable to form any usable episodic memories after the brain injury. This may result in the patient appearing 'stuck in the past', as nothing that has occurred since the brain injury can be recalled. 'HM', the patient mentioned above, also had a profound anterograde amnesia and, despite extensive testing by psychologists, was able to learn almost no new information in the years that followed his brain operation. This memory impairment was also evident in his everyday life and would be apparent to relatively simple bedside tests. He was, for example, unable to recall the names of the physicians with whom he was in regular contact in the months and years following his injury and could recall neither what he had eaten at his last meal, nor even if he had eaten at all. Notably, this loss of memories applies only to episodic memories and other forms of memory may still be intact. Thus, patients may still have intact semantic memories that will allow them to converse normally on matters of general knowledge. Procedural learning may also be intact, so that patients may learn new skills, although they will have no episodic memory of how they acquired them. For example, a patient given the same jigsaw puzzle to do each day will gradually learn to complete the jigsaw more quickly, but will have no recollection of ever doing this jigsaw before.

Organic amnesia will normally have a clear cause in the sense that it is likely to follow a relatively severe precipitating event, for example traffic accident, stroke or viral illness (such as encephalitis). However, occasionally a patient may suffer from an acute and severe amnesia with no obvious precipitating injury. This is known as *transient global amnesia* (TGA). The major features of TGA are sudden onset of a severe anterograde amnesia with a retrograde amnesia for the proceeding days or even weeks. As in organic amnesia, the patient with TGA will have a normal digit span, revealing that STS is unaffected. Patients may, perhaps understandably, be disorientated and a little confused but retain good insight into the disorder and so may present themselves at a hospital aware that 'something is wrong'. Patients also retain a knowledge of personal identity at all times and so they will be able to give accurate personal details and may be capable of driving themselves home to seek help. Fortunately, TGA will resolve, an attack lasting only from a few minutes to a few days. Transient global amnesia is probably caused by transient cerebral ischemia causing a temporary lack of blood supply to the regions of the brain concerned with memory functions. In support of this view, attacks often follow physical stress such as sport or cold showers in those over 50 years old. It is also much more common in those with a history of migraine attacks, again suggesting a vascular cause (Markowitsch, 1983).

Both organic amnesia and TGA have a clear underlying organic cause. Yet, amnesic episodes also occur in those who have had no brain injury but who have suffered a traumatic or emotionally disturbing event. Such an amnesia is known as *hysterical amnesia* or *fugue*. However, the characteristics of a hysterical amnesia are quite unlike those of organic amnesia. In a fugue state, patients have a severe retrograde amnesia as they are unable to recall any recent events or to give names of friends or family. They may be found wandering, lost and helpless, unable to recall how they came to be there or where they might have been going. In contrast, they do not usually have anterograde amnesia, so they have memories of the events that occurred since they were found wandering. Importantly though, and in complete contrast to those suffering from organic amnesias, they have lost memory of their personal identity, so are unable to give their name, address or any personal information. This amnesia for personal information essentially cuts them off from their previous life. In some cases, the fugue state will clear over a few days. However, where the patient does not spontaneously regain memories and relatives cannot be traced, the patient may have to adopt a new name and identity and begin a new life. As in organic amnesia, fugue patients will normally retain their procedural and semantic memories. These may, for example, allow a patient with hysteric amnesia to successfully work as a secretary, while having no memory of where and when the secretarial skills were acquired.

Summary

This chapter has suggested that memory or remembering cannot be considered as a single entity. Short-term store and LTS operate in very different ways. A summary of some of the major differences between LTS and STS discussed in this chapter is shown in Figure 4.1. Equally there are different types of memories within LTS (as shown in Figure 4.2). As they operate in different ways, these different memory systems will break down in different ways. A summary of the different types of memory loss discussed in this chapter is shown in Figure 4.3. By carefully choosing a memory test, one can specifically test the operation of each of these components of memory. However, by understanding the operation of different types of memory, one can use them efficiently to store and retrieve information when required.

| | Type of memory | |
Property	STS	LTS
Length of retention	up to 30 seconds unless rehearsed	> 80 years
Storage capacity	7 ± 2 chunks	vast, possibly infinite
Coding	mainly phonological but visual also possible	mainly semantic
Forgetting by	a) interference b) decay	a) interference b) retrieval failures
Memory aided by	(maintenance) rehearsal	deep encoding elaborative rehearsal

Figure 4.1: Summary table of some major differences between short-term store (STS) and long-term store (LTS).

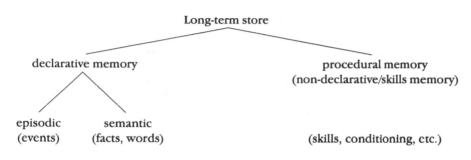

Figure 4.2: Subdivisions within LTS.

	STM	LTM			PI	Duration
		episodic	semantic	procedural		
Korsakoff's amnesia	intact	RA + AA	intact	intact	intact	permanent
TGA	intact	RA + AA	intact	intact	intact	transient
other organic amnesias	intact	RA + AA	intact	intact	intact	permanent RA may shrink
hysterical amnesias	intact	RA only	intact	intact	lost	Mainly transient

RA = retrograde amnesia; AA = anterograde amnesia; PI = knowledge of personal identity. For other abreviations see text.

Figure 4.3: A summary of types of amnesia.

References

Atkinson RC, Shiffrin RM (1968) Human memory: a proposed system and its control processes. In KW Spence (ed.) The Psychology of Learning and Motivation: Advances in Research and Theory, Vol 2. New York: Academic Press.

Baddeley AD (1966) The influence of acoustic and semantic similarity on long-term memory for word sequences. Quarterly Journal of Experimental Psychology 18: 302–9.

Baddeley AD (1992) Is working memory working? The fifteenth Bartlett lecture. Quarterly Journal of Experimental Psychology 44A: 1–31.

Baddeley AD, Hitch G (1974) Working memory. In GH Bower (ed.) The Psychology of Learning and Motivation, Vol. 8. New York: Academic Press, pp. 47–89.

Bahrick HP (1984) Semantic memory content in permastore: Fifty years of memory for Spanish learned in school. Journal of Experimental Psychology: General 113: 1–29.

Bartlett FC (1932) Remembering. Cambridge: Cambridge University Press.

Bower GH (1981) Mood and memory. American Psychologist 36: 129–48.

Carmichael L, Hogan HP, Walter AA (1932) An experimental study of language on the reproduction of visually perceived forms. Journal of Experimental Psychology 15: 73–86.

Conrad R (1964) Accoustic confusion in immediate memory. British Journal of Psychology 55: 75–84.

Craik FIM, Lockhart RS (1972) Levels of processing: a framework for memory research. Journal of Verbal Learning and Verbal Behaviour 11: 671–84.

Craik FIM, Tulving E (1975) Depth of processing and the retention of words in episodic memory. Journal of Experimental Psychology: General 104: 268–294.

Craik FIM, Watkins MJ (1973) The role of rehearsal in short-term memory. Journal of Verbal Learning and Verbal Behaviour 12: 599–607.

Godden D, Baddeley AD (1975) Context-dependent memory in two natural environments: on land and under water. British Journal of Psychology 66: 325–31.

Goodwin DW, Powell B, Bremer D, Hoine H, Stern J (1969) Alcohol and recall: state dependent effects in man. Science 163: 1358.

James W (1890) Principles of Psychology. New York: Holt, pp. 89–195.

Ley P (1979) Memory for medical information. British Journal of Social and Clinical Psychology 18: 245–55.

Linton M (1975) Memory for real-world events. In DA Norman, DE Rumelhart (eds) Explorations in Cognition. San Francisco: Freeman.

Loftus EF, Miller DG, Burns HJ (1978) Semantic integration of verbal information into visual memory. Journal of Experimental Psychology: Human Learning and Memory 4: 19–31.

McGeoch JA, McDonald WT (1931) Meaningful relation and retroactive inhibition. American Journal of Psychology 43: 579–88.

Markowitsch HJ (1983) Transient global amnesia. Neuroscience and Biobehavioural Reviews 7: 35–43.

Miller GA (1956) The magical number seven, plus or minus two: Some limits on our capacity for processing information. Psychological Review 63: 81–97.

Peterson LR, Peterson MJ (1959) Short-term retention of individual verbal items. Journal of Experimental Psychology 58: 193-8.

Postman L, Phillips LW (1965) Short-term temporal changes in free recall. Quarterly Journal of Experimental Psychology 17: 132–8.

Schachter DL (1987) Implicit memory: history and current status. Journal of Experimental Psychology: Learning, Memory and Cognition 13: 501–18.

Scoville WB, Milner B (1957) Loss of recent memory after bilateral hippocampal lesions. Journal of Neurology, Neurosurgery and Psychiatry 20: 11–21.

Smith SM (1979) Remembering in and out of context. Journal of Experimental Psychology: Human Learning and Memory 5: 460–71.

Thorndike EL (1914) The Psychology of Learning. New York: Teachers College.

Tulving E (1985) Memory and consciousness. Canadian Psychologist 26: 1–12.

Tulving E, Thompson DM (1973) Encoding specificity and retrieval processes in episodic memory. Psychological Review 80: 352–73.

Other reading

A full but readable account of human memory can be found in:

Baddeley A (1990) Human Memory: Theory and Practice. Needham Heights: Allyn & Bacon.

Another readable account of many of the issues introduced in this chapter can be found in:

Parkin A (1987) Memory and Amnesia: An Introduction. Oxford: Blackwell.

Chapter 5
The development of cognition, moral reasoning and language

KIERON SHEEHY

Key concepts	Key names
Genetic epistemology	
Adaptation and assimilation	
Schemata	
Stages of development	
Sensorimotor	
Preoperational	
Concrete operations	
Formal operations	Piaget
Object permanence	
Conservation	
Syncretic reasoning	
Deductive reasoning	
Hypothetico-deductive reasoning	
Propositional thought	
Thought–language	Vygotsky
Moral development	Piaget, Kohlberg
Language development	Skinner, Chomsky
LAD–language acquisition device	

The process by which children come to understand and make judgements about their world is a fascinating one. This chapter focuses on four topics that outline how children's thinking develops over time and with experience. These topics are:

- cognitive development;
- the relationship between thinking and language;
- moral reasoning; and
- language development.

Each area is considered from the viewpoint of the major theorists involved with the topic.

Cognitive development

The term cognitive development refers to the psychological processes involved in thinking and how these processes change over time. The best known theorist in this subject is *Jean Piaget*. His ideas form the basis of much of this chapter. Piaget coined the term *genetic epistemology* to describe his study of how children develop their knowledge and understanding of the world (from the Greek *episteme,* meaning 'knowledge').

Piaget's theory is concerned with the process by which innate motor reflexes are gradually transformed and develop into mature, psychological structures of adults, capable of abstract thinking and reasoning.

Basic concepts of Piaget's theory of cognitive development

Children have an inherent drive to adapt to the world and to organize what they learn from their experiences. It is this *adaptation* that results in cognitive development.

Development is an active process rather than purely the result of biological maturation or environmental shaping. Thus, Piaget's theory is *constructivist.* Children construct their own development through their actions.

The psychological structures that change through this adaptation are known as *schemata* (from the Greek, *skhema,* meaning 'form' – *schema* in the singular). These established patterns of physical or mental action can be regarded as ways of doing things, organized sequences of action and thought, which are altered as our experience of the world grows. Schemata are psychological constructs that direct our behaviour and thought processes. Adaptation occurs when schemata change. This change is brought about by two processes. The first process, *assimilation*, occurs when new information or responses are taken into existing schemata. Assimilation is seen when a schema can be successfully applied to a new situation.

For example, the young infant will try out the grasping reflex in different situations. A grasping schema is built that may be used successfully on different objects.

In contrast, the second process, *accommodation*, occurs when a schema needs to be altered to meet the demands of a new situation.

When the schema doesn't work in a situation and adaptive changes need to be made, then accommodation has occurred.

For example, where the basic grasping technique fails to pick up a particular object a new hand position is needed. If a young child has conceptualized drinks into two categories; milk and juice, he or she might apply this categorization to a new sparkling drink and call it juice.

However, when this categorization fails to elicit the correct responses from others when asking for a drink, the child will accommodate his or her drink concept to contain three categories: milk, juice and fizzy.

It is through accommodation and assimilation that all cognitive structures, ideas, concepts and language, grow and develop. Even concepts that appear to be fundamental to human thought need to be discovered through adaptation. For example; the awareness and understanding of causation, time, space and even that objects continue to exist when out of sight need to be learned by the child through their own investigations. Assimilation and accommodation occur throughout life and result in all adult cognitive abilities. For example, in hypothesis testing, if our theory can explain a new phenomenon then assimilation occurs; if theory needs to be changed in order to explain a phenomenon then accommodation occurs.

The processes of assimilation and accommodation work together in an interacting dynamic way to produce cognitive growth. This dynamic interaction is an *equilibration* between states of equilibrium and disequilibrium. When a state of equilibration is reached the cognitive functions can become integrated with one another. This process is illustrated in Figure 5.1.

Equilibrium ----------➤ Assimilation ---------➤ Novel experience schema
                                                cannot assimilate -------
------------------➤ Accommodation --------➤ Equilibrium
                                                re-established

Figure 5.1: The process of equilibration.

Piaget proposed that each schema that is created contains within it an intrinsic motivation for its future use. In other words, children are inherently motivated to use their schemata.

Stages of cognitive development

Piaget's theory of cognitive development is a *stage theory*. Children are seen as passing through a sequence of stages, a predetermined hierarchy, in an invariant order. Each stage represents a qualitatively different way of viewing the world and is developed as a result of the child's active exploration of the environment. Each stage has a characteristic age span, although there may be considerable variation between individuals.

As children grow and adapt to their world the result is not simply an additive accumulation of knowledge and responses. At certain points in the child's development, changes will occur in which the child's view of the world will alter qualitatively. It is these qualitative changes that give rise to the four main stages of cognitive development proposed by Piaget. Each of these stages is outlined below and the substages of the first and second stages are described.

Stage one: the sensorimotor stage (before 2 years)

In this first stage the world is known through action and sensory information. A characteristic feature of the sensorimotor stage is a lack of *object permanence*. Until the child possesses an internal representational system (a combination of language and memory development) 'out of sight is out of mind'. For example, a 7-month-old child will expend considerable effort to reach for and pick up a favourite toy. However if the child watches as the toy is covered, the child will give up and behave as if the toy has ceased to exist (Piaget, 1963). Later, at around 9 months, the child may learn to uncover the hidden object from the cloth. However, if he or she watches the toy hidden underneath a second, adjacent, cloth, the child will continue to look for the toy under the original cloth.

The ability to hold on to an image of an object once it is removed from view develops progressively during the sensorimotor stage.

There are six substages within the sensorimotor period:

- Reflex activity (below 1 month). Innate reflexes are exercised and become more fluent during this time. Note that even at this early stage accommodation can be occurring.
- Self-investigation (1–4 months). *Primary circular reactions* are seen. These reactions are simple repetitive acts that centre upon the infant's own body, e.g. thumb sucking, hand or foot clasping.
- Co-ordination and reaching out (4–8 months). *Secondary circular reactions* are developed where the child reproduces actions whose effects are focused away from their own bodies. The new technique may be stumbled upon accidentally but the child is able to reproduce it. Piaget described this as 'making interesting sights last' (Piaget, 1936, cited in Crain, 1992). An example is kicking legs to move a hanging object.
- The co-ordination of secondary schemata/goal directed behaviour (8–12 months). In the previous substage, the infant could use a single action to produce a result, for example striking a tower of blocks to knock them over. In the current substage, the child becomes able to co-ordinate separate schemata to obtain an end point. Piaget views this as the first time that purposeful sequential behaviour is seen. Piaget observed his own son Laurent at 7 months and noted that the child would move one object out of the way to obtain another (Piaget, 1936, cited in Crain, 1992), co-ordinating striking an obstacle out of the way in order to grab a desired object
- Experimentation (12–18 months). *Tertiary circular reactions* arise which consist of active experimentation to find out how acts will affect objects or outcomes. For example, dropping food items and noticing how they react when hitting the floor. Schemata are being actively built by the child through experimentation.

- Problem solving and mental combinations (18 month–2 years). The development of language and memory enables the child to solve problems using signs, symbols or images. Direct physical exploration of the environment is no longer essential. The use of internal representations allows imaginative play and symbolic thought to emerge. Object permanence is now established.

Stage two: the preoperational stage (2–7 years)

Operations are mental sequences of actions that follow a logical pattern. The preoperational child has not developed this logical ability. Preoperational children have acquired language and are able to articulate their beliefs about the world and how it functions. However, the illogical nature that characterizes preoperational children can be seen in their idiosyncratic explanations for events or definitions (Sheehy, 1993, 1995).

Piaget saw preoperational children as *egocentric*, being unable to consider the world from any viewpoint other than their own.

Evidence supporting this idea came from the *three mountains task*, which is illustrated in Figure 5.2. In this task, Piaget and Inhelder (1972) presented individual children with a small model of three mountains.

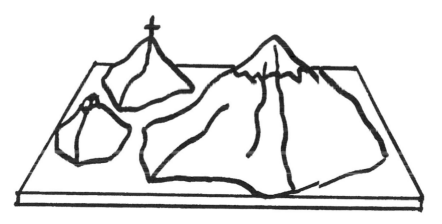

(Based on Smith and Cowie, 1991)

Figure 5.2: The three mountains task. A test of egocentricity.

A doll was placed within the display. The children were shown some cards depicting different views of the three mountains and asked to pick one that showed the view as seen from the doll's point of view. Other tasks were given to the children to assess how well they could imagine the doll's perspective.

Typically, 4- and 5-year-olds chose answers that reflected their own perspective. In contrast, children older than 9 years were able to cope successfully with the task. The performance of the younger children was attributed by Piaget to their egocentric thinking. These children were unable to imagine someone else's perspective.

Other examples of children's pre-logical thinking can be seen in how they perform on *conservation tasks*. Children master the concept of conservation when they realize that the quantity or amount of a substance or group of objects remains unchanged when nothing has been added or taken away from it. For example Figure 5.3 shows a conservation of volume test.

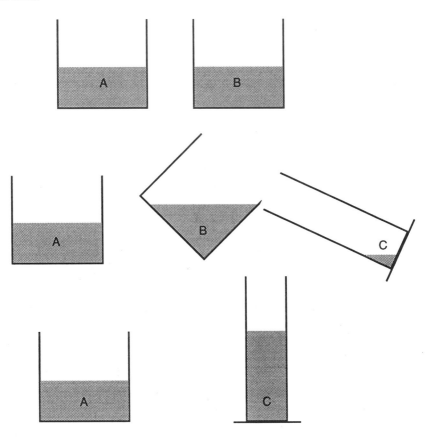

A child identifies that A and B contain the same amount of liquid. The child watches as the liquid is transferred from B to C. Preoperational children may now judge the amounts of liquid in A and C to be different.

Figure 5.3: Testing conservation of volume.

If children watch as liquid is poured from a tall container into a short wide container, children who can conserve volume will realize that the amount of liquid remains the same regardless of the shape of the container. In contrast, preoperational children perform poorly on conservation tasks and cannot conserve properties such as volume, mass, length or even number. For example; the length of a piece of rope is not changed by an alteration in configuration of the rope (length). The mass of a ball of Plasticine remains the same when it is rolled into a sausage shape (mass). The number of marbles in a line remain the same after they have been spread out (number).

Two types of reasoning are seen during this time:

* syncretic reasoning, where items are classified by a single and changing criterion. For example, in sorting out a mixture of toy hats and boats: 'Boat goes with boat because they are boats . . . hat goes with boat because they are both green';
* transductive reasoning. Inferences are made about relationships based on a single attribute. This may also influence the development of *animistic thinking.* In animistic thinking inanimate objects are seen as being alive. An illustration of this is 'things that move are alive, the wind moves – it's alive'.

Preoperational children also have difficulty with *reversibility* and so they are unable to reverse mental operations. This can be seen in the following interaction.

Teacher: Do you have a brother?
Boy: Yes.
Teacher: Does he have a brother?
Boy: No!

In the conservation experiments children cannot mentally return substances to their original states by reversing the transformations.

During the second half of the preoperational stage (sometimes referred to as the intuitive stage, from 4 to 7 years), the child can classify and order a few items systematically in terms of a single attribute; for example length or membership of a particular group. However, children are unable to describe their own classification or move beyond a single attribute, as illustrated below.

Experimenter: Are the pigeons birds?
Child: Yes.
Experimenter: Are the robins birds?
Child: Yes.
Experimenter: If all the robins fly away, will there be any birds left?
Child: No, they'll all have gone away.
(Smith and Cowie, 1988: 290)

The child cannot deal with both dimensions at once and thus the whole–parts relationship is beyond their understanding.

Stage three: the concrete operational stage (7–12 years)

Children can now deal with different perspectives, resulting in a loss of egocentric thinking. Reversibility and conservation begin. They are now flexible logical thinkers when considering real-life concrete issues. However, they are not yet able to think about abstract propositions. Piaget's experiments into conservation revealed that children at the concrete operational stage master some aspects of conservation before others. This successive mastery is known as *horizontal decalage*. For example, conservation of number is achieved (at the age of 5–6 years) before mass; mass is conserved before weight (7–8 years); and finally volume is conserved.

The concrete operational stage is also characterized by the child's ability to co-ordinate two dimensions of an object simultaneously and, arrange structures in sequence. Now the child is able to *classify items into hierarchies* and sort items according to several dimensions or features. *Transitive inference* problems can now be mastered. For example, if told that A is greater than B, and B is greater than C, the child can correctly infer the relationship between A and C. However, in order to arrive at this conclusion, the child relies on physical prompts or reference to real-life examples.

Stage four: the formal operational stage (11 plus years)

The formal operational stage is the fourth and final stage in Piaget's theory. It begins at approximately 11 to 12 years of age, and continues throughout adulthood. This stage is characterized by the ability to formulate hypotheses and systematically test them to arrive at answers to problems that are posed at a purely verbal level. Children's thinking is no longer tied to the concrete situation and *hypothetico-deductive reasoning* emerges. Systematic analysis and scientific thought begin here and hypotheses can be tested. The child can examine a series of possible influences on a given problem and work through these systematically to identify the prime issues (Piaget and Inhelder, 1972)

Children develop the ability to apply logical rules to situations that are contrary to fact and that violate the principles of reality and reason. For example, they can cope with discussions such as 'what would happen if water ran uphill?' or 'what would technology be like if all people had five arms?'

Further, the arguments used in such discussions can be evaluated in terms of the internal consistency of the statements used. This is an example of *propositional thought*. The logic of a statement is being evaluated without a check against a real-life situation.

Table 5.1 presents a summary of Piaget's stages. It illustrates the divide between those who can and cannot use operational thought. The latter having the ability to use words and symbols to solve problems as a mental activity. Preoperational thought requires physical actions. Children at this stage are influenced by their senses. Older operational children can go beyond physical appearance and are able to perform the mental transformations necessary to conserve properties such as number or mass and they are less egocentric. Although concrete operational children are logical thinkers tied to the here and now, formal operational thinkers are able to go beyond direct experience and hypothesize. Formal operational thinking is not reached by all adults, neither is it always used by those who are capable of it. It has been suggested that adults primarily use this level of thinking in areas that are of special and particular interest to them (Crain, 1992; Hayslip and Panek, 1989).

Table 5.1: Summary of Piaget's developmental stages

Name of stage	Typical age	Key features
Sensorimotor stage	Birth to 2 years	Intelligence takes the form of motor actions. The child 'thinks' through action and action schemata are primarily developed. Learns to act intentionally to achieve a result. Object permanence and symbolic representation emerge.
Preoperational stage	2 to 7 years	Egocentric. Uses language to represent objects and actions. Classifies on a single feature. Animistic thinking.
Concrete operational stage	7 to 11 years	Logical thought can be applied to objects and events. Conservation is mastered. Objects classified by several features or ordered by a single attribute (length, weight).
Formal operational stage	11 to 15 years	Logical thought can be applied to abstract ideas. Hypothetical events, ideals and the future become issues for consideration. Hypothesis testing begins.

The implications of Piaget's theory

In order to facilitate child development, a child-orientated approach is suggested by Piaget's theory. Children should be given opportunities to actively explore and investigate. The problems that are presented to children should be appropriate in terms of the motor and mental schemata established by the child. The focus should not be on the end product of correct responses. The name or word given by a young child may be the same as an adult but the underlying concept is often different (Kozulin, 1990; Sheehy, 1993). Therefore emphasis should be given to developing the child's underlying thinking. Teaching should encourage self-initiated and directed investigation rather than a superficial understanding which imitates adult performance.

Children will express and comprehend different explanations of reality at different stages of cognitive development. The practical implications of this are seen, for example, when informing young children about illness. The cognitive abilities of the child should be considered to ensure an appropriate level of explanation is given (Eiser, 1985). It has been suggested that children's concepts of illness parallel Piaget's stages (Bibace and Walsh, 1981). Two to four year olds are influenced by their perceptual impressions. The commonest explanation of illness causation is that of contagion, although the mechanism of transfer though is not understood.

Later, concrete explanations of illness identify contamination through physical contact or internalization through swallowing or inhaling something.

When explaining illness to young children, simple and concrete information should be used. Metaphors may be useful to concrete operational children, if they liken the child's illness to events and structures with which they are already familiar. For example, the nervous system likened to a telephone system to explain how messages can be 'lost', or white blood cells as 'good guys' getting rid of 'baddies'.

At the formal stage, the child is able to consider both psychological and physical explanations. Initially the child may refer to specific structures and processes but as children mature they are able to consider the way in which thoughts and feelings can affect an individual's health. (For an excellent review of this area see Eiser, 1985.)

Beyond Piaget – the social nature of knowledge

Piaget was concerned with how knowledge developed, and obtained evidence that supported his stage theory. However, later experiments revealed that under certain conditions young children could operate at levels above that predicted by Piaget. Concerning very young children, the development of new experimental procedures has shown that infants are more cognitively competent than predicted by Piaget with respect to object permanence and simple problem solving (Slater, 1990).

With regard to older children, Piaget's 'three mountains' experiment showed how the egocentric preoperational child was unable to adopt the perspective of another person. However, Donaldson and Hughes (Donaldson, 1978) gave young children a perspective task involving hiding a toy from two toy policemen within walls forming a simple cross, as shown in Figure 5.4. They found that the children could successfully adopt the viewpoints of the policemen and hide the toy, in the example shown, at location C. This skill revealed that the children could decentre and were less egocentric than predicted by Piaget.

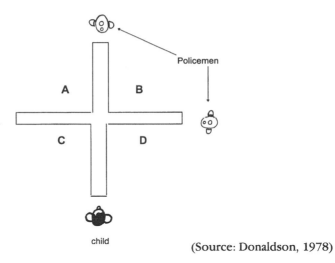

(Source: Donaldson, 1978)

Figure 5.4: Hughes and Donaldson's 'hiding from policemen' experiment.

Light, Buckingham and Robbins (1979) produced a Piagetian-type conservation task where pasta was moved between two beakers of different sizes. As predicted by Piaget's theory, 6-year-old children were unable to realize that the amount of pasta remained the same (was conserved) when transferred to a beaker of a different size. However, Light et al. (1979) subsequently gave a reason for the transfer to the children, telling them that the beaker was chipped and therefore the pasta needed to be moved. With this simple addition the majority of children were able to conserve and realize that the amount of pasta remained the same.

There are numerous other examples where simple changes in the experimental environment enable children to perform at levels that should be cognitively beyond them in Piagetian terms (Lloyd and Freeman, 1986 cited in Slater, 1990; Yates and Bremner, 1988 cited by Slater, 1990)

Why does this occur? One explanation is that the newer experiments made *human sense*. This term expresses an important feature of child development that is not considered sufficiently in Piaget's theory: the relationship between social interaction and cognitive/intellectual functioning. Experiments such as those of Light et al. (1979) and Donaldson (1978) show how important the social situation is for the child's cognitive development. Children's cognitive development takes place within a social situation and is supported by the social situation. The child's knowledge is *embedded* within this social context. Other experiments (Donaldson and McGarrigle, cited in Donaldson, 1978) reveal how the understanding of the meanings of words, such as 'more', is strongly influenced by the situation in which they occur. The young child's understanding of language is inextricably linked to the context in which the language is presented. Language and cognition are only disembedded from the social situation later in development as a result of formal education (Donaldson, 1978; Kahney, 1990).

Piaget assumed that intelligence and cognition occurred in parallel with social development and therefore that the children's functioning in his experiments would reflect a general cognitive level of functioning. Because of this assumption Piaget's experiments underestimated how the social environment (including the experimental situation itself) affects language and cognition. This relationship is highlighted when the links between thought and language are considered.

The relationship between thought and language

Of the many psychologists who have considered the topic only two are considered here: Piaget and Vygotsky.

Piaget's view

Piaget proposed that both thought and language depend on underlying intelligence, language being a reflection of cognition. Language can enable symbolic thinking to occur but depends on an underlying intelligence. This deeper construct originates from internalized actions that are transformed into cognitive operations. Schemata develop first as adaptive responses. Language develops later and may be able to reflect on these responses. Therefore intelligence precedes language and is independent of it.

Vygotsky's view

In the book *Thought and Language* (1962) Vygotsky proposed an alternative view to that of Piaget. Language is seen as having two functions; *inner speech*, our self-talk, and *external speech* to communicate with other people.

The internal and social functions of language arise separately. Up until around the age of two, the young child uses words purely as social acts of communication without internal thought. At this time the child's internal cognition is without language. The child has internal thoughts without language and an external language without thought (see Table 5.2).

At around two years of age these two separate function join together. Words, which were originally social in function are internalized and become capable of representing thought. Children can now begin to consider their own and other people's thoughts and this ability enables the child's social development to advance (Roth, 1993).

Thus, for Vygotsky, language and social development occur in partnership and interact intimately in the development of each other.

The language that once accompanied a purely social interaction is internalized to give a language for thought. This internalized language is used to guide the child's actions and thinking (Vygotsky, 1978 [1931]). The social environment fundamentally shapes the way in which children think and act. Vygotsky states that:

> Every function in the child's cultural development appears twice: first, on the social level, and later, on the individual level; first, between people (interpsychological) and then inside the child (intrapsychological). This applies equally to voluntary attention, to logical memory, and to the formation of concepts. All the higher functions (thought and language) originate as actual relationships between individuals. (Vygotsky, 1978 [1931]: 57)

The process by which intellect and speech come together at around two years of age is characterized by four stages. These are outlined in Table 5.2.

Table 5.2: A Vygotskian perspective on early thought and language (after Kozulin, 1990)

Stage	Speech characteristics	Thought characteristics	Comments
Primitive	Speech is pre-intellectual	Non-verbal Sensory motor problem solving	
Practical intelligence	Some grammar may be used but this is not underpinned by logical thinking, e.g. child uses 'because' but unaware of the causality the term implies	Embedded in concrete communication	Notice how the syntax of speech comes before the syntax of thought
External symbolic cues	Egocentric speech, transitory between primitive and more mature forms of controlling behaviour and thinking	External symbols are used to represent problems; e.g. finger counting, mnemonic aids	Egocentric speech arises and increases in frequency
Internalization	Internalized to silent inner speech.	Internalizing external operators, e.g. arithmetic solved mentally rather than on fingers	Egocentric speech decreases

Young preoperational children (around three or four years of age) talk to themselves. Investigation of this has helped to explain the relationship between thought and language. Piaget and Vygotsky give different explanations of this phenomenon (Piaget, 1923; Vygotsky, 1978 [1931]).

For Piaget such speech suggests egocentricity (not adjusting their talk to the presence of others) and is a sign of immaturity. Egocentric speech disappears as children get older and Piaget assumed that it ceases to exist because the child matures and becomes less egocentric.

In contrast Vygotsky asserts that to believe that such speech disappears totally is akin to saying that a child stops counting when they ceases to use their fingers and begin mental arithmetic. Self-talk does not disappear but becomes internalized and is used to guide the child's actions. Evidence from a range of studies supports this view (Roth, 1993). When children are presented with tasks of increasing difficulty their conscious use of self-talk is seen to increase in order to guide their efforts. Further, this type of speech is seen most frequently in the more cognitively mature and socially competent of children rather than in immature children.

Piaget's *internal schema* and Vygotsky's *socialized knowledge* views are in conflict. However, Piaget did support a social transmission view to some extent (Piaget, 1970) and Vygotsky considered the child's active construction of knowledge to be a vital part of child development (Vygotsky, 1978 [1931]).

Practical applications

Vygotsky's ideas have been applied to the remediation of the developmental problems encountered by a wide variety of children, most notably children who are deaf and blind and those having learning disabilities. By developing the language abilities of these children (often through using sign language or alternative communication systems) the children are enabled to develop higher order psychological skills, which can be used to manage their lower level sensory ones (Sheehy, 1992a). The social environment is used to support the child's learning and the children's potential is indicated by the levels they can reach with adult guidance. The difference between unaided and aided performance levels is referred to as the *zone of proximal development*. Teaching occurs within this zone. The social interaction that forms the zone supports the child's cognition and develops a higher level of functioning than could be achieved alone. These higher processes are later internalized by the child.

Echoes of Vygotsky's ideas are seen in the practice of *conductive education* in which children with motor disorders such as cerebral palsy are taught using methods that develop the internalization of language in order to control motor responses (Sheehy, 1992b). Impressive claims have been made for these types of approaches, which are not typically found in western rehabilitation techniques.

Moral development

As the cognitive abilities of children develop, their understanding of social issues – such as what is right and wrong – also changes. The reasoning that underpins such moral development was considered by Piaget. For Piaget, moral reasoning divided into two stages, before and after approximately 11 years of age.

- The *stage of moral reasoning*. Before 11 years, the child views moral codes as unchanging and unchangeable laws, handed down by their parents or God. The child is able to consider the consequences of actions and the relative benefit or harm produced a specific action.
- The *stage of moral co-operation*. After 11 years of age, the child considers the motives of the person involved to be of primary importance. This change revolves around the development of formal operational thinking. For a detailed review of Piaget's ideas see Crain (1992). The reciprocal nature of fair and just behaviour is emphasized by the child.

Kohlberg's stage theory of moral development

Lawrence Kohlberg developed Piaget's ideas from the premise that, at birth, all humans have no moral or ethical stance. As our intellect and social behaviour matures, so our understanding of what constitutes moral behaviour is changed. Kohlberg presented a moral dilemma to a range of participants and noted the types of reasoning that were used in their responses. His most well-known dilemma was 'Heinz steals the drug'. This dilemma describes the predicament of a man named Heinz. His wife is dying. She can only be saved by a particular medicine, which has been invented by a chemist in the town. Unfortunately, the medicine costs more money than Heinz is able to raise and so he breaks into the chemist's shop and takes it.

Participants were asked what Heinz should have done in this situation. Their responses, and the type of reasoning they applied to such questions, led Kohlberg to suggest that moral reasoning develops in stages. This is not to say that all children will reach the same conclusions for given dilemmas, but rather that similar reasoning will be revealed in reaching possibly opposing views. Kohlberg formulated three main levels of moral development (with substages). Levels one and two occur most commonly until adolescence.

Level one: pre-conventional morality

Morality is externally governed by the consequences of the action. Actions that are punished are seen as bad because they are punished. Children conform to the rules imposed on them by adults, who are more powerful than they are.

- Stage one: obedience and punishment orientation. Avoidance of punishment is the key factor in the child's understanding of right and wrong. In response to the Heinz dilemma, children at this stage focus their responses on 'not getting into trouble'. A child may take off wellington boots before entering the kitchen to avoid the consequences of breaking a strict family rule.

- Stage two: individualism and exchange. Here children can express different opinions about the right and wrong things to do; however, this is still a very concrete view based around the return of favours or exchanges. 'Fairness is an equal exchange of favours' (Berk, 1994). There is no identification with, or reference to, the codes of family or society. Children may moderate their behaviour in order to receive a later gain. A child might let her brother choose the music in the car going to school, in order to have her own choice on the way home. She would become upset if her brother had the return journey choice as well.

Level two: conventional morality

Social norms are seen as the mainstay of ethical action. Social order is taken into account at the expense of immediate concrete outcomes and is typical of young teenagers.

- Stage three: good interpersonal relationships. Children can see their own actions from the perspective of another person. Their actions illustrate a wish to maintain a good relationship with the person. Their concern in making judgements centres around 'what other people will think' should particular actions occur. People should behave in accordance with 'good' motives or intentions. Sometimes referred to as the 'good boy/nice girl orientation', a child may help his or her mother or teacher in order to be seen as a particular type of child by that person. In answering the Heinz dilemma, children will focus on who is behaving fairly or acting on the basis of good intent – for example, the chemist is being unfair charging so much and Heinz wants to save his wife.
- Stage four: maintaining the social order. The child now expands the idea of fair behaviour or just motives and sees just laws and judgements as those that are applied equally to all members of society. Morally just people uphold these laws and judgements. There are no exceptions to these laws. For example; children may believe that Heinz is wrong in his actions because theft of private property is socially wrong. The morality of an action is defined with reference to society as a whole and in particular conforming with laws. These laws are seen as preventing chaos and being fair for all members of society. Moral behaviour obeys these laws.

Level three: post-conventional morality

The guidance of abstract principles and ideals develops here. There is a search for guiding principles that can be applied to all situations and people and that go beyond the simple law-and-order view of the previous stage. A society ruled by a totalitarian government may satisfy the ideas of stage four, but such a situation may present problems for individuals.

- Stage five: social contract and individual rights. Rules are seen as judgements produced by a particular society and the person is aware that alternative rules can be developed which will produce a different type of society. People should abide by laws that protect basic human rights such as life or freedom of speech and develop mechanisms to change unjust laws. There is a balance to consider between moral justice and the upholding of generally workable laws. With regard to Heinz, people at this stage of development may support Heinz's theft because of a basic moral imperative to save life yet he has broken the law and therefore should be punished, albeit to the minimum legal level permissible. In a sense, respondents at this stage are working out and ranking a set of priorities for society.

Stage six: universal principles

This is the 'peak' of moral development in Kohlberg's model. People are governed by abstract principles that they have considered and developed for themselves. These principles are the means by which justice can be achieved. Such principles are universal, being valid for everyone, and can transcend the laws of society. For example, in the Heinz example, the right to life not only overrides the financial and legal arguments against theft but may be seen as giving Heinz a moral duty to break the law. If Heinz does not steal the drug he is not following his own standards of morality in placing finance and the law above the life of another human being. Moral values exist that apply across all situations and transcend societal norms.

An evaluation of Kohlberg's theory

There is support for the concept that people move through the stages in the order Kohlberg's predicted (Walker and Taylor, 1991) although few people appear to move as far as stage five and therefore the existence of stage six has been questioned. As with Piaget's experiments, Kohlberg's methodology underestimates the power of context in developing reasoning. Rather than a one-way, invariate progression, it is suggested that as people mature they can use an increasing range of moral reasoning but that this is influenced by the environment in which the dilemma exists. It has been argued that Kohlberg's theory is culturally biased in that it does not consider traditions that do not have large infrastructures to resolve conflict. Early involvement in the social institutions of a society can lead to a more rapid development of stages four and five. For example children reared in *kibbutzim* are taught about the governing of their community. At adolescence these children are more advanced on Kohlberg's measures than children from outside the system (Snarey, Reimer and Kohlberg, 1985). At a more general level there is also evidence to suggest that the ability to think in abstract terms is a by-product of a particular type of educational system (Kahney, 1997) and certainly moral reasoning ability correlates with years of completed schooling (Rest and Narvaes, 1991 cited in Berk, 1996). The key factor here is the opportunity to interact with others about moral concerns.

Kohlberg's original research interviews were conducted with males. It has been suggested that any differences that exist in moral reasoning between males and females are not considered (see Gilligan, 1982; Crain, 1992; Berk, 1994). Carol Gilligan argues that by focusing on the 'masculine' ideals of rights and justice, Kohlberg misses out on the more 'feminine' qualities of responsiveness and caring (Gilligan, 1982).

Other criticisms are more general ones and concern issues as to whether moral development actually occurs in discrete stages, the degree to which progression is automatic, the reliability of Kohlberg's procedures, and the degree to which reasoning influences behaviour in the real world.

Practical applications

Kohlberg's work extended Piaget's original ideas and suggests that if children are to develop their moral thinking they must actively consider issues and develop their own conclusions. Telling children an adult's moral judgements produces little change (Tureil, 1996, cited in Crain, 1992). Individual moral development occurs as the outcome of interactions in which issues are debated and alternative views considered.

The development of language

The process by which the smiles and gurgles of an infant are transformed into the rich language of adulthood is a fascinating one. Language requires the use of signs or symbols within a grammar (a set of rules) and by combining these symbols, previously unknown, novel expressions can be constructed. The process of language development is outlined in Table 5.3, which shows the typical language milestones achieved by children at approximate ages.

The sequence of language development is agreed to be similar globally (Dworetsky, 1981) but there are conflicting ideas about the process by which language is learned. Historically, the two views that have stood in starkest contrast are those of B.F. Skinner and Noam Chomsky.

In 1957 Skinner published *Verbal Behaviour*. In this book he proposed that the spontaneous babbling of infants becomes reinforced and shaped into approximations of speech. The reinforcement comes from the reactions of the infant's caregivers. These approximations are gradually reinforced to shaped up adult speech patterns through operant conditioning.

Table 5.3: Milestones of language development

Year 1	From birth *crying* to express hunger, anger or pain. *Cooing* at 1 month. The 'oooh' sound.
6–9 months	*Babbling*. Deaf babies also babble. Reinforcement cannot change the nature of early babbling but can change the frequency (rate of occurrence).
9–12 months	*Phonemic contraction*. The babbling sounds reduce in variety and begin to correspond with those found in the child's language environment. *Turn taking* is not unusual here between the carer and the infant, both in gaze and verbal interactions. The *intonation* of language develops and children appear to be talking without words when they make sounds.
12 months	The *first word* is spoken at about 12 months. A one-word phrase or *holophrase* is used where one word can stand for a complete sentence.
18–21 months	The first few words are used for several months before a period of rapid vocabulary growth. Typically child at 18 months has approximately 20 words and this grows rapidly to around 200 at 21 months. Mainly *nouns*. From 18 months onwards, two-word sentences can be produced.
2–3 years	By 2 years of age most children have established vocabularies of about 250–300 words. *Two word phase* is established. These often form *telegraphic speech* for example 'go car, more cake'. A considerable variety of meanings/concepts is possible. The development of grammatical rules begins. Plurals, prepositions and verb endings. Questions can be constructed by changing the order of a sentence. The child learns to produce three and four word sentences. The errors of applying grammatical rules are seen here. Grammatical morphemes are acquired in a highly regular order by English-speaking children.
3–4 years	1000 word vocabulary established. Conversations quite sophisticated but may be rooted in present. Children, however, use *syntactically correct* sentences by the age of 3 and highly *complex constructions* by the age of 5. Relative clauses can be used, e.g. 'the cake I ate was a thunderbirds one'. but children still struggle with passive verbs (Smith and Cowie, 1988). *Metalinguistic awareness* The ability to think about and reflect on language itself. The child begins to understand jokes, puns and double entendres to some extent.
6–8 years	Approximately 2600 words have been learned.

However, to learn language in this way would be an immensely complex task if each word and sound needed to be built up gradually through reinforcement. It would be more complicated still if word combinations needed to be reinforced into sentences.

There is little evidence to support a skilled shaping process by mothers (Smith and Cowie, 1988). Mothers appear to respond to the meaning of an expression, not its precise form. Parents do not spend time large amounts of time shaping individual aspects of grammar. Further, the novel sentences generated as children master grammar suggests that they are constructing completely new sentences. Although the size of children's vocabulary is greater if they are exposed to a wide range of words (Smith and Cowie, 1988) this exposure does not appear to affect the *generative* aspect of the child's language. In 1957 Noam Chomsky published *Syntactic Structures*. This work advanced a nativist explanation of language development. Children appear to develop the use of rules in a way that is greater than the amount of environmental contact, or parental training, that they receive. Chomsky suggested that this phenomenon would only be possible if there were an innate, inherited mechanism for noticing and developing grammar. He proposed that children are born with a *language acquisition device* (LAD). This is an innate human faculty, a universal innate grammar that is unique to humans and underpins all languages. Chomsky set out to delineate the parts of language learning that were innate and those that were cultural. He developed a theory of *transformational-generative grammar* to show how the grammatically diverse language systems that exist can be rapidly acquired by young children around the world.

Language is seen as having two levels of structure: a *surface structure* – the actual speech one produces – and a *deep structure*, the underlying meaning of that speech. The relationship between speech and meaning is not simple but the surface structure and deep structure are linked together via the rules of transformational grammar. The implication of this is that the *deep structures are universal* and apply to all languages and the transformational rules and the surface structure are responsible for the differences between languages of different cultures. For Chomsky it is the syntax (see Table 5.4) of language (its grammatical rules) that allows meaning to emerge

When a person hears diverse surface structures these can be translated into deep ones through transformational grammar – rules that are contained within the LAD. The translation, via transformational grammar, is also the means by which children can understand the changes in meaning resulting from changes in surface structure. For example the phrase 'consulting psychiatrists can cause problems' has one surface structure and the possibility of two deep structures.

When a child encounters words, the LAD is able to pick out the regularities between the words and generate hypotheses about them. For example, adding 's' to form a plural. Sometimes these hypotheses may be inaccurate and this is observed when children produce words such as 'sheeps' or 'runned'. These words are the result of the application of a generated rule. This explains how children can produce words that have not been modelled or reinforced by adults. Berko (1958) presented children with picture cards showing a man wielding a strange club. The children were told that the man was 'ricking' Later when discussing the cards, the children stated that man had 'ricked'. This is a good example of *over-regularization*, requiring the active use of rules to produce new words. This capability is too generative to be explicable by environmental conditioning or modelling alone. Language development is a controversial research area. Table 5.5 compares, in summary form, the views of several theorists who have been discussed in this chapter.

Table 5.4: Language: some key terms

Phonology – how we understand and produce speech sounds. **Grammar** – consists of two parts; 1) **Syntax**, rules that delineate how sentences are constructed. 2) **Morphology**, grammatical markers denoting number or tense (e.g. 's' or 'ed'.) **Phonemes** – the smallest units of speech that can be discriminated. Distinct units of sound.	**Semantics** – the meaning of words and concepts expressed in words. **Pragmatics** – communicative actions and processes including taking turns, and paralanguage (tone or voice, rate of speech).

The regular nature of the pattern of language development (see Table 5.5) and young children's incredible sensitivity to speech sounds tend to support the idea of an innate language programme of some kind. However, the single grammatical system that underpins all language has yet to be identified and children's language development is neither as fast nor as perfect as Chomsky's view proposes (Berk, 1996). Most modern views adopt an *interactive* model in which innate and environmental influences interact to develop language (Berk, 1996).

Research into early language development suggests that strong individual differences may occur. For example, two groups of children are noted – those who initially acquire a large number of object names are termed *referential*. Such children are in contrast with those whose initial language consists primarily of social words ('ta', 'hiya', 'please') and the names of persons and actions. These infants are known as *expressive* infants (Barret, 1989, cited in Slater, 1990). It has also been discovered that the development of early language recognition responses between mother and child begins *in utero*, far earlier than previously expected.

Table 5.5: A comparison of Chomsky's, Piaget's, Skinner's and Vygotsky's view on language development

Chomsky	Piaget	Skinner	Vygotsky	Comments
Language develops via the genetic LAD	Language develops as children build their own schemata	Reinforcement and shaping of responses produce language	Language arises and is embedded within social relationships	C, P & S stressed innate origins to differing degrees. The LAD is 'hard-wired'. Schematic and reinforcement theories see language developing from innate responses. For Piaget the child is active in this construction. For Skinner the environment is more strongly emphasized.
Learning is guided by the LAD	Children build their own sche-mata through exploration of the environment	Shaping of behaviour and imitation of adult responses	Internalization of social interactions	Chomsky's LAD is a specific structure for language acquisition. Piaget's view is more closely related to a reflection of general intelligence.
Grammar is developed as a surface structure translated from a deeper innate universal grammar	Grammar development is a reflection of underlying general cognitive development	Grammar development is achieved through differential reinforcement	Grammar is internalized from social interactions and actively develops cognition. The syntax of speech comes before the syntax of thought	Notice how Piaget's and Vygotsky's ideas here are in conflict. For Chomsky and Skinner the child is relatively passive in this process. For Piaget the child is an active construc-tor. For Vygotsky the child's social world determines his or her cognition.

Practical applications

Although Skinner's views seem unwieldy today as an explanation of language development, programmes that are based on his behaviourist principles have become effective tools in language remediation programmes (Rhodes and Sheehy, 1999). As with cognitive development, however, an emphasis on the simple production of 'correct responses' is inappropriate, language development being the culmination of several processes.

Chomsky's work has less direct practical application and yet has sparked much research, including experiments with primates and sign language, which question the human specificity of the LAD, and computer modelling of language skills.

One noticeable feature of early parent–child interaction is the way in which adults modify their own speech when talking to the infant. The term *motherese* (or baby-talk register) has been coined to describe this pattern (Gleitman and Gleitman, 1986; Greene, 1990). The adult uses very simple, grammatically correct phrases. Words are simplified for the child to pronounce – for example, tummy (stomach) and bot-bot (bottle). Phrases are repeated and represented to help the child's understanding. The following example is between Janis and her son Rory (21 months) as they get ready to go to Granny's house:

Janis: Go see Granny now.
Rory: Ganny how.
Janis: That's right. Go to Granny's house in the car.
Rory: Dodie tum?
Janis: No Dodie stay with Daddy, Mummy and Rory go to Granny's.
Rory: Bot bot, bot bot. Bot bot.
Janis: Take your bot bot in the car?
Rory: (looks around the room)
Janis: There's bot bot, on the chair.
Rory: Bot bot. (picks up bottle)
Janis: Good boy, let's go see . . .
Rory: Ganny!
Janis: That's right!

This type of interaction can be seen as operating at two levels. Firstly motherese models simple and effective communication for the child to copy. Secondly, by adopting a more 'childlike' language, the adult is taking into account the child's level of cognitive and social development. This achieves a mutual understanding and by 5 months children are more emotionally responsive to motherese than other kinds of adult talk (Fernald, 1993, cited in Berk, 1996). As with cognition (mentioned previously), by moving closer to the child's level of development a *zone of proximal development* is created. This responsive social environment supports and accelerates early language development (Crain, 1992). In contrast, impatience and overcorrection of children's early language productions can hamper the child's linguistic development and result in immature language skills (Nelson, 1973, cited in Berk, 1996).

Summary

The development of cognition, moral reasoning and language is a complex matter in which the developing processes interact within a social environment. Piaget's constructivist viewpoint has been developed by other theorists to highlight the social nature of developing functions and the influence of language on development. Whilst the stages of language development are well documented, and its influence on cognition established, the underlying mechanisms of language development have yet to be fully explained.

References

Berk LE (1994) Child Development. London: Allyn & Bacon.

Berk LE (1996) Infants, Children and Adolescence (2 edn). London: Allyn & Bacon.

Berko J (1958) The child's learning of English morphology. Word 14: 150–77.

Bibace R, Walsh ME (1981) Children's conceptions of illness. In R Bibace, ME Wallace (eds) New Directions for Child Development, vol. 14. San Francisco: Jossey-Bass, pp. 31–8.

Chomsky N (1957) Syntactic Structures. The Hague: Mouton.

Crain W (1992) Theories of Development. Concepts and Applications. London: Prentice-Hall.

Donaldson M (1978) Children's Minds. London: Fontana/Collins.

Dworetsky JP (1981) Introduction to Child Development. New York: West Publishing Company.

Eiser C (1985) The Psychology of Childhood Illness. New York: Springer-Verlag.

Gilligan CF (1982) In a Different Voice. Cambridge MA: Harvard University Press.

Gleitman LR, Gleitman H (1986) Language. In H Gleitman, Psychology (2 edn). New York: WW Norton.

Greene J (1990) Topics in Language and Communication. In I Roth (ed.) Introduction to Psychology, vol 2. Hillsdale: Erlbaum.

Hayslip G, Panek C (1989) Adult Development and Ageing. New York: Harper & Row.

Kahney H (1997) Problem Solving: Current Issues. Milton Keynes: Open University Press.

Kozulin A (1990) Vygotsky's Psychology. A Biography of Ideas. Exeter: Harvester Wheatsheaf.

Light PH, Buckingham N, Robbins H (1979) The development of communication: competence as a function of age. Child Development 40: 255–66.

Piaget J (1923) The Language and Thought of the Child (translated M Gabian, 1959). London: Routledge & Kegan Paul.

Piaget J (1936) The Origins of Intelligence in Children (translated M Cook, 1974). New York: International Universities Press.

Piaget J (1963) The Origins of Intelligence in Children. New York: Norton.

Piaget J, Inhelder B (1972) (trans. H Weaver) The Psychology of the Child. New York: Basic Books.

Piaget J (1970) Piaget's Theory. In PA Mussen (ed.) (1983) Handbook of Child Psychology (4 edn). New York: John Wiley.

Rest JR, Narvaes D (1991) The college experience and moral development. In WM Kurtiness, JL Gewirtz (eds) Handbook of Moral Behaviour and Development, vol. 2. Hillsdale NJ: Erlbaum, pp. 333–64.

Rhodes S, Sheehy K (1999) Teaching language and socialisation skills to a young child with autism. Journal of Special Needs Education in Ireland 12, 2: 94–102.

Roth I (ed.) (1993) Introduction to Psychology. Volume 1. Hillsdale: Lawrence Erlbaum/Open University.

Sheehy K (1992) The Moscow initiative. Therapy 18 (November): 20.

Sheehy K (1993) Words fail me. Special Children (Nov/Dec) 5: 12–15.

Sheehy K (1995) Teaching word recognition to children with severe learning disabilities: the quick word technique. In G Shiel, U Ni Dhalaigh, B O'Reilly (eds) Reading Development to Age 15: Overcoming Reading Difficulties. Reading Association of Ireland, pp. 64–70.

Skinner BF (1957) Verbal Behaviour. New York: Appleton Century Crofts.

Slater A (1990) Infant development: The origins of competence. The Psychologist 3 (March): 109–13.

Smith PK, Cowic H (1988) Understanding Children's Development. Oxford: Blackwell.

Smith PK, Cowie H (1991) Understanding Children's Development (2 edn) Oxford: Blackwell.

Snarey JR, Reimer J, Kohlberg L (1985) The development of social-moral reasoning among kibbutz adolescents. A longitudinal cross-cultural study. Developmental Psychology 21: 3–17.

Vygotsky LS (1978 [1931]) The history of the development of the higher mental functions (translated M Coles). In M Cole, V John-Steiner, S Scribner, E Souberman (eds) LS Vygotsky: Mind in Society. Cambridge MA: Harvard University Press.

Vygotsky LS (1962) Thought and Language (translated A Kozulin). Cambridge MA: MIT Press. (Original work (1934) Mshlenie I Rech. Moscow and Leningrad: Sotezekgiz.)

Walker LJ, Taylor JH (1991) Sex differences in moral reasoning. In WM Kurtiness, JL Gewirtz (eds) Handbook of Moral Behaviour and Development, vol. 2. Hillsdale: Erlbaum, pp. 333–64.

Chapter 6
Understanding the psychology of personality

MAN CHEUNG CHUNG

Key concepts	Key names
Psychoanalytic	Freud
Psychosexual stages	
Libido, conscious, unconscious	
Ego, id, superego	
Pleasure principle, Reality principle	
Ego ideal	
Defence mechanisms	Freud and Anna Freud
Neopsychoanalytic	Jung, Adler, Erikson, Horney, Sullivan, Fromm
Behaviouristic	Watson, Skinner, Bandura
Humanistic	Maslow, Rogers
Cognitive	Kelly
Psychic energy, ego	Jung
Personal unconscious, Complexes	
Collective unconscious, Extraversion	
Introversion, Archetypes	
Operant and respondent behaviour	Skinner
Superstitious behaviour	
Self-control of behaviour	
Modelling	Bandura
Observational learning	
Self-reinforcement, Self-efficacy	
Hierarchy of needs	
Cripple psychology	Maslow
Incongruent self-concept	
Ideal self, Positive regard	Rogers
Positive self-regard	
Person-centred therapy	
Personal-construct theory	Kelly
Man as scientist	
Traits	Allport, Cattell, Eysenck

Introduction

The present chapter is an attempt to provide an introduction to the psychological understanding of personality. However, due to limited space this introduction is by no means a comprehensive account of all that we need to know about the psychology of personality. Instead, it provides a brief outline of significant theories of some psychologists who represent six main approaches to personality, namely, the psychoanalytic, neopsychoanalytic, behaviouristic, humanistic, cognitive and the trait approaches. The chapter will conclude by giving small examples of personality tests that are currently used in measuring personality. Finally, in order to facilitate further reading, the reference section contains suggested readings that cover the general ground of personality theory and the original writings of the psychologists outlined in the above six approaches.

The psychoanalytic approach to personality

It is commonly thought that the first formal theory of personality originated with Sigmund Freud (1856–1939), the founder of *psychoanalysis*. Freud (1917/1991) believed that instincts are the basic elements or units of personality. They motivate and drive our behaviour and determine its direction. He postulated that *libido* is the basic sexual force or energy behind all instinctual drives, and all pleasure-seeking activities. The term *sexual* is used in a broader sense and implies not only genital sex but also pleasurable sensations derived from activities such as chewing, defecation, thumb-sucking, and talking. In addition, pleasurable sensations include satisfaction associated with intellectual endeavour and aesthetic expression. In other words, the libido provides energy not only for psychosexual growth but for all creative activities, for example, poetry, art, music, and science.

In his earliest attempt to understand personality structure, Freud pointed out that the human mind is like an iceberg. The part that is above the surface of the water symbolizes the *conscious*, our current awareness, and the *pre-conscious*, the information of which we are not currently aware, but which can be brought into consciousness when necessary (for example the names of our parents). The part that is below the surface of the water, a much larger mass of the iceberg, symbolizes the *unconscious*. The latter consists of impulses, wishes and inaccessible memories that affect our thoughts and behaviours.

In later years, Freud developed his theory further by dividing personality structure into three major components: the *id*, the *ego* and the *superego*. The id is the most primitive part of personality, while the ego and superego later develop from the id. The id is usually found in newborn infants and consists of basic biological needs, drives or impulses, for example, eating, drinking, avoiding pain, gaining sensual pleasure as well as being aggressive. In other words, the id seeks immediate gratification of impulses and operates on what Freud called the *pleasure principle*. This principle indicates that the organism wants to obtain pleasure, but avoid pain, regardless of external circumstances.

The ego, on the other hand, operates on the *reality principle*, which indicates that the organism delays the gratification of impulses until the situation is appropriate. While children want to satisfy their impulses, they learn that they cannot always simply do so at once. For example, when they are hungry, they may have to wait for food; when they want to defecate, they need to wait until they reach the toilet. When children learn to consider the demands of reality, they then develop the ego, a new part of personality. In other words, the ego decides for us which action is appropriate or inappropriate, and which id impulses can be satisfied or need to be suppressed, as well as in what manner we can satisfy or suppress them. The ego constantly tries to mediate the demands of the id, the realities of the world and the demands of the superego.

The superego informs us whether or not our actions are right or wrong. In other words, it has internalized the values and morals of society; it consists of human conscience and an image of the morally ideal person, sometimes called the *ego ideal*. The superego develops as a result of responding to parental teaching, rewards and punishments, through which children learn to control their behaviour. As time goes by, they no longer need their parents or others to tell them the right or wrong things to do. Instead, the superego tells them. If they violate the standards of the superego, they experience anxiety, which originates from the fear of losing parental love. This anxiety is largely unconscious and might be experienced as guilt.

The above three components of personality structure do not exist independently, but interact intimately. In fact, they are often in opposition, in that the id wants certain immediate gratification that the ego wants to postpone. Meanwhile the superego struggles with both the id and ego and urges morality above all. However, people with a well-integrated personality will have a firm ego, but will exercise flexible control. To understand these three components in the light of the iceberg model outlined previously, Freud postulated that the entire id and most of the ego and superego are submerged in the unconscious. Meanwhile, there are small parts of the ego and superego in either the conscious or the pre-conscious (see Figure 6.1).

It was mentioned earlier that when people violate the standards of the superego, they experience anxiety. Such a phenomenon is common because people often have a desire to do something that they are forbidden to do. In order to reduce this anxiety, people employ what Freud called the *ego mechanism of defence*, a concept that was later extended by his daughter, Anna Freud. Briefly, the strategies of this defence mechanism are as follows:

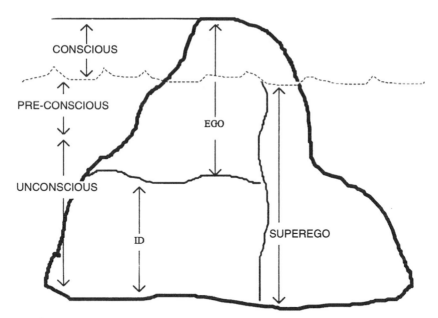

CONSCIOUS

PRE-CONSCIOUS

UNCONSCIOUS

EGO

ID

SUPEREGO

Figure 6.1: Freud's 'iceberg' model of the mind.

- Repression. By means of selective, motivated forgetting, we repress certain ideas and emotions and keep them forcefully from consciousness. Amnesia is one example of repression.
- Isolation. This defence refers to our splitting off ideas from feelings. In other words, it is a partial repression, i.e. repressing merely emotions. For example, a soldier might describe his war experience without manifesting the guilt of failing to protect his wounded fellow soldier from being killed.
- Reaction formation. We repress a threatening idea by substituting it with an idea representing the opposite extreme. For example, people might control their sexual desires or fantasies by becoming excessively moralistic and believing that sexual activity is dirty and immoral.
- Projection. Our personal drive-related fantasy is attributed to another person. For example, a husband, who wishes to develop an extramarital relationship with another woman, might become jealous and project adulterous desires on to his wife.
- Undoing. We take back, or make amends for, an impulse or guilt-ridden thought or action. A husband, who experiences strain in his relationship with his wife and consequently experiences some aggressive fantasies, 'spontaneously' decides to give his wife flowers.
- Displacement. Our unconscious fantasy is directed away from the original object toward a relatively neutral one. For example, children who hate their parents but are afraid to become hostile towards them, due to the fear of punishment, might displace their aggression on to someone who is not a threat to them, such as a younger sibling.

- Turning against the self. Our impulse, usually aggressive in nature, is displaced from the external object toward the self, hence, self-denigration, self-blame or self-harm.
- Rationalization. We use emotionally neutral, objective reasoning to explain certain behaviour or the avoidance of it, when a drive-related idea is really the motivating factor. For example, people might rationalize their reading of pornography by claiming the importance of aesthetic appreciation, when they are actually trying to fulfil their sexual desires.
- Denial. We block out aspects of reality to avoid painful consequences. Refusal to accept one's terminal illness is one example of denial.
- Identification. We adopt the characteristics of a significant other in order to defend against, for example, the pain of separation or the loss of love. For example, when the father has gone away, the little boy might behave like the father in looking after the mother.

Freud believed that our unique character type develops in childhood from the nature of the parent–child relationship. According to Freud, during the first five years of our lives, we progress through what he called *psychosexual stages*, which ultimately shape and crystallize personality type. There are five stages to this psychosexual development. However, some people are unable to move from one stage to the next because the conflict in the stage from which they cannot move has not been resolved or the satisfaction of the needs from that stage is too great for them to want to move on. Consequently, they are *fixated* at this stage of development, thus affecting their behaviour even in adulthood.

The first stage is called the *oral* stage (from birth to sometime in the second year of life). During this stage, infants gain pleasure from sucking, biting and swallowing and indeed putting anything they can reach into their mouths. They also depend completely on the mother who then becomes the primary object of the infants' libido. There are two oral behaviours happening at this stage: *oral incorporative behaviour* and *oral aggressive behaviour*. The former involves the pleasurable stimulation of the mouth by others and by food. The latter occurs during the painful eruption of teeth. As a result, the infants might develop hatred toward their mothers. Adults who are fixated at the oral incorporative stage tend to be those who are excessively concerned with eating, drinking, smoking and the like. Adults who are fixated at the oral aggressive stage tend to be those who are excessively pessimistic, hostile and aggressive.

The second stage is called the *anal stage* (around the age of two years). During this stage, children are thought to gain pleasure from withholding and expelling faeces. However this pleasure often conflicts with parents' expectations, when attempting toilet training. In other words, this is the stage where they first experience imposed control. If toilet training goes badly, in that children have difficulty in learning, or parents are being too harsh and demanding, children will become frustrated and react to this frustration in two ways. One way is to defecate whenever and wherever the parents forbid them to. If they find that this is a satisfactory way of reducing frustration, they will use it on a regular basis and will consequently develop what Freud called an *anal aggressive personality*, the basis for hostile and sadistic behaviour, cruelty, destructiveness and temper tantrums. The other way of reacting is to hold back or retain the faeces. The parents might consequently become overly concerned over the long period of time when their children do not defecate. This is one way to secure attention and affection from parents. If they find this strategy satisfactory, they will develop an *anal retentive personality* in that they become hoarders, rigid and compulsively neat.

The third stage is called the *phallic stage* (from three to five years of age). During this stage, children gain pleasure by fondling their genitals. They also observe gender differences, and begin to direct their sexual impulses towards the parent of the opposite sex. Two types of conflict will occur at this stage. One is called the *Oedipal conflict*, in which the boy would direct his sexual impulses towards the mother. Consequently, he perceives his father as a rival for his mother's affection. At the same time, however, the boy is fearful that his father will retaliate against the boy's sexual impulses by castrating him. Freud calls this *castration anxiety*. This fear may cause the boy to reduce his anxiety by identifying himself with his father – that is by internalizing his father's attitudes and values.

Another conflict is called the *Electra conflict*, in which the girl's first object of love is her mother but later the father becomes the girl's new love object, apparently because he possesses a protruding and highly valued organ, a penis. Freud called this *penis envy*. Eventually, to resolve the conflict, the girl comes to identify with her mother and to repress her love for her father. If people develop a phallic personality, they develop strong narcissism, experience difficulties in establishing mature heterosexual relationships, and need continual appreciation of their attractive and unique qualities.

The fourth stage is called the *latency stage* (from six years of age through puberty). During this stage, children become less concerned with their bodies, but begin to pay attention to coping with the environment. The sex instinct becomes largely inactive. Children become sublimated in school activities, hobbies and sports and developing friendships. The final stage is called the *genital stage*, which is basically a stage of adolescents' and adults' sexuality and functioning.

The neopsychoanalytic approach to personality

After having established his reputation and his school of psychoanalysis, Freud began to be confronted by opposition. Many of his followers, who were committed and loyal to Freud's ideas and to the man himself, began to develop theories that deviated from Freud's orthodox psychoanalysis, although they did not entirely escape the influence of Freud's work. For example, instead of emphasizing the importance of sexuality, many of his followers emphasized the importance of motivational processes. The growing differences eventually led them to break away from psychoanalysis. Some examples of these people were Carl Jung, Alfred Adler, Erik Erikson, Karen Horney, Harry Stack Sullivan and Erich Fromm.

To demonstrate the differences between the neopsychoanalytic thinking and Freud's orthodox psychoanalysis, Carl Jung's theory is selected. Carl Jung (1875–1961), who was a close associate with Freud and was thought by Freud to be his spiritual heir, disagreed with Freud on the role of sexuality. He broadened Freud's concept of libido by redefining it as a more generalized dynamic force of personality. Also, Jung investigated, more deeply than Freud, the unconscious, and added some new understanding of the world of the unconscious. In addition, Jung believed that human beings are shaped by the future as well as the past, not merely the past events and processes as Freud postulated.

Let us consider briefly each of the above disagreements. Instead of looking at libido as sexual energy, like Freud, Jung investigated the functioning of libido as *psychic energy* in three principles: *opposites*, *equivalence* and *entropy*. These principles represent the dynamic mechanisms for the operation of personality and are thought to be the prime movers of behaviour and, indeed, the generators of all energy.

The principle of opposites indicates that every wish or feeling has its opposite, for example love and hate. Because of the existence of polarities or extremes, there is a process or tendency toward equalization, and that process is energy. The sharper the conflict between polarities, the greater the energy produced.

The principle of equivalence indicates that psychic energy is not lost to the personality but is shifted from one part to another. Thus, if one has lost interest in a person or a hobby, one has in fact shifted the psychic energy, formerly invested in that person and hobby, to a new area or several different areas.

The principle of entropy indicates that there is equalization of energy differences. In other words, there is a tendency toward a balance or equilibrium in personality. Thus, if two desires or beliefs differ greatly, psychic energy will flow from the more strongly held to the weaker. Ideally, our personality should have an equal distribution of psychic energy over all its systems and over all aspects of personality, but this complete state of equilibrium is never totally achieved.

In studying the personality structure, Jung refers to three major systems: the *ego*, the *personal unconscious* and the *collective unconscious*. The ego is our conscious mind, awareness of ourselves, and is responsible for carrying out normal day-to-day activities. Our conscious perception of reality is determined by the attitudes of *extraversion* (for example, people are open, sociable and socially aggressive) and *introversion* (for example, people are somewhat withdrawn, shy and focus on themselves). Jung believed that while we are able to have both attitudes, one tends to be more dominant than the other. The dominant attitude rules our behaviour and consciousness, while the non-dominant attitude becomes part of the personal unconscious.

The personal unconscious is similar to Freud's pre-conscious – it consists of trivial or distressing materials that have been forgotten or suppressed. However, when we are asked to remember them, we can take the materials out of the personal unconscious, examine them, and then put them back in the personal unconscious. Jung believed that, as we store more and more materials in the personal unconscious, we begin to group them into clusters called *complexes*. These complexes are composed of emotions, memories, perceptions and wishes, clustering around a common theme. They affect behaviour, determine the way in which we perceive the world and interfere with our consciousness. For example, if one has a complex about power, one might try to associate oneself with power by driving a motorcycle or a powerful car.

The collective unconscious refers to humankind as a whole. As human beings accumulate and store past experience in the personal unconscious, humankind as a whole can also accumulate the experience of the human and prehuman (animal ancestry) species in the collective unconscious and pass this experience on to each generation. In other words, the collective unconscious consists of all the experience of humankind transmitted to each one of us. The above universal experience becomes part of each individual's personality. That is to say, Jung believed that the personality of each individual is connected with not only the person's childhood and early years, but also the entire history of humankind.

The manifestation or expression of the above universal experience, contained in the collective unconscious, is in the form of images, which Jung called *archetypes*. The latter are not memories or pictures of past events or people in our lives. They are, for example, *persona*, the *anima* and *animus*, the *shadow* and the *self*. Simply put, the persona is a mask or a public face that we wear in order to present ourselves as someone other than who we really are. The anima and animus refer to the idea that we are essentially bisexual beings, both masculine and feminine at the same time. Biologically, humans secrete the hormones of both sexes. Psychologically, each sex manifests characteristics, temperaments and attitudes of the other sex. The shadow has the deepest roots of all the archetypes and consists of the basic, primitive animal instincts. Society tends to consider the primitive impulses contained in the shadow as evil and immoral. We need to suppress and overcome them, otherwise we would probably be punished by society.

The self is Jung's most important archetype. It represents the wholeness and integration of the total personality. The full realization of the self involves a future orientation – plans, goals and purpose – and an accurate perception and full knowledge of self. Thus, Jung believed that our personality is determined by what we want, and hope to be, in the future (i.e. teleological), not merely what we have been in the past (i.e. causal). We are constantly developing and growing, moving towards a more complete human level of development. Jung called this *progression*, although he also talked about the possibility of *regression* (how we quietly retreat into ourselves in order to foster creativity).

Thus, Jung did not believe that the development of personality would stop, as long as we live. He did not concentrate on childhood and think that the early years were the most important in fixing our personality pattern. Initially, children are governed by physical instincts and their consciousness begins to emerge when they can use the word 'I'. In puberty, they find themselves having to adapt to many problems and to stop fantasizing as they need to confront reality. From the teenage years through young adulthood, they are concerned with education, career, getting married and starting a family. In other words, the focus is external, i.e. extraversion. Then, the second half of their lives begins, between age 35 and 40. They become more introspective and introverted. This is the period when the self, the important archetype, begins to emerge; hence, they might begin to realize their capacities and live with a fully harmonious and integrated personality. Of course, such progress is not achievable for everybody and can be hindered by environmental factors.

The behaviouristic approach to personality

In the early 1900s, US culture engaged in a modern technological industrial revolution, which meant that Americans were primarily concerned with the practical use of science and technology. This undoubtedly paved the way for the new movement of *behaviourism*, which was led by John B. Watson (1878–1958) (Richards, 1996). In this movement of behaviourism, Watson proposed that one should take a natural science approach to study psychological topics such as personality, i.e. to base study on careful experimental research and precise quantification of stimuli and responses. To behaviourists, the notions of conscious and unconscious forces were not important because they could not be seen, manipulated, measured and quantified. They also undermined the importance of internal entities such as anxiety, drives, motives, needs and defence mechanisms. Instead, they believed that personality was simply an accumulation of learned responses to stimuli or habit systems. Personality referred merely to what could be objectively observed and manipulated.

To demonstrate how personality can be understood in the light of behaviourism, two influential representatives are selected, namely,

B.F. Skinner and Albert Bandura. B.F. Skinner's (1904–90) work reflects the original form of behaviourism and follows the tradition of J.B. Watson. He attempted to explain behaviour, rather than merely personality, in purely factual and descriptive terms, and believed that psychology should be about measuring what we can see and manipulate in a laboratory – a reaction against the psychoanalytic approach to personality.

All behaviour, according to Skinner, could be controlled by the extent and nature of the *reinforcement* that follows the behaviour. In other words, when one can control the reinforcement available to us, one would be able to change and control our behaviour. Skinner distinguished two kinds of behaviour: *respondent* and *operant behaviour.* Respondent behaviour involves a response made to, or elicited by, specific stimuli in the environment – for example, a knee jerk. Such a response is unlearned and is elicited automatically and involuntarily. However, some respondent behaviours are learned through a process called *conditioning.* This concept originated from the work of Ivan Pavlov (1849–1936) who sounded a bell shortly before feeding a dog. Initially, the dog salivated only to food but it eventually salivated at the sound of the bell. Thus, the dog had been conditioned to respond to the bell. However, it is noteworthy that the dog would not have remained conditioned to respond to the bell if it had not received food in return. In other words, conditioned responses cannot be established when reinforcement is absent. By the same token, after a conditioned response is established, one can gradually extinguish that response by withdrawing reinforcement.

However, Skinner believed that operant behaviour is more important than respondent behaviour. Operant behaviour operates on the environment and consequently changes it. For example, when an infant cries, the parents go to pick up the infant and consequently change the infant's environment. If the environmental changes brought about by the behaviour are reinforced, for example, with food, then the chance of that behaviour occurring again will be increased. On the other hand, if the environmental changes brought about by the behaviour are not reinforcing, then that behaviour is less likely to occur again. Indeed, Skinner believed that, starting from infancy, we engage in a great deal of random, spontaneous behaviour, and that which is reinforced will grow stronger and form into networks or patterns. Many of our complex human behaviours are *shaped* through successive reinforcements, and personality is simply a pattern or collection of operant behaviours.

Sometimes, however, we behave in a certain way and our behaviour is reinforced by accident. When we learn a few times that the performance of our behaviour is followed by the occurrence of accidental reinforcement, we might develop what Skinner called *superstitious behaviour* – we think that there is a causal relationship there. For example, a football player might wear a particular pair of football boots and find himself or herself scoring goals. When this happens a few times, this football player might never go to a match unless he or she is wearing the lucky pair of football boots.

Obviously, according to Skinner, our behaviour is caused and changed by external environmental factors. No internal activity will determine our behaviour. However, he did not deny that although external stimuli and reinforcers shape our behaviour, we can act to change them. He called this *self-control of behaviour*, by which he meant that we exercise control over the external factors that determine our behaviour. For example, if my neighbours are screaming at each other so much that I cannot concentrate on writing this chapter, I can go to my office, to remove myself from an external factor that affects my behaviour.

There are different techniques of self-control: *satiation, aversive stimulation* and *reinforcement of oneself*. Satiation means that we can, for example, overcome bad habits by overdoing the habit. Aversive stimulation means that if we want to stop drinking, we need to declare our intention to friends. If we break the resolution, we will need to face up to the unpleasant consequences, such as severe criticism from friends. Reinforcing oneself simply means that we reinforce ourselves when we have displayed a good or desirable behaviour.

The above principles of respondent and operant conditioning set the wheels of *behaviour therapy* or *behaviour modification* in motion. It has been applied in prisons, school classrooms, reform schools and institutions for people with mental illness and learning difficulty.

Albert Bandura (1925) criticized Skinner's theory on the basis that Skinner concentrated on studying individual subjects in isolation, rather than on how individuals interact with each other. Bandura believes that one should investigate how behaviour is formed and modified in a social context. He recognizes the fact that learning can take place due to reinforcement, but he also recognizes that some learning can take place when we do not directly experience reinforcement. Instead, we learn by means of observation and *modelling*. That is, we learn to observe other people's behaviour and model our behaviour on theirs. He believes that much of our good, bad, normal and abnormal behaviour is learned by imitation. From infancy, we respond to the many models that society offers us, and we consequently develop our behaviour.

Bandura points out that there are three factors that can influence modelling: *the characteristics of the models, the attributes of the observers*, and the *reward consequences associated with the behaviour*. The characteristics of the models will certainly affect whether or not we want to imitate their behaviour, as we are more inclined to imitate the people who are like us rather than those who are different from us in obvious and significant ways. These characteristics include age, sex, status and prestige. The attributes of the observers can also determine the effectiveness of modelling. People with low self-confidence and self-esteem will be more likely to imitate a model's behaviour than those with high self-confidence and self-esteem. The reward consequences associated with behaviour may also affect the effectiveness of modelling. That is, if the reward consequences associated with the behaviour are not sufficient, the person might discontinue modelling that behaviour, and will be less likely to use that as a model in the future.

Bandura explains that the nature of observational learning is governed by four processes or mechanisms: *attentional processes, retention processes, motor reproduction processes* and *incentive and motivational processes.* Attentional processes mean that observational learning will not take place if we do not attend to the model – mere exposure to the model will not guarantee the imitation of the model. Retention processes indicate that we must retain or remember all significant aspects of the behaviour, unless we are imitating a model's behaviour as it is taking place or immediately afterwards. We encode and represent symbolically what we have seen, in order to retain the behaviour to which we have attended. We store or retain the observed events and rehearse them internally for later performance.

The motor reproduction processes indicate that, while we are imitating the behaviour, we might not be able to perform the behaviour correctly, especially highly skilful behaviour. In such a situation, we will need to actually practise and perform the motor movements, and we will need feedback about their correctness. The incentive and motivational processes indicate that we need to have sufficient incentive or motivation in order to perform the behaviour, no matter how precisely we attend to and retain the behaviour of a model. One way to influence the level of our incentive and motivational processes is through the anticipation of reinforcement or punishment.

Unlike Skinner, Bandura does not disregard the importance of looking at some internal variables about an individual. He believes that our cognition and thought processes can influence observational learning. That is, one does not automatically model other people's behaviour; rather, one makes a deliberate and conscious decision to behave. One can somehow regulate and guide one's own behaviour by visualizing or imagining the consequences of the behaviour, even when the consequences are not experienced.

In viewing the self, Bandura looks at two important aspects: *self-reinforcement* and *self-efficacy.* Self-reinforcement indicates that we often set standards of behaviour or achievement for ourselves in various activities. We reward or punish ourselves for meeting or failing to meet the standards. The rewards could include feelings of pride or satisfaction; the punishments could include shame, guilt or depression. Self-efficacy refers to our self-esteem and self-worth, our feeling of adequacy and efficiency in dealing with life. It is derived from past experiences and accomplishments. We enhance or reduce our self-efficacy by meeting and maintaining, or failing to meet and maintain, our performance standards respectively.

The humanistic approach to personality

Humanistic psychology is often described as the *third-force psychology*, which is derived from a reaction against the psychoanalytic and behaviouristic approaches to psychology. The humanistic approach to personality focuses on the individual's subjective experience, i.e. his or her own personal view of the world. Humanistic psychologists emphasize four main principles about humans. Firstly, humans are not simply objects of study. Rather, we have our own subjective views of the world and our subjective perception and feelings of self-worth. Secondly, the topics of investigation into humans should include human choice, creativity and self-actualization – humans should be seen as developing and expressing their potential and capabilities. Thirdly, while psychological researchers should be objective in collecting data and interpreting observations, their choice of research topics should be guided by values – research is not value free. Finally, humans are essentially good and psychology should be about understanding them rather than predicting or controlling them.

Abraham Maslow (1908–70) and Carl Rogers (1902–87) were the central figures in the movement of humanistic psychology. Let us consider each briefly in turn. Abraham Maslow was an active spokesman and leader for the movement of humanistic psychology. He found Freud's approach to personality to be problematic, in the sense that emphasis is placed on the crippled side of humans, such as the neurotics, which consequently generates what Maslow called *cripple psychology*. According to Maslow, the positive side of humans is largely ignored – happiness, contentment, satisfaction and peace of mind. Psychologists should focus on the creative, and the healthiest side of humans. He believed that each person is born with certain innate needs, which motivate the person to choose to grow, develop and actualize himself or herself – to fulfil his or her potential.

Maslow postulated that there is a *hierarchy of innate needs*, a ladder of motivations, which activate and direct our behaviour. Our behaviour to satisfy needs, however, is not innate but learned, and differs from person to person. The hierarchy of needs is structured as follows:

5. The need for self-actualization
4. The need for self-esteem
3. The need for belongingness and love
2. The need for safety
1. The physiological needs

The physiological needs must be satisfied before those at the top can be satisfied. In fact, the needs at the top will not even appear if we have not fulfilled, at least partially, the lower order ones. For example, if we are hungry and feel no safety in life, we are then concerned with bread, rather than love. However, when we are fed and feel safe in our surrounding, we then come to feel the needs for belongingness and love. When the latter needs are satisfied, we then begin to long for self-esteem. When we achieve that, we then desire *self-actualization.* In other words, people are not driven by all of the above needs simultaneously. Instead, only one need is dominant at a time, and the nature of that need depends upon which other needs have been satisfied or not satisfied.

Focusing on the highest need in the hierarchy, Maslow described in detail the characteristics of self-actualizers who have made extraordinary use of their potential.

• They have a highly efficient perception of reality and can tolerate uncertainty.
• They can accept themselves, others and nature for what they are.
• They are spontaneous, simplistic and natural in thought and behaviour.
• They focus on problems rather than on self.
• They have a need for privacy and independence.
• They have an ability to perceive and experience the world with freshness, wonder and awe.
• They have moments of mystical or *peak experience* in that they experience intense ecstasy, wonder, awe and delight.
• They are concerned with the welfare of humanity.
• They have deep, intense and satisfying friendships.
• They are highly creative.
• They are tolerant, accepting everyone and have no racial, religious or social prejudice.
• They are free to resist social and cultural pressures to think and behave in certain ways.

One of the characteristics on the list is that self-actualizers experience transient moments of peak experience. Maslow further explained that happiness and fulfilment characterize this peak experience. It may occur at different intensities and in different circumstances, such as when engaging in creative activities, appreciating nature, having an intimate relationship with others, participating in athletic activities and the like.

Going along with the notion of self-actualization, Carl Rogers believed that we have an innate tendency to head towards the direction of growth, maturity and positive change. The basic force that motivates us is the actualizing tendency – a tendency towards fulfilment or actualization of all the capacities of the person. He believed that we always choose to grow rather than regress. A growing person is someone who seeks to fulfil his or her potential within the limits of his or her heredity.

In viewing the concept of self, Rogers believed that it consists of all the ideas, perceptions and values that characterize 'I' or 'me'. It also consists of the awareness of what I am, and what I can do. In other words, the self can perceive itself, which in turn influences the person's perception of the world, and his or her behaviour. For example, those who perceive themselves as competent would perceive and act upon the world quite differently from those who consider themselves as ineffectual.

Rogers believed that we do evaluate every area of our experience in relation to our concept of self. We want to behave in a way that is consistent with the way in which we perceive our concept of self. On the other hand, an experience that is not consistent with the concept of self would be threatening to us. We would therefore try to repress it. According to Rogers, the more areas of experience that we deny, the wider the gap becomes between our concept of self and reality and, as a result, the greater the potential maladjustment. That is, when our self-concept is *incongruent* with our personal experience, we must defend ourselves against the truth, because the truth will result in anxiety. However if the incongruence becomes too great, our defence may break down, resulting in severe anxiety or other forms of emotional disturbance.

Rogers put forward another concept of self called the *ideal self*. That is, we have a perception of the kind of person we would like to be. The closer the ideal self is to the real self, the more fulfilled and content we become. On the other hand, the greater the discrepancy between the ideal self and the real self, the more unhappiness and dissatisfaction we experience. In other words, he believed that there are two kinds of incongruence that can develop in us. The first is the incongruence between the self and the experience of reality and the second is that between the self and the ideal self.

Rogers believed that the self starts to develop from infancy. It develops a need for what he called *positive regard*, which is found in all humans and which includes acceptance, love and approval from others. It is satisfying for the infant to experience positive regard, but frustrating not to experience it. If the infant does not receive positive regard, its tendency toward actualization and enhancement of the self would be restricted. In fact, the infant would stop striving toward actualizing the self, because it would instead work towards securing positive regard. Ideally, the infant should receive *unconditional positive regard*, in that the mother's love for the child is not conditional. The child can then freely and fully grow to become a person. Gradually, the child would learn to internalize the unconditional positive regard. Consequently, the positive regard would come from within the child, which Rogers called *positive self-regard*.

Well-adjusted individuals have positive self-regard, which is always consistent with personal experience, thought and behaviour. The concept of self is not rigid but flexible and can change by incorporating new experiences and ideas. People with this positive self-regard are free to utilize experience, and to fulfil their potential. In other words, they are free to become self-actualizing and eventually become what Rogers called *fully functioning individuals.*

Rogers described the characteristics of fully functioning individuals as follows. They have the ability to be aware of all experience and do not need to distort or deny experience in any way. There is no defensiveness or threat to their self-concept and they are free and open to both positive and negative feelings. They have the tendency or ability to live fully and richly in each and every moment. Each moment and the experience associated with it is fresh and new. There is no rigidity and tight organization or structure imposed on their experience.

Fully functioning individuals can also trust the feeling of their own reaction, rather than rely on the guidance and judgement of others. They can choose to move freely in any direction that they wish. Consequently, they experience a sense of personal power over their lives, because they know that the future depends on themselves rather than circumstances, past events or others.

Fully functioning individuals are creative people who can flexibly adapt to, and find, new experiences and challenges. They are spontaneous, enriching, exciting, rewarding, challenging and meaningful. They are constantly changing and growing as they are striving to actualize all of their potentialities.

According to Rogers, actualization forms the basis of his *person-centred therapy.* This therapy assumes that humans are motivated and able to change, and that humans are in the best position to decide the direction that changes should take. The therapy role is to act as a sounding board, while trying to explore and analyse the problems of clients.

The cognitive approach to personality

The cognitive approach focuses on conscious mental activities, the ways in which we know our environment and ourselves – how we perceive, evaluate, think, make decisions and solve problems. To cognitivists, personality can be understood in terms of cognitive processes. These processes are not seen as elements of personality. Instead, they are the entire personality. George Kelly is the representative of the above approach for the present chapter.

George Kelly (1905–67) postulated a theory called *personal-construct theory*, in which he believed that we can engage in conscious mental activities and consequently know something about the world and ourselves. He believed that we can construct our lives, or reconstruct the progress in our lives, rather than just follow our impulses. We are like formal scientists, who observe the world, formulate and test hypotheses against the world and consequently make up theories about it. We can construct behaviour by categorizing, interpreting, labelling and judging our world and ourselves. We can also identify invalid theories that might hinder us in daily life, and which would lead us to distort our interpretations of events and people around us.

According to Kelly, throughout our lives, we develop many constructs in order to deal with all kinds of situations or events or people that we contact. We create a construct and test that against reality. If it works, this construct is a useful one and might be used again in the future. However, if it does not work, we must create a new construct and test that against reality. We always want to improve our constructs so that they will fit reality better. In other words, there is always room for people to freely revise constructs, or replace them with alternative ones. Kelly called this *constructive alternativism.*

Personal-construct theory forms the basis of a therapy that aims to help people construct more effective interpretations and theories of the world. For example, if clients have certain negative claims about themselves, the therapists would not try to find out if these claims are valid, but would encourage the clients to see how these claims affect the way in which they perceive themselves and their behaviour in daily life. The therapists will then encourage the clients to consider alternative constructs about their behaviour.

Kelly developed the Role Construct Repertory Test, which aims to identify the constructs of the person – how he or she interprets or constructs his or her interpersonal world. For example, subjects are asked to compile a list of people and give each of them a role (for example, father, mother, friend, neighbour, teacher and so forth) that is thought to be important to all people. Subjects usually arrive at 20 to 30 roles and are subsequently asked to name a person they know who can fit each role. Subjects are then asked to pick three specific people from the list and to indicate the way in which two of the figures are similar and different from the third. In so doing, subjects might conclude that mother and neighbour are similar in that they are both outgoing and different from father, who is introverted. Consequently, the construct of outgoing–introverted is formed. Subjects will then be asked to consider other groups of three, and arrive at more constructs. These constructs could be the same as previous ones, or could be new ones. This test ultimately aims to generate people's constructs, or different ways in which they perceive the world, based on their perception of the way in which two things are similar and different from a third.

The trait approach to personality

Unlike all of the above approaches, the trait approach has a common-sense appeal. Even in daily discourse, we find ourselves sharing with one another our understanding of personality types or traits or temperament. In the media, for example, we recognize the traits of bashful, grumpy, dopey and the like, among the Seven Dwarfs in the Snow White story. These traits are only some of the many traits that we daily mention. By the same token, Gordon Allport (1897–1967) believed that personality is contained within us, and so we should look at personality traits rather than social roles or environmental influences. By doing that, we would be able to differentiate between people with regard to how they respond to the same situation. He came up with 18 000 adjectives that describe people's personality characteristics. These include, for example, cheerful, lazy, mean, honest and the like. They are called *trait labels.*

Specifically, Allport postulated three types of traits: *cardinal, central* and *secondary traits.* The cardinal trait is pervasive, general, extremely influential and touches every aspect of our lives. In other words, we are truly dominated by it and every single one of our acts is influenced by it. For example, if we have achievement as the cardinal trait, we would build life around competitiveness and success. The central traits are less general and pervasive. We all possess them in small numbers – about five to ten. These traits are themes that characterize our behaviour, such as energetic, easy, friendly, reliable and competent. The secondary trait is the least important and least general. It is displayed less conspicuously and less consistently than the other types. Personal preferences, for example, are secondary traits. Consequently, they are only something that a very close friend might notice.

Allport believed that we can observe traits through how frequently we display a particular kind of behaviour, and the range of situations in which the same kind of behaviour occurs, and the intensities of the responses. We can also observe traits by interviewing people and asking them directly about themselves and their plans and intentions. He believed that traits are not fully present at birth, but develop as we learn in a complex environment. However, he did not deny that our physique and temperament and intelligence are the bases upon which individual traits can develop, in interaction with the environment.

Allport believed that, to understand personality, one has to emphasize the whole personality of the individual, the whole and unique person. In other words, to Allport, it is mistaken to measure isolated aspects of personality. Instead, the whole person should be measured as a *living synthesis* – the combination of traits. This would then give us a sense of the whole person, rather than specific concepts of traits.

Allport also believed that we should explain behaviour in terms of the present motives and intentions of the individual rather than in terms of the past. Conscious intention, which is essentially directed by the self, should be at the centre of the theory. In other words, although personality may result from the interaction between genetic dispositions and social learning, it is the here and now that is most important, in order to understand the personality of the whole individual. Due to the fact that Allport focused on the present, personality to him is always growing – it is something that is becoming different and always changing.

Allport developed theories of personality around the concept of traits, but Raymond B. Cattell (1905–) provided a detailed scientific analysis and classification of traits by means of *factor analysis*. The latter form of analysis assesses the relationship between each possible pair of measurements (for example, scores on two different personality tests or on two subscales of the same test) taken from a group of people. The aim is to find out how highly the measures correlate with each other. A high correlation assumes that they must be measuring related aspects of personality. For example, if there is a high correlation between the happiness and extraversion subscales of a personality test, one can assume that they both provide information on the same aspect or factor of personality. If one uses the same technique and analyses statistically a large amount of data, one should then uncover more factors of person-ality. Cattell called these factors *personality traits*. These traits are permanent parts of our personality. In order to understand an individual fully, one needs to arrive at the entire pattern of traits of that individual. One can then begin to predict what he or she will do in any given situation.

According to Cattell, there are different ways of classifying or grouping personality traits. Firstly, traits can be classified in terms of *surface traits* and *source traits*. Surface traits refer to a set of personality characteristics that are correlated with one another. For example, anxiety, indecision and irritability may cluster together to constitute the surface trait of neuroticism. That is, the trait of neuroticism is derived from a cluster of several characteristics rather than a single source. Cattell believed that surface traits are less stable and permanent in nature; therefore he did not consider them as important in understanding personality. On the other hand, source traits are the underlying individual factors, derived from factor analysis, which control the variation in the clustering of surface traits. According to Cattell, there are 16 basic personality factors (known as *16 PF*) or source traits that constitute the building blocks of personality. These traits are dichotomized or organized in bipolar form (see Table 6.1).

Secondly, Cattell classified and grouped traits into *common traits* and *unique traits*. The former are those that we all possess, such as general mental ability, introversion and extraversion – although the degree to which we possess them differs from one individual to the next. The latter are those that only a few or perhaps no other people share. One tends to find these traits in the areas of interests and attitudes.

Thirdly, Cattell classified traits in terms of *ability traits*, *temperament traits* and *dynamic traits*. Ability traits refer to how efficiently we are able to work toward a particular goal. One example is intelligence. Temperament traits refer to the general style or tempo of behaviour, such as how bold, easygoing or irritable we are. Dynamic traits refer to the motivations or driving forces of behaviour such as ambition.

Table 6.1: Cattell's 16 personality factors

Factors	People with a low score on this factor are described as:	People with a high score on this factor are described as:
A	Reserved	Outgoing
B	Less intelligent	More intelligent
C	Emotional	Stable
E	Humble	Assertive
F	Sober	Happy-go-lucky
G	Expedient	Conscientious
H	Shy	Venturesome
I	Tough-minded	Tender-minded
L	Trusting	Suspicious
M	Practical	Imaginative
N	Forthright	Shrewd
O	Placid	Apprehensive
Q_1	Conservative	Experimenting
Q_2	Group-tied	Self-sufficient
Q_3	Casual	Controlled
Q_4	Relaxed	Tense

To focus on dynamic traits, Cattell thought that these traits can be divided into *ergs*, *sentiments* and *attitudes*. Ergs mean work or energy that replace the concept of instinct or drive. They are an innate energy source for all behaviour; they are the basic units of motivation and are directed towards specific goals. They are permanent and can weaken or intensify but cannot disappear altogether. Sentiment traits are learned attitudes that focus on important objects in our lives, such as spouse and job. They can be unlearned and can thus disappear. That is, a particular sentiment would not be forever important in one's life. Attitudes refer to our interest in some areas, objects or people. This interest is usually manifested in some overt behaviours. They do not mean opinions for or against something. Instead, they encompass all of our emotions and actions towards an event or object or person.

Ergs, sentiments and attitudes exist in relation to each other through the concept of *subsidiation*, which means that some elements are subsidiary to others in the system. For example, attitudes are subsidiary to sentiments, which, in turn, are subsidiary to ergs. One attitude (for example receiving university education) can be subsidiary to a second attitude (such as getting a good job and earning a living), which, in turn, is subsidiary to a third attitude (for example having a family).

In addition to the above ways of classifying and grouping personality traits, Cattell emphasizes the importance of *anxiety* as one aspect of personality. It is both a state of being and a personality trait. For example, we experience a state of anxiety when we find ourselves in a life-threatening or stressful situation. On the other hand, some of us are chronically anxious – anxiety is a personality trait for us. These people would be affected easily by feelings, and may be suspicious of other people, apprehensive and self-reproaching, tense and excitable, and would not have a well-developed self-concept.

In terms of the development of personality, Cattell believed that it could be divided into six stages. The first stage is *infancy* (from birth to 6 years of age) which is the major formative period in developing personality. During this stage, individuals are strongly influenced by parents, siblings and their weaning and toilet-training experiences. As a result of these influences, they form primary social attitudes, the stability and strength of the superego, secure or insecure feelings, their attitude toward authority and tendency to neuroticism.

The second stage is that of *childhood* (between 6 and 14 years of age) in which children experience a few psychological problems. This is the time of what Cattell called *consolidation* in which they begin to become independent from parents and to increasingly identify themselves with peers. The third stage is called *adolescence* (between 14 and 23 years old) and is the most troublesome and stressful stage of development. During this stage, one might experience mental disorders or neuroses, or become delinquent. One may also have conflicts around the drives for independence, self-assertion and sex.

The fourth stage is called *maturity* (between 23 and 50 years of age) and is a busy, happy and productive time for most people. During this stage, they begin their careers, and marital and family lives. Their personality, interests and attitudes tend to become more stabilized and less changeable. The fifth stage is called *middle age* in which they shift and adjust their personality in order to respond to physical, social and psychological changes. During this stage, their health, physical and mental energy and attractiveness are not as good as before. Their children also leave home. Their values and goals in life would usually be re-examined.

The last stage is called *senility*. This involves adjustment to a number of losses, the loss of relatives, friends as well as of work (i.e. retirement) and status. People experience loneliness and insecurity.

Briefly, let us describe the work of Hans Eysenck (1916–97), who undoubtedly expanded the scope of trait theory by claiming that, in order to understand the personality trait, we need to consider *personality dimensions* or *dimensional traits* that vary from person to person. He focused on three personality dimensions: extraversion–introversion, neuroticism–stability, and psychoticism. Each dimension is associated with personality traits that determine habitual responses. Extraversion–introversion refers to the degree to which a person's orientation is turned inward toward the self, or outward toward the external world. The traits for extraversion are impulsiveness, lack of reflection, risk taking, activity, sociability, lack of responsibility and expressiveness, while the traits for introversion include persistence, rigidity, subjectivity, shyness and irritability. Neuroticism–stability refers to people's emotionality. The traits for neuroticism are anxiety, low self-esteem, obsessiveness, lack of autonomy, hypochondriasis, unhappiness and guilt. The traits for psychoticism refer to aggression, coldness, egocentricity, impersonalness, impulsiveness, antisocial and unempathic behaviour, creativity, and tough-mindedness (see Figure 6.2).

Measuring personality

Some tests that are available for measuring personality conclude the chapter. Again, due to space limitations, only some of the tests are briefly mentioned. They take the form of personality questionnaires and inventories, as well as projective tests (where subjects are presented with unstructured material of ambiguous pictures or inkblots and asked to respond to them. The idea is that they will reveal their character traits, feelings, attitudes and behaviour patterns through these responses).

Personality questionnaires and inventories include:

- The Eysenck Personality Questionnaire (EPQ) (Eysenck and Eysenck, 1975) measures four scales: neuroticism, extraversion, psychoticism and the lie scale or social desirability.
- The Sixteen Personality Factor Questionnaire (16PF) (Cattell et al., 1970) was developed to measure 16 basic factors or traits that constitute the building blocks of personality. The traits are in dichotomized or bipolar forms as shown in Table 6.1 on page 123.
- The Minnesota Multiphasic Personality Inventory (MMPI) (Hathaway and McKinley, 1951) provides scores on 10 clinical scales: hypochondriasis, depression, hysteria, psychopathic deviate, masculinity–femininity, paranoia, psychasthenia, schizophrenia, hypomania, and social introversion.

Projective tests include:

- Rorschach test (Rorschach, 1921). This consists of 10 symmetrical inkblots and subjects have to describe them. From the descriptions, one would make assumptions about aspects of the subject's personality and ability.
- Thematic Apperception Test (TAT) (Murray, 1938). This consists of 19 cards presenting vague pictures in black and white and one blank card. Subjects are asked to create a story in order to fit each picture, explaining what led up to the event in the picture, describing what is happening at present and what the figures on the picture are feeling and thinking. In terms of the blank card, subjects are asked to imagine

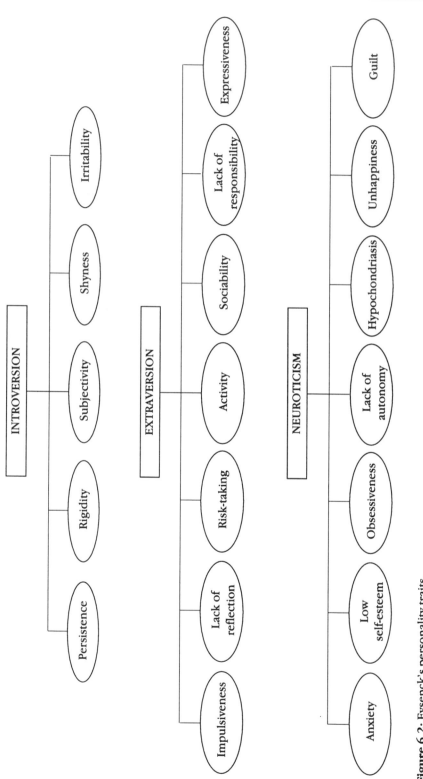

Figure 6.2: Eysenck's personality traits.

a picture on the card, describe it and tell a story about it. The content of the stories is then analysed according to Murray's list of *needs* (for example, achievement, affiliation, aggression) and *presses* – environmental forces that might facilitate or interfere with the satisfaction of needs (for example, being attacked or criticized).

Summary

Personality is a complex concept. This chapter merely glimpses at that complexity by means of outlining some personality theories characterized by the psychoanalytic, neopsychoanalytic, behavioural, humanistic, cognitive and trait approaches. It is at readers' discretion to tease out similarities and differences between them. One can, for example, compare and contrast the theories in terms of two general perspectives, namely, ideographic or nomothetic perspectives (see Figure 6.3). It is also at their discretion to conclude which approach or aspects of approaches bear relevance to their clinical or academic work. While various theoreticians have been chosen with the specific aim of demonstrating the above approaches, others have not been mentioned. This by no means reflects the significance or otherwise of their work; rather, it reflects the limitation of space.

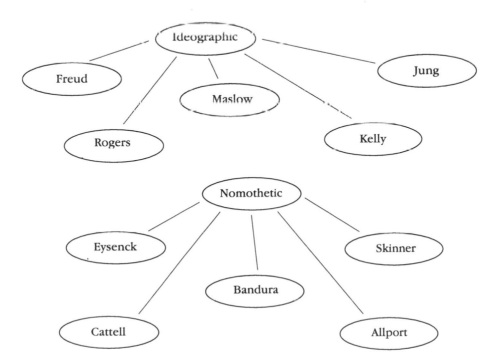

Figure 6.3: Personality theories in ideographic and nomothetic perspectives.

References and further reading

Allport GW (1955) Becoming: Basic Considerations for a Psychology of Personality. New Haven: Yale University Press.

Allport GW (1937) Personality: A Psychological Interpretation. New York: Henry Holt & Company.

Bandura A (1974a) Behavior theory and the models of man. American Psychologist 29: 859–69.

Bandura A (1974b) Psychological Modeling: Conflicting Theories. Chicago: Atherton.

Cattell RB (1964) Personality and Social Psychology. San Diego: Knapp.

Cattell RB (1965) The Scientific Analysis of Personality. Baltimore: Penguin.

Cattell RB, Eber HW, Tatsuoka MM (1970) Handbook for the Sixteen Personality Factor Questionnaire. Champaign IL: Institute for Personality and Ability Testing.

Eysenck HJ (1970) The Structure of Human Personality. London: Methuen.

Eysenck HJ, Eysenck SGB (1975) The Eysenck Personality Questionnaire. Sevenoaks: Hodder & Stoughton.

Freud S (1917/1991). Introductory Lectures on Psychoanalysis. Volume One. London: Penguin Books.

Gay P (1988) Freud: A Life for Our Time. London: Papermac.

Hampson SE, Colman AM (1995). Individual Differences and Personality. London: Longman.

Hathaway SR, McKinley JC (1951) The Minnesota Multiphasic Personality Inventory Manual. New York: Psychological Corporation.

Jung CG (1964) Man and His Symbols. London: Aldus Books.

Jung CG (1965) Memories, Dreams, Reflections. New York: Vintage Books.

Kelly GA (1963) A Theory of Personality. New York: WW Norton & Company.

Kirschenbaum H, Henderson VL (eds) (1989). The Carl Rogers Reader. London: Constable.

Maslow AH (1968) Toward a Psychology of Being. New York: Van Nostrand Reinhold Company Inc.

Maslow AH (1971) The Farther Reaches of Human Nature. New York: Viking.

Mischel W (1993) Introduction to Personality. London: Harcourt Brace Jovanovich.

Murray HA (1938) Explorations in Personality. New York: Oxford University Press.

Pervin LA, John OP (1997) Personality: Theory and Research. New York: Wiley.

Richards G (1996) Putting Psychology in Its Place. London: Routledge.

Rogers CR (1965) Client-Centered Therapy. London: Constable.

Rorschach H (1921) Psychodiagnostics. Berne: Hans Huber.

Skinner BF (1953) Science and Human Behavior. Toronto: The Macmillan Company.

Skinner BF (1974) About Behaviorism. New York: Alfred A Knopf.

Chapter 7
Motivation

RICHARD TOOGOOD

Key concepts	Key names
Functional autonomy	Allport
Dual-centre theory	Anand and Brobeck
Rational being	Aristotle/Plato
Social learning theory	Bandura and Walters
Drive theory	Cannon
Intrinsic motivation	Darwin/McDougall
Instincts/Evolution	Darwin
Cognitive dissonance	Festinger
Psychoanalysis/Developmental theories	Freud
Proximity seeking	Harlow
Selfish being	Hobbes
Imprinting	Lorenz
Achievement motivation (n-Ach)	McClelland
Instincts (Intrinsic motivation)	McDougall
Hierarchy of needs	Maslow
Psychogenic needs	Murray
Social motivation	
Developmental theories, curiosity and	Piaget
stimulus seeking	
Ethology	Tinbergen

What is motivation?

One of the key quests in psychology is to reach an explanation for the
behaviour of individuals, groups and societies as much of Man's behaviour
is directed to the completion of tasks, satisfaction of wants or improvement of personal situations. Over the ages philosophical interpretations of
the *reasons* for our behaviours have led writers and thinkers to the ascription of *motives*. The motive for a particular piece of behaviour is usually

assumed to be an internal state. We will say 'he was motivated to run by fear' or 'the reason for her behaviour was that she wanted to achieve', with the primary cause for the behaviour viewed as a state or trait of the individual rather than an environmental one. Motivational theory in psychology is very much a case of nature rather than nurture. The challenge for modern psychology is to integrate long-established theories and philosophical viewpoints of Man's nature with more recent findings from the psychological laboratory and social observations.

Ancient philosophers including Plato and Aristotle viewed Man as a rational being who identifies what he wants and how he can get it. More recent writers such as the seventeenth-century English philosopher, Thomas Hobbes, believed that man is a selfish being. Around the same time, John Locke believed that Man is essentially peaceful with feelings of good will towards his neighbours. This concept of will was influential in these and related theories at this time. It was deemed that as man had free will he was responsible for what he did. He was not the pawn of fate or a reactive physiological machine – 'will' means having purpose.

Another philosophical strand explaining man's behaviour was the concept of *hedonism*. The notion that man seeks pleasure and avoids pain was prominent in the eighteenth and nineteenth centuries and although discarded by many writers in the twentieth century has re-emerged in some *social drive theories* such as the concept of *achievement motivation* developed by David C. McClelland (1961). Achieving is all about maximizing pleasurable experiences and minimizing painful or punishing events. Although the route to achievement is socially determined, the energy required is assumed to be within the person.

The influence of Darwinian theory on the concept of motivation is also important. Darwin argued that certain complex actions are inherited and the role of instincts, through the process of natural selection, became influential in the developing discipline of psychology. Several theorists including William McDougall (1908) and Sigmund Freud (1938) developed the concept of *instincts* as fundamental to our understanding of man and other animals, a notion that is still popular to this day. For Freud, much of our behaviour was rooted in sexual and aggressive instinctual behaviour (such as the struggle between id, ego and super-ego) whereas theorists such as McDougall produced lists of instincts that included curiosity and constructiveness as well as hunger and reproduction.

The instinct-based theories of motivation have been superseded by theories evolving from the psychological laboratory but they still enjoy much popularity. This has been reinforced by *ethological theorists* such as Tinbergen (1951) and Lorenz (1937) in the development of the concept of *imprinting* where particular behaviour patterns can be observed in certain species. For example, baby ducks become imprinted upon and follow a particular stimulus if this appears within a critical period after birth. This is usually one of their parents, but ethologists have shown that if substituted by other birds, models, or even human beings, the same following and attachment behaviours are observed. Such theories have fuelled the development of *attachment theory* in child psychology and the notion of *critical periods* during which the organism 'must' develop certain attributes. This philosophical thread is backed up by some empirical evidence and gives support to the concept of instinctive behaviours and internal, genetically determined motivational states.

The concept of *unconscious motivation* is also worthy of brief exploration. This is a popular and influential concept in the search for our reasons for doing things. There is an assumption of *unconscious need* and a separation of the *unconscious life* from the *conscious life*, a view made popular by Freud and the psychoanalytic school. The notion of unconscious motivation grew in popularity at the same time that more learning-based and goal-directed theorists were developing views on motivation from experimental work in the psychological and physiological laboratories. Although still popular, the notion of *unconscious motivation* has largely been eclipsed by concepts of *needs* and *drives* and the development of *drive theory*.

Needs and drives

The ascription of an internal state as the reason for behaviour had been well established long before the development of drive theory. *Drives* refer to purposeful activity initially produced to satisfy an internal *need*. This is linked to a state of deprivation and the desire to achieve a balanced existence, or in the case of primary needs such as food and water, the desire by the organism to survive.

Drives are commonly divided into *primary* and *secondary* drives. Some examples are given in Table 7.1. Secondary drives acquire their value or importance very often through social learning processes and their association with primary drives. For example, affection and socialization are often built upon the satisfaction of primary drives for food and contact. This can have clinical implications where the socialization processes are maladaptive or deviant.

Table 7.1: Examples of primary and secondary drives

Primary drives	Secondary drives
Eating	Affection
Drinking	Socialization
Sex	Comfort
Aggression	Achievement
Avoidance	Dominance

Drive theory was advanced by the concept of *homeostasis* introduced by Cannon (1932) to refer to a state of physiological and psychological equilibrium of the body and the tendency of all living things to keep on restoring this equilibrium. For example, most diurnal organisms wake up in the morning and fall asleep at night without any required or observable learning process. Most animals become hungry, eat, and become hungry again. Sexual activity is cyclic and linked to physiological changes that pattern themselves differently across the species. These cycles can be described as endogenous rhythms and if disturbed can result in the organism engaging in behaviours aimed at restoring the natural balance. Cannon argued that this 'homeostatic' drive is fundamental to our functioning, a view taken up by the learning theorist Clark Hull in 1943. Hull assumed that all behaviour is motivated by primary homeostatic drives or secondary drives based upon them. He also argued that rewards assume their power by their ability to reduce a primary homeostatic need. For example, a reward of food will reduce the imbalance in the homeostatic mechanism produced by hunger (see Figure 7.1).

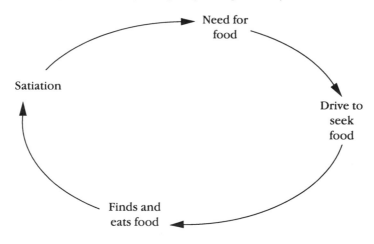

Figure 7.1: Example of homeostatic cycle of need arousal and reduction.

In addition to maintaining a sense of physical homeostasis most social groupings seek a sense of homeostasis in the social environment. Society is a system consisting of a complex pattern of interactions amongst people that are 'self-regulating'. Most nations and other organizations have an established governmental system, which, if disrupted, leads to conflict and to the eventual restoration of law and order. In a homeostatic social environment, the community takes care of most of the essentials for survival. Water is piped to our homes, food is available in shops and communication is provided by telephone, fax and the Internet. When a 'natural disaster' occurs such as flood or storm and these essentials are no longer provided, our deficiencies are made conscious and more primary drives become employed. In this sense there is a natural hierarchy of physical and social drives that have been integrated by more recent theorists such as Maslow (1971).

Physiology and motivation

Many of the scientific findings supporting homeostatic theory derive from physiological rather than psychological experimentation. Much work has focused upon thirst and hunger and the role that various internal stimuli have in the maintenance of the homeostatic systems. For example, apart from lack of water, thirst is affected by the salt needs of the animal and by its hunger. General dehydration of body tissues rather than, for example, a dry throat seems to be the main stimulus to elicit a search for water and drinking behaviour. With respect to hunger, nutrients are released from various store sites (such as the liver) until a point is reached that triggers the animal to be hungry. It seeks and eats food and so replenishes the supply of nutrients, achieving physiological homeostasis again.

In recent years, as physiological techniques of neural stimulation and ablation have became more precise, most physiological research on thirst and hunger has focused upon brain structures in general and upon the hypothalamus in particular. The hypothalamus and its associated structures have primary control of automatic functions. Associated with the hypothalamus are the pituitary gland and the amygdala and it is known that neural impulses are received from a number of different sources including the cerebral hemispheres and the visceral organs of the body. Similarly, the hypothalamus sends messages to various bodily areas and the higher centres of the brain. Physiologically speaking, the hypothalamus is the principal homeostatic mechanism or structure. It maintains very fine balances in various functions including heart activity, breathing, temperature regulation and blood pressure. It is also known to have a role in the regulation of eating, drinking and emotional behaviour. The distinct role of the hypothalamus is not in producing specific autonomic effects but in integrating them into patterns of activity. For example, body temperature is restored by the hypothalamus via increased sweating, respiration and the lowering of metabolism. The hypothalamus also has an important regulatory function with respect to sexual behaviour and sexual drives in particular.

Electrical stimulation of the ventromedial nucleus of the hypothalamus will result in a decrease in food consumption whereas bilateral lesions in the area will result in the animal doubling or trebling its food intake – hyperphagia. Stimulation to the lateral hyperthalamic nuclei also produces increased food consumption whereas lesions in this area cause aphagia in which animals refuse to eat (see Figure 7.2).

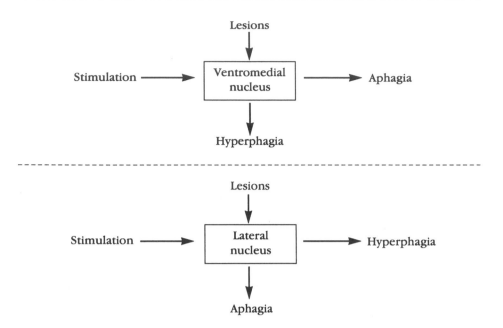

Figure 7.2: The effects of stimulation and lesions on hypothalamic nuclei.

The lateral hypothalamus also appears to regulate drinking behaviour, although Anderson (1955) reported that injection of a microscopic amount of a salt solution directly into the supraoptic nucleus of the hypothalamus of a goat caused immediate drinking. The same injection into other parts of the brain failed to have the same effect. Of note too, was that animals who were stimulated in the ventromedial nucleus or had their ventromedial nucleus ablated produced rage and aggression towards their handlers in addition to acquiring voracious appetites. Because the destruction of the ventromedial nucleus produces overeating, its normal function is thought to be to inhibit or stop this response. It has thus become known as the satiety centre, there being a corresponding centre in lateral hypothalamus known as the feeding centre. When those centres are stimulated, the expected effect occurs – eating is inhibited when the ventromedial nucleus is stimulated and increased when the lateral hypothalamic nucleus is stimulated. When these centres are ablated the opposite effects occur with hyperphagia resulting from ablation of the ventromedial area and aphagia resulting from ablation of the lateral area (see Figure 7.3).

These findings have been brought together as the *dual-centre theory* by Anand and Brobeck (1951) and have been developed in respect of *biological drives* by Stellar (1954) who postulated that both inhibitory and excitatory centres exist in the hypothalamus for each of the biological drives. When behaviour results in the need being satisfied, neural transmissions relay messages to both the excitatory and inhibitory centres to react in opposite directions.

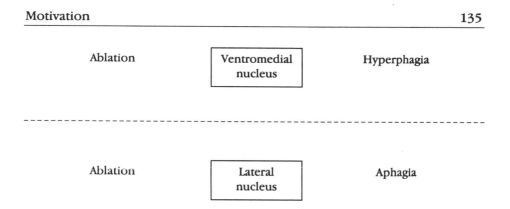

Figure 7.3: The effects of ablation on hypothalamic nuclei.

Different physiological and anatomical factors clearly affect the functioning of hypothalamic systems. Blood-borne hormones or their synthetic equivalents are clearly important, as is sensory information such as the sight, smell and tastes of food and drink. The hypothalamus is also affected by learning and it is presumed that food preferences and dietary differences are laid down very early in life.

Intrinsic motivation

Although drive theory and its physiological foundations have made an enormous contribution to the study of motivation, observation studies and laboratory experiments indicate that many behaviours are performed because they are of value in themselves – the activity is *intrinsically motivating* to the organism. The instinct theorists, including Darwin and McDougall, recognized that certain kinds of sensory experience were innately rewarding and that other activities gave inherent pleasure and satisfaction. Curiosity was listed as a basic instinct and play was added to that list also. An attempt was made by some theorists to consider these phenomena as 'derived drives' from more basic or primary drives. Sigmund Freud argued that sexual and aggressive motives are sublimated into culturally specific areas. Allport (1937) advanced the concept of *functional autonomy* where some motives separate from their primary drives. Miller (1948) put forward the notion that drives and rewards can be acquired because of their association with primary drives of food, water and sex.

As explained above, exploration, play, curiosity and stimulus seeking may well occur for their own sake, for some inherent satisfaction. Examples of drives already in early development are closeness, proximity or comfort seeking. Earlier reference was made to imprinting, where young baby ducks would follow the first stimulus object. Studies of young primates have shown proximity seeking to be a similar phenomenon that is probably innate. Harlow (1959) studying affection behaviour in rhesus monkeys found that certain textures of cloth, which mimicked adult fur, appeared intrinsically rewarding to the young. Human babies do not show the same behaviour but they appear to persistently seek stimulation and appear to be programmed to do so.

Classic theories of motivation have assumed that people seek to reduce excessive stimulation and inner tension. We all like to escape, to 'get away from it all' and enjoy periods of 'time out' and relaxation, enabling our minds and bodies to regenerate. After a period, however, we are eager again for stimulation. Most organisms seem to need to engage in *purposeful behaviour.* Long periods without any stimulation are known to be psychologically damaging. The desire for stimulation is dramatically illustrated by sensory deprivation studies. Volunteers are requested to lie down on comfortable beds. They wear translucent goggles, cardboard circles prevent touch, and earmuffs mask sounds. Except for brief 'time outs' to eat and go to the toilet and undertake psychological tests, volunteers were instructed to do absolutely nothing. Although paid by the hour, most subjects could not remain in these conditions for more than two or three days. Subjective reports indicated that although the situation was quite pleasant at first, most students experienced visual and auditory hallucinations that disappeared after the experiments ended. It would therefore appear to be the case that stimulus-seeking behaviour, of a moderate level, is an innate motivational state.

Stimulus seeking is not random; there is clearly some selectivity based upon learning. Yet all organisms must deal with new and previously unencountered stimuli. The concept of *curiosity* has been used to explain this process. To the extent that a stimulus is novel, it arouses curiosity in the organism. Laboratory rats demonstrate a great deal of exploratory behaviour when there seems to be no pressing internal drive and where the only 'reward' is to explore a new maze. Monkeys will eagerly solve problems where there is no extrinsic reward. Jean Piaget, the developmental psychologist, suspended a rattle above the cot of his three-month-old son who spent 15 minutes shaking the rattle and laughing. There were no extrinsic rewards here, nor any indication of primary and secondary drives to explain this behaviour.

In addition to there being motives for sensory stimulation and curiosity, children and adults seem motivated to do things. The achievement of developmental milestones in the child seems to be genetically programmed but children can be seen to struggle to achieve these. The applications of rewards by parents do not seem to be the main influence. The child wants to do it. Harlow (1959), in his experiments with baby rhesus monkeys, underlined the child's desire to manipulate objects in its environment. Monkeys in cages gradually learned a mechanized puzzle with increasing rates of success until error-free performance was attained. There were no extrinsic rewards and the curiosity or novelty effect must have worn off. The monkeys seemed motivated to engage in the task simply to solve the problem and manipulate the puzzle. Young children also seem eager to learn for its own sake and the notion of 'intellectual motivation' has been viewed by educationalists keen to harness this in the formal education system.

Problem solving is, then, an area that seems to merit study from a motivational viewpoint and may provide further examples of intrinsic motivation. Thinking about and symbolizing the world are cognitive functions best studied in humans. Many of us like 'playing' with puzzles, verbal and non-verbal, and seem to derive satisfaction from engaging in a range of occupational or artistic pursuits for their own sake. We also appear to have a need to be logical and cognitively consistent, removing from our thought processes many of the ambiguities that conflicting information creates. This notion has been best developed by Festinger (1957) in the concept of *cognitive dissonance*. He offers various experimental demonstrations that, when there is perceived inconsistency between ideas or bits of information, then a state of dissonance occurs that is uncomfortable and motivates the person to reduce dissonance and regain consonance. Festinger gives the example of the person who knows smoking is bad for him but continues to smoke. The smoker will 'rationalize' his behaviour by pointing to other health risks in which he does not engage, the source of other environmental pollutants, or that the damage that has already been done. Festinger believes that however the thoughts are acquired, the dissonance between thoughts is as basic a motive as any other.

Intrinsic motivational theories have also been extended to consider concepts such as fear and aggression. People describe themselves and others doing things 'out of fear' or because they 'felt aggressive'. The 'fight or flight' response is also well known. The phenomenon of 'freezing' has been observed in animals and is hypothesized in human behaviour as a survival instinct or response. The notion of being motivated by fear reduction as an intrinsic motive rather than a drive is an interesting one. Anxiety and fear reactions arise in more ways than one. Some are programmed, some are learned, but some may be intrinsic to the organism as a mechanism for maintaining emotional and cognitive consistency. *Agonistic behaviour*, referring to aggression against or withdrawing from other individuals may also be intrinsically motivated and linked to the emotions of fear and anger. *Predatory behaviour* is basic in some species and the notion of 'man the hunter' still exists. Individuals compete for territory and to reproduce the species. Darwin emphasized these behaviours in his theories of natural selection. Freud linked aggressive behaviour to the concept of frustration and thwarted goal-oriented behaviour but it is clear that aggressive behaviour does not always arise from frustration. There is evidence from social learning theory (Bandura and Walters, 1959) that aggression and antisocial behaviour in adolescent boys is partly linked to parental reinforcement of this type of behaviour. Yet some aggressive acts feature as play amongst young animals and children, almost as if they were being rehearsed for appearance at a later development stage. In this sense there is evidence of aggressive behaviour being intrinsically motivated.

It may be that intrinsic motives have some homeostatic consequences. That social learning and cognitive consistency theories have a role in maintaining psychological and physiological consistency for the organism. Are certain levels of stimulation necessary for brain functioning? Sensory deprivation in infancy seems to have devastating consequences for the rest of life. If brain mechanisms trigger intrinsic motives then their role may be to ensure proper development thereby ensuring adjustment to the environment.

Motivation and social behaviour

Many motives involve other people in social settings. Not only do we compete against others but we live with them in families or communes and seek approval, love and affection from them. *Social behaviour* and all its complexities cannot be explained solely by drive theories or inherited intrinsic motivational states. There is wide recognition that we are prepared for social functioning but that our learning experiences can dramatically alter our capacity to function in social ways. Whether innate, learned or both, social motives dominate our everyday behaviour.

Numerous lists of *social motives* have been constructed. Murray (1938) produced a list of 'psychogenic needs' that come from intensive clinical and experimental study and framed the basis for the Thematic Apperception Test, a widely used test of personality. They include affection, aggression, dominance, order, play and rejection, each of which is highly socially charged. In a sense Murray was beginning to define human personality as well as motivation in social terms.

McClelland et al. (1953) has postulated a popular theory of *social motivation* in his description of the achievement motive. This theory diminished in appeal in the late 1960s and 1970s but has been enjoying a revival recently. This is perhaps indicative of the relationship between psychological theories and current social trends. McClelland argues that people learn in early childhood that certain behaviours lead to fulfilment and achievement and hence they develop a need for achievement. He states three basic needs, achievement, affiliation and power. There are usually referred to as 'n-Ach', 'n-Aff' and 'n-Power', with 'n-Ach' being the most important. McClelland and his associates suggest that 'n-Ach' is encouraged by parents who set high achievement goals for their children but who are non-authoritarian in helping them achieve these goals. Entrepreneurs are primarily driven by the achievement motive being organizers, risk takers and the economic builders of the world. McClelland linked this theory to the relationship between entrepreneurial behaviour and the development of modern industrial capitalism. He argued that those societies that encouraged achievement amongst their children would be economically more successful. He set out to measure this by obtaining two folk stories from a range of nations as symbolic of cultural heritage. These were analysed for evidence of achievement motivation and correlated with rates of economic growth. He did, in fact, find such a positive relationship using indices of economic growth as a comparison amongst nations. Despite many corrections and re-analyses, the level of achievement motivation seems productive of a subsequent rise in the rate of economic growth of a nation.

An opposite and complementary social motive is the *affiliation motive*. Those with a strong affiliation motive prefer to work co-operatively for the common good of the group. Murray (1938) defined affiliation as the motive to 'draw nearer and enjoyably co-operate or reciprocate with an allied other, to adhere or remain loyal to a friend'. McClelland (1961) found that some of the major figures in industry did not, as he first expected, score highly on 'n-Ach'. They did, however, have high 'n-Aff' scores and were able to relate well with subordinates and superiors. There is less clear evidence of how the affiliation motive develops. Some observations suggest that the parents of affiliation motivated children put more emphasis on close family ties and conformity to parental authority. They seem to encourage dependence rather than independence. However, these facts have not yet been established on a firm basis. There is some evidence that affiliation is related to anxiety. In an experiment, groups of students were asked to take part in a study and then told they would be subject to painful electric shocks. They could wait alone or within groups. Most of the students who waited in groups expressed higher anxiety scores than those who waited alone. Anxiety thus tended to increase affiliation, underlying finding from animal studies such as those undertaken by Harlow (1959).

More recently there has been a move to build integrated models of motivation, recognizing that the different strands of drive theory, physiological need and social motivation all form part of a complex explanation of human motives. Abraham Maslow (1971) made the first comprehensive attempt. He suggested that needs can be classified in a hierarchy and that the relationship between the needs is in the form of a pyramid structure as shown in Figure 7.4.

According to Maslow, individuals work their way up the pyramid, having to satisfy needs at one level before progressing to the next. Thus basic physiological needs of hunger and thirst must be satisfied before safety and social needs. Prestige, self-respect and self-esteem can only then be satisfied. Only then can you 'self-actualize' and reach your full potential. Unfortunately, the theory does have some flaws. Some levels of the pyramid do not seem to exist for some individuals and some analyses of important historical self-actualizers show that it is possible to reach this level and maintain it whilst losing some of the assumed social needs. Nevertheless the theory is an important pointer to the possible hierarchical organization of human needs and motives.

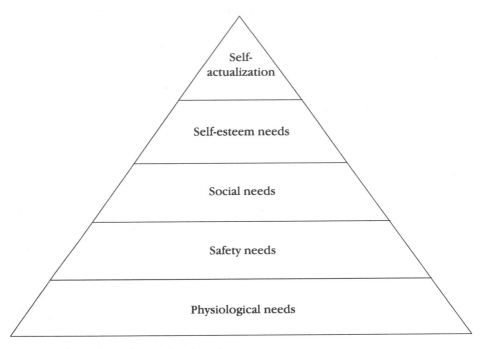

Figure 7.4: Maslow's hierarchy of needs.

Clinical implications

The contributions of motivational theories to our understanding of psychological and psychiatric disorders cannot be underemphasized. Drive theories, in one form or another, still stand at the centre of modern thinking about motivation and learning and can easily be extended to the analysis of most major psychiatric problems.

If emotional states are subject to homeostatic theory then *anxiety* can be perceived as a state of disequilibrium created by anticipations of fear or failure with avoidance behaviour being produced by a drive to reduce the anxiety being experienced. Similarly *frustration* can be linked to feelings of anger and their reduction by engaging in aggressive behaviour. *Depression* is manifested by a reduction in 'driven' behaviour, which often creates and maintains disequilibrium in physical and emotional systems. Many related disorders such as *obsessive/compulsive* states can be understood by reference to drive theories. Such patients can engage in increased rates of checking or validating behaviours and thoughts often linked to a goal of reducing anxieties or uncertainties. *Eating disorders*, including anorexia and bulimia can be understood by the patient being 'driven' to lose or maintain low body weight to achieve a psychological perception that is not matched by the perception of others.

The relevance of drive theory to *addictive behaviours* requires further research. Some animals, including human beings will often demonstrate strong drives that are physiologically harmful, such as drives for drugs or even self-injury. Psychological drive in such cases is stronger than physiological need. Similarly the *avoidance behaviour* observed in phobic states can be interpreted as driven by the need to reduce fear aroused by a conditioned stimulus such as a spider or a snake, which does not pose a real threat to the person.

Whilst motivational theories including physiological models can be seen to have relevance to *neurotic states*, the implications for *psychotic behaviour* are less clear. We are aware that hypothalamic damage produces primary drive behaviours at the extremes, and clearly damage to associated pathways may alter perceptions and produce phenonema such as *hallucinations*. Experiments on animals indicate that both reserpine and chlorpromazine inhibit the action of the hypothalamus and may also have an effect upon the reticular formation. The clinical impact of these drugs on *schizophrenia* is well known so there are some clear links between psychopharmacology and the psychology of motivations yet to be explored.

Aggressive behaviour as a clinical phenomenon may be linked to drive theories or intrinsic theories of motivation. *Psychopathic behaviour* is characterized by impulsive, goal-oriented, self-satisfying acts without regard to consequences. There is a failure to learn from experience or to take account of the needs of others. Whatever the origins of this personality type, motivational theories can help understand and predict current and future actions.

Many of the psychological therapies are geared towards helping individuals understand, develop and improve their motivation. *Cognitive behaviour therapies* are essentially goal directed with patients rewarding themselves for gradually enlarging their behavioural repertoires and thinking processes. They have been shown to be particularly helpful in the treatment of depression, obsessive/compulsive and anxiety-based disorders. *Psychoanalytic approaches*, although focusing upon previous experience, help the patient explore motivational influences from the past that are affecting current behaviours and creating blockages to further development. Much current *group therapy* relies heavily on social motivations, peer pressure and the need to conform. Thus our understanding and treatment of clinical phenonema is rooted in the psychology of motivation.

Summary

The study of human motives has its roots in ancient philosophies concerned with the nature of Man. As the division and classification of human behaviour progressed, so did the reasons or motives for it. The study of motivation is at the heart of the 'nature versus nurture' debate within psychology, with inherited characteristics and learned responses both providing evidence for genetic and environmental influences. The growth of physiological knowledge has provided some of the answers to the questions about the relationship between brain function and behaviour. Drive theory has been enormously influential in adding to our understanding of motives for basic needs and desires. We maintain intrinsic motives for stimulation, curiosity and novelty, however, and seem to have developed motives that enable us to operate successfully in a social environment. Achievement and affiliation motives help explain our competitive and co-operative styles of social functioning. Maslow's theory is one explanation of how these complex motives interact and have some internal consistency and cohesiveness. The study of motivation helps inform and understand normal and abnormal behaviour in both the general and clinical populations.

References

Allport GW (1937) Personality. New York: Holt.
Anand BD, Brobeck JR (1951) Hypothalmic control and food intake. Yale J Biol Med 24: 123–40.
Anderson B (1955) Polydipsia caused by intra hypothalamic injections of hypertive NaCl solutions. Expereintia 8: 157.
Bandura A, Walters RH (1959) Adolescent Aggression. New York: Ronald Press.
Cannon WB (1932) The Wisdom of the Body. New York: Norton.
Festinger L (1957) A Theory of Cognitive Dissonance. Evanston: Peterson.
Freud S (1938) The Basic Writings of Sigmund Freud. New York: Rinehart.
Harlow HF (1959) Love in infant monkeys. Scient American 200: 68–74.
Hull CL (1943) Principles of Behavior. New York: Appleton Century Crofts.
Lorenz KZ (1937) Imprinting. The Auk 54: 245–73.
McClelland DC (1961) The Achieving Society. Princeton: Van Nostrand.
McClelland DC, Atkinson JW, Clark RA, Lowell EL (1953) The Achievement Motive. New York: Appleton Century Crofts.
McDougall W (1908) An Introduction to Social Psychology. New York: Barnes & Noble.
Maslow A H (1971) The Farther Reaches of Human Nature. New York: Viking.
Miller NE (1948) Fear as an acquired drive. J Exp Psychol 38: 89–101.
Murray AH (1938) Explorations in Personality. New York: Oxford University Press.
Stellar E (1954) The physiology of motivation. Psychol Review 61: 5–22.
Tinbergen N (1951) The Study of Instincts. London: Oxford University Press.

Chapter 8
Stress and emotion: physiology, cognition and health

GERALD MATTHEWS

Key concepts	Key names
Trait-state theory	Spielberger
Neuroticism	H.J. Eysenck
Life events	Holmes and Rahe
Transactional theory of stress	Lazarus and Folkman
General adaptation syndrome	Selye
Arousal theory	Duffy
Animal models of stress	Gray
Centralist theory of emotion	Cannon, Bard
Peripheralist theory of emotion	James, Lange
Cognitive labelling of emotion	Schachter and Singer
Appraisal theories	Leventhal and Scherer
Coping strategies	Lazarus and Folkman
Learned helplessness	Seligman
Type A/B personality	Rosenman
Cognitive patterning	Hockey
Attentional resources	Norman and Bobrow
Attentional selectivity	Easterbrook
Mood congruence	Bower
Emotional Stroop test	Mathews and MacLeod
Cognitive behaviour therapy	Beck
Self-referent executive function	Wells and Matthews

Introduction

Most or all of the important events of a person's life are accompanied by emotion. Many events also provoke feelings of 'stress'. This chapter reviews the psychology of emotion and stress. It begins with some of the basic issues, such as definitions of the two terms, and introduces three key themes, developed in subsequent sections. The first is the role of physiology: is emotion simply the subjective expression of neural processes?

The second is the role of cognition: emotions depend critically on the person's interpretation of events. The third theme is that people participate actively in emotional events. *Relational* approaches to emotion emphasize their place in the individual's ongoing management of external events. The chapter lays out some of the main theoretical issues relating to these themes, and then reviews the consequences of states of emotion and stress, focusing especially on (a) health and (b) attention and cognition. Finally, clinical applications of the research to stress management and psychotherapy are examined.

Definitions of emotion

Emotions refer to subjective feeling states, such as joy, surprise, anxiety and unhappiness. The term *affect* is sometimes used as an umbrella term for various aspects of the person's feelings. Emotion is studied over various time scales. On the one hand, emotionality may relate to personality *traits*, stable dispositions such as *extraversion–introversion*, which, typically, may not change much over years or even decades (Costa and McCrae, 1994). It is generally agreed that *neuroticism* or negative affectivity is one of the basic personality traits which differentiates individuals in all cultures (Matthews and Deary, 1998). Individuals high in neuroticism are generally prone to negative emotions such as anxiety and depression. Neuroticism is influenced by both genes and environment (Loehlin, 1992). It seems that our genetic makeup and early experiences may predispose us to happiness or sadness throughout our lives, although, of course, our successes and failures as adults are important too.

Traits may be contrasted with more transient *states*, the person's immediate experience of emotion. Traits are only predispositions to states. Someone with an anxious personality (trait anxiety) is more vulnerable to feeling anxious (state anxiety), and may experience anxiety more acutely. However, the trait-anxious person is not anxious all the time, and may feel calm and relaxed in secure surroundings: state anxiety depends on an interaction between personality and external events. States are usually seen as more powerful and more direct influences on behaviour than are traits. A contrast is sometimes made between *emotional states* and *mood states*. Moods refer to basic feeling states such as energy and tension, which are not necessarily tied to any particular event and may persist over several hours. Some days a person might feel somewhat grouchy all day for no particular reason. Emotions are more tightly linked to specific events, and may be as brief as the event itself. Emotions may also be quite complex, as expressed by terms such as the German *schadenfreude*: pleasure at the misfortunes of others. Often, however, the distinction between moods and emotions is fuzzy, especially in dealing with basic states such as anxious and depressed moods.

Definitions of stress

'Stress' is both a narrower and a wider term than 'emotion'. It is narrower in that it may refer simply to emotional reactions to unpleasant or demanding events. Anxiety, depression, anger and tiredness might all be seen as stress-induced emotions. Relational theories of emotion see positive and negative emotions as being generated by the same underlying processes of interaction between person and environment. However, 'stress' is also a wider term, in that it is not tied as closely to subjective feeling states as 'emotion'. Stress may refer to event-driven disturbances of the organism expressed physiologically or behaviourally, rather than through subjective experience. Of course, unpleasant events such as bereavement, divorce or loss of job normally provoke subjective affect. Sometimes, though, and perhaps especially in clinical cases, the troubled person may deny or repress subjective symptoms. Freud described cases of 'hysterias' such as glove-like anaesthesias in which patients denied any particular problems of living, and attributed their symptoms to physiological causes. Freud's attribution of such symptoms to sexual fantasy is highly suspect, but they nevertheless appear to be psychological in nature (glove-like anaesthesia is neurologically impossible). A more modern example might be anorexia nervosa, in which the physically emaciated patient may claim to be content, and even pleased with her slim appearance. A possible explanation is that the patient is unconsciously rejecting the demands of female roles relating to appearance and food. Similarly, stress may perhaps be experienced through acute (for example, racing heart) and chronic (health problems) physiological reactions, even though the person denies any significant emotional upset.

The upshot is that there has been much debate over definitions of stress. Cox (1978) distinguishes stimulus, response and transactional definitions. *Stimulus definitions* attempt to describe the external events or 'stressors' that provoke stress (such as bereavement). For example, Holmes and Rahe's (1967) Social Readjustment Rating Scale assigned a points score to a variety of events, ranging from severe stressors such as death of spouse (100 points) and divorce (73) to more trivial events such as Christmas (12) and minor violations of the law (11). The problem here is that reactions to disturbing events depend on the individual and the circumstances. For example, a bereavement might be experienced with relief if the dead person had suffered a long and debilitating illness, or with indifference if the bereaved person did not actually care about the deceased. Thus, life event measures are reliably correlated with stress symptoms, but often the correlations are quite small in magnitude (Lazarus and Folkman, 1984). It seems, too, that relatively minor disruptions or *hassles* can have similar adverse effects to major life events (Kohn, 1996). There have been attempts to investigate positive *uplifts* that have beneficial effects on well-being, although it is difficult to distinguish uplifts from the absence of hassles.

Response definitions try to pick out physiological or psychological markers for stress reactions, such as arousal of the autonomic nervous system, or subjective anxiety. These are more successful, especially at the psychological level, as there is little doubt that a person experiencing acute anxiety or depression has a genuine problem in dealing with life events, as shown by impaired social functioning (see, for example, Brown and Harris, 1978). Again, such definitions fail to accommodate individual variability in that, as described above, reactions to demanding events vary from person to person, and even from occasion to occasion. Hence, measures of different types of stress response are often poorly correlated, so we cannot assess any overall stress response with confidence.

The *transactional definition of stress* attempts to circumvent these difficulties by relating stress to the interaction between external events and internal reactions. According to Lazarus and Folkman (1984: 21), stress is 'a relationship between the person and the environment that is appraised by the person as taxing or exceeding his or her resources and endangering his or her well-being'. Furthermore, stress varies dynamically as the person attempts to deal with the external source of stress over a period of time. During the course of an academic year, people will feel differently about examinations, according to the progress of their studies and revision. The transactional approach to stress identifies people's evaluation or *cognitive appraisal* of events, and their *coping* efforts, as causal influences on stress outcomes, as further discussed below.

Physiological bases for emotion and stress

We experience important events somatically as well as emotionally; typical reactions might include a racing heart, tightness in the stomach, perspiration and so forth. There seems to be a correlation between somatic activity and emotion, which raises two basic questions. First, how specific are the physiological correlates of different emotions? Cardiac acceleration might accompany the very different emotions associated with falling in love and being threatened by a mugger, but perhaps we can find other physiological indices that differentiate these conditions. Second, what is the causal explanation for the correlation between physiology and subjective experience? Is emotion the direct result of physiological processes, or is something more subtle taking place?

The general adaptation syndrome

Selye (1976) proposed the influential idea that there is a general physiological stress response (the *general adaptation syndrome* or GAS) provoked by noxious or challenging stimuli. Its purpose is to maintain the biological functioning of the organism. Table 8.1 shows the concomitants of the three stages described by Selye. Initially (alarm reaction) the organism experiences shock and then reacts with the 'fight or flight' response, which prepares it for energetic activity. The sympathetic branch of the autonomic nervous system (ANS) is activated, leading to raised heart rate, blood pressure and respiration rate, diversion of blood to the skeletal muscles, and decreased gastrointestinal activity. Hormones such as adrenaline are released, and more glucose is made available, supported by physiological changes such as enlargement of the adrenal cortex. With prolonged stress, the organism moves into the resistance stage during which hormone levels remain high, but the underlying physiological changes are reversed. The immune system is initially active but becomes progressively impaired. The person attempts to resist the chronic stressor behaviourally, but resistance becomes more difficult over time. Eventually, if the source of stress persists, the person may move into the exhaustion stage, at which physiological systems start to break down, leading to severe illness, collapse and even death.

Table 8.1: Physiological and behavioural stages of the general adaptation syndrome

Stage	Physiological	Behavioural
1. Alarm reaction	Sympathetic activation Enlargement of adrenal cortex and lymphatic system	Energization of response
2. Resistance	Parasympathetic branch of ANS counteracts sympathetic activation Shrinkage of adrenal cortex and lymphatic system Progressive immune impairment	Prolonged behavioural compensation Vulnerability to illness
3. Exhaustion	Various systems overwhelmed	Collapse or serious illness

It might be inferred from the GAS hypothesis that the particular emotions felt by the stressed person are not very significant; what is important is the underlying generalized physiological reaction. In fact, the physiological concomitants of different emotions do seem to vary: fine-grained analyses of physiological response have succeeded in differentiating emotions, at least to some degree (for example, Ekman, Levenson and Friesen, 1983). Futhermore, different styles of coping with negative emotions are associated with different patterns of response. Active coping correlates with cardiovascular activity and catecholamine releases, whereas passive withdrawal is associated with corticosteroid secretion (Steptoe, 1991).

Arousal theory of stress

The GAS is primarily concerned with chronic stress reactions. Another theory, *arousal theory*, attempts to relate acute stress reactions to a generalized physiological response (Duffy, 1962). Arousal refers to a spectrum of states of organismic activation. It is measured most directly through the electroencephalogram (EEG). As the person becomes more aroused, the waveforms of the EEG become lower in amplitude but higher in frequency (smaller, more tightly spaced waves). Arousal may also be expressed through autonomic nervous system responses, and a predominance of sympathetic over parasympathetic activity, giving rise to the fight or flight reactions previously described. In general, moderate levels of arousal are most adaptive. Emotion may be seen as a concomitant of arousal. There is indeed some correspondence between emotional and physiological arousal, though associations are rarely very strong, perhaps because of the complexity of the underlying neural processes (Thayer, 1996).

Arousal theory also has its difficulties. Experimental studies show that the different arousal responses do not in fact tend to correlate well with one another: a person might seem aroused with respect to high heart rate, but de-aroused according to their skin conductance (Fahrenberg et al., 1983). In addition, it is unlikely that arousal states are 'non-specific' – that all emotions of equal strength are associated with the same physiological state. There is however a grain of truth in the non-specificity idea. States of both pleasurable excitation and unpleasant tension are similarly related to ANS measures such as skin conductance (Thayer, 1978). However, more detailed analyses reveal differences in the patterning of psychophysiological response.

Many physiological psychologists have reacted to these difficulties by retreating from arousal theory. In contemporary theory, both the emotional and physiological expressions of arousal are seen as the consequence of several interacting systems. One of the best known theories of this kind is Gray's (1987) animal model of stress. From studies of drug effects and brain lesions, Gray describes a number of circuits which control behaviour. For example, anxiety is one of the outputs of a 'behavioural inhibition system', associated with the hippocampus and septum, whose function is to interrupt activity and reorient attention when the organism is exposed to signals of punishment or non-reward ('threat'), novelty or fear. Theories of this kind provide a rationale for drug treatments. Gray argues for correspondences between the behavioural effects of anxiolytic drugs in animals and humans. This approach seems likely to be more successful than arousal theory in describing the biological bases of emotion, although there are considerable difficulties in extrapolating animal models to human emotions (for example, Eysenck, 1992). Stimulating or lesioning another cortical structure, the amygdala, also consistently influences emotional behaviour, and this structure seems especially important in emotion (LeDoux, 1994).

Gray (1987) also links personality to brain systems. Chronically anxious individuals (high trait anxiety) have a high sensitivity behavioural inhibition system. Extraverts differ from introverts in having a more sensitive behavioural activation system. The psychophysiological and behavioural evidence for these hypotheses is rather weak though (Matthews and Gilliland, 1998).

Does physiology cause emotion?

Most psychologists wish to distinguish emotion from physiological constructs such as arousal, even if there is some overlap. In this case, we must address the causality question, one of the big questions of scientific psychology since its inception. There are two traditional answers. The first, *centralist*, theory (see Figure 8.1), proposed by Bard and by Cannon (1932) argues that physiology is causal. Significant stimuli activate a brain structure called the thalamus, which, in turn, generates both subjective responses and the physiological signs of stress. The second, opposing view, was independently proposed by William James (1890) and Carl Lange towards the end of the nineteenth century. According to this *peripheralist* view, emotion is inferred or constructed from instinctive peripheral physiological responses. Events provoke reflex bodily responses, and emotion results from the perception of those changes. Reversing everyday logic, we do not cry because we are unhappy; we are unhappy because we cry.

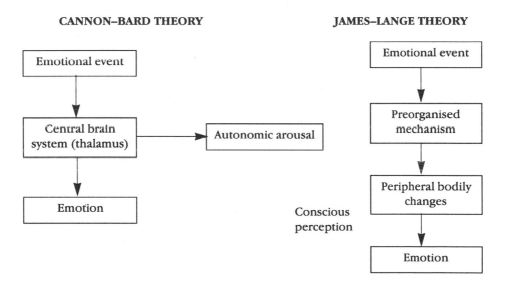

Figure 8.1: Schematic representation of the Cannon–Bard and James–Lange theories of emotion.

It has subsequently become clear that both views have some merit, but neither provides a full explanation of emotion. The James–Lange hypothesis is supported by studies showing that manipulation of physiological systems may generate emotion. For example, artificial manipulation of facial expression to produce smiles and frowns seems to generate the appropriate emotion (Zajonc, Murphy and Inglehart, 1989). However, feedback from the ANS is less critical than James suggested. Individuals with spinal injuries which reduce autonomic feedback seem to experience normal emotional responses (Chwalisz, Diener and Gallagher, 1988).

The Cannon–Bard view is supported by evidence that stimulation of various areas of the brain provokes emotional reactions in animals. It is wrong in supposing that the thalamus is the 'emotion centre' of the brain. In fact, various structures are implicated, of which the most important seems to be the amygdala (LeDoux, 1994). Drug studies also demonstrate the existence of central brain mechanisms. For example, the euphoria induced by opioid drugs such as heroin may be associated with a type of neurotransmitter called endorphins. Therapeutic studies allow clinical conditions to be linked to abnormality of neurotransmitter functions. Antidepressants such as Prozac may compensate for a reduced level of serotonin activity.

However, drug studies also show the limitations of the hypothesis. In general, drug effects on emotion are not as straightforward as the hypothesis predicts. For example, the nicotine in cigarettes is known to affect a neurotransmitter called acetylcholine. However, some people find smoking relaxing, whereas others use cigarettes for stimulation and increased energy. These individual differences may reflect not just variation in inhalation of nicotine, but also differing perceptions of smoking effects (O'Connor, 1985). Schachter and Singer (1962) conducted a classic experiment that showed that drug effects depend on the person's cognitions. Their subjects were injected with adrenaline, and provided with various contexts for experiencing its stimulant effects. Subjects told that the drug would make increase their heart rate and so forth (an appropriate explanation) did not experience these physiological responses as emotion. In other conditions, subjects were not given any explanation. Instead, they were exposed to a confederate of the experimenter, who posed as an additional subject. The confederate pretended either to feel happy or angry. The true subjects tended to pick up these emotions from the confederate. The key finding was that subjects injected with adrenaline experienced either the happiness or the anger more intensely – adrenaline was not linked to any particular emotion. Schachter and Singer's (1962) *cognitive labelling theory* explained this finding as follows. Like James and Lange, they propose that people label emotions using their perceptions of their own somatic activity. However, labelling is a cognitive process that is affected by the person's beliefs about the situation. If people believe they have reason to be angry, they will experience their bodily symptoms as anger, and so forth. Movie makers capitalize on this process by incorporating rhythms resembling cardiac acceleration into the soundtrack when something exciting or frightening is about to happen.

Subsequently, there have been various criticisms of Schachter and Singer's work, and it seems that drug-induced emotion is not quite as plastic as at first suggested. Nevertheless, most emotion researchers accept that cognitions of somatic activity influence emotion, although they disagree on how important they are. The Schachter and Singer study also opens up the whole question of how cognitions may influence emotion, which is explored in the next section.

Cognitive theories of stress and emotion

Appraisal and emotion

A radically different approach is to put the physiological correlates of emotion to one side, and to explore the cognitive basis of emotion. Lazarus (1966) conducted a series of studies in which he had volunteers watch a threatening film (a tribal penis incision ritual). Experimental manipulations that affected the viewer's orientation towards the film affected both autonomic and subjective responses. For example, denial statements saying that the surgical procedure was not actually very painful reduced emotion. Conversely, emotion was heightened by identification with the victim. Evidence of this kind supports appraisal theories of stress and emotion, which see emotion as a product of the person's interpretation and evaluation of stimuli and events. It also suggests why the link between life events and stress outcomes is relatively weak: what is important is not so much the event, but the way the person evaluates it (Lazarus and Folkman, 1984). It is useful to distinguish two types of appraisal. *Primary appraisal* refers to the immediate personal significance of an event, which might, for example, be threatening or challenging. *Secondary appraisal* describes evaluation of one's coping options, and whether coping is likely to be successful. The transactional definition of stress above refers to the secondary appraisal that one lacks the coping resources to deal with a problem straightforwardly. Appraisals that one lacks control over important events seem to be particularly potent in inducing stress symptoms.

Appraisal theories make fairly detailed statements about correspondences between specific appraisals and emotions. Events appraised as dangerous lead to anxiety and so forth. Links between appraisal and emotion seem similar across different cultures (Mauro et al., 1992). Cultures differ in how they appraise particular events, and in how emotions are expressed behaviourally. A criticism of appraisal theories is that they 'over-cognitivize' emotion, which often seems to develop rapidly and unconsciously, implying that emotion and cognition constitute separate systems (Zajonc, 1984). However, the inference is false, resulting from a confusion of cognition and consciousness (cf. Lazarus, 1984, 1991). It is true that emotion does not depend on conscious cognition: people may become anxious when presented with masked 'subliminal' threat stimuli, which they cannot consciously identify (Kemp-Wheeler and Hill,

1987). Generally, it seems that the mind has some capability for the rapid, 'automatic' analysis of the emotional content and personal significance of stimuli (e.g. Kitayama, 1997). However, this analysis is still a form of cognition, requiring the processing of information. The correct inference is that there are different levels of cognitive appraisal, some of which are more consciously accessible than others (Leventhal and Scherer, 1987).

We should not underestimate people's capriciousness, but, in general, they do not pluck their appraisals from thin air. Instead, appraisals are strongly influenced by the person's pre-existing knowledge and beliefs (Lazarus, 1991). The strongest evidence for this view comes from the clinical domain. Emotional disorders are usually associated with *irrational beliefs* (Ellis, 1962). Depressed individuals are typically characterized by negative 'core beliefs' that they are worthless and the future is hopeless (Beck, 1987). These beliefs seem to feed into irrational appraisals, such as interpreting a minor setback as a personal disaster. Beck (1967) has argued that the basis for depression is the person's *self-schema*, or organized store of self-knowledge. The schema biases people's cognitions of their interactions with the outside world, and leads to various errors in thinking, such as inferring one's worthlessness from an isolated instance of failure (overgeneralization). Other forms of schematized knowledge seem to influence appraisal and abnormality in other emotional disorders. Anxiety seems to relate to overestimation of personal vulnerability to danger, whereas panic disorder patients often believe that physical symptoms are a sign of an impending medical catastrophe (Wells, 1997). In normal individuals too, appraisals may be bound up with more general sets of beliefs about the world and one's place within it.

Coping and stress

The limitation of appraisal theories is that they present a rather passive view of the person. The relational perspective on stress emphasizes that people are not just passive victims of the events they perceive as threatening, harmful or uncontrollable. Instead, the stressful encounter unfolds dynamically as the person seeks to manage environmental demands actively, or to *cope* with them. Lazarus and Folkman (1984) discriminated two basic strategies for coping. *Problem-focused* coping refers to attempts to deal with the perceived problem through dealing directly with the external demand. The person sacked from his or her job might seek new employment, the divorced person might seek a new intimate relationship, and so forth. Such strategies are also described as *task focused*, because the person takes on tasks directed towards changing external reality. Alternatively, coping may be *emotion focused* – directed towards changing internal feelings and thoughts about the problem. Such attempts may be broadly constructive, such as looking for a silver lining to the situation, trying to learn from events, or coming to terms with loss. They may also be maladaptive, as when people brood perseveratively on the problem without resolving it (rumination), or blame themselves to an excessive degree. Two more types of strategy are frequently observed. *Avoidance* refers to attempts to evade the problem altogether, often by diverting oneself with activities such as shopping or watching television (Endler and Parker, 1990). People also cope by *seeking social support* from others. Social support may relate to problem-focus, when other people can provide material aid, to emotion-focus, when they offer sympathy, and to avoidance, where they are a source of diversion. Table 8.2 summarizes some common coping strategies.

Table 8.2: Examples of coping strategies

Type of coping	Example strategy
Task-focused	Make a determined effort to deal with the problem Work out a plan of action Try different solutions to the problem
Emotion-focused	Blame oneself for difficulties Try to come to terms with what has happened Wish things had turned out differently
Avoidance	Go for a walk Try not to think about the problem Watch TV
Social support	Get practical advice from an expert Talk to someone sympathetic Spend some leisure time with friends

'Coping' is a somewhat ambiguous term, as it can refer either to attempts to deal with a problem, or to attempts that actually succeed. The former usage is to be preferred, as coping attempts do not always achieve their intended aims: coping may be adaptive or maladaptive. There is some tendency for problem-focused coping to be more successful than the more negative forms of emotion-focus (self-blame, rumination) and avoidance. However, all forms of coping may be useful in particular circumstances: what is important is what works for the individual in particular circumstances. The best form of coping varies from person to person and occasion to occasion (Zeidner and Saklofske, 1996).

Like appraisal, choice of coping strategies is influenced by prior knowledge and experience, but people also seem generally disposed to choose different styles of coping.

Several personality factors relate to coping (see Matthews et al., 1998, for a review). Individuals high in neuroticism favour emotion-focus, whereas extraversion and conscientiousness relate to use of problem-focus (Deary et al., 1996). A variety of traits related to beliefs in one's effectiveness in mastering external challenges also relate to active or problem-focused coping. They include *hardiness*, *self-efficacy*, *internal locus of control*, and *learned resourcefulness*. Internal locus of control refers to beliefs that one's actions control the outcome of significant events, as opposed to external factors such as luck. Learned resourcefulness is based on self-control skills that facilitate active coping: it contrasts with *learned helplessness* – beliefs that one cannot deflect or mitigate unpleasant events. Unfortunately, these various 'active coping' traits tend to correlate with one another, and with low neuroticism, so it is unclear whether they really represent distinct constructs or not (Hurrell and Murphy, 1991).

Deciding how to cope is a fundamentally rational activity, but the choice may be maladaptive if the individual's appraisal of the nature of demands and of personal competence in coping is faulty. Problem-focus reflects individuals' confidence in their ability to influence the situation through taking action. Hence, it is more likely when the situation is perceived as changeable, and when the person believes in their power to effect change (Lazarus and Folkman, 1984). Emotion-focus may sometimes derive from the realization that the external situation cannot be changed, following bereavement for example. The more damaging forms of emotion-focus may stem from misconceived beliefs about the person's own thoughts, which are described as *metacognitions*. Generalized anxiety patients often seem to believe that worrying helps them to be prepared for sources of danger, although, in fact, such beliefs tend to be counterproductive (Wells, 1997).

The final aspect of cognitive theories is their emphasis on the dynamic nature of the stress process (Lazarus and Folkman, 1984). As the stressful encounter unfolds, people *reappraise* the success or failure of their coping efforts, which may reduce or increase stress symptoms such as negative emotion. One of the problems experienced by emotional disorder patients is that 'vicious circles' may tend to develop, in which negative cognitions and emotions are mutually reinforcing over time (Wells and Matthews, 1994). Depressives often believe they make a poor impression on other people. They tend to be rather unresponsive to others, who find them unrewarding to talk to, and so may withdraw from the conversation, perpetuating the vicious circle. Similarly, depressives and some anxiety patients may tend to *ruminate* or worry perseveratively over their problems, which keeps the problem in the forefront of awareness, and maintains negative emotion. Conversely, support from others may counter negative beliefs, preventing the vicious circle from developing.

Consequences of stress

Stress may have many consequences, which vary from person to person and occasion to occasion. These are not necessarily harmful: demanding circumstances may provide opportunities for material success, or for personal growth and learning. We cannot expect to forge lasting intimate relationships or to achieve job success without some degree of stress. For example, Mughal, Walsh and Wilding (1996) showed that anxious insurance sales executives worked longer hours and closed more sales. However, stress may also have various consequences that are harmful to a greater or lesser degree:

- Discomfort. Emotions and physiological sensations may be disturbing or distracting, even if they are not otherwise harmful, especially when prolonged or severe. Worry about stress symptoms may be more damaging than the symptoms themselves. Discomfort is not necessarily closely related to behaviour, because some people cope better with the experience of stress than others.
- Disruption of social functioning. Stress reactions may hinder a person's pursuit of their everyday activities and maintenance of social relationships. It may be socially unacceptable to display strong emotions in some circumstances. The socially anxious person seems preoccupied with other people's reactions, which interferes with social skills. Stress may also affect motivation and application deleteriously. The *burnout* syndrome (Maslach, 1982) combines negative emotions, fatigue, cognitions of overload and helplessness, and a tendency to withdraw from work activities. It is common in human service professions, and even dedicated individuals may fall victim to it when exposed to chronic job stress.
- Health problems. The relationship between stress and health is one of the more controversial topics. Stress often accompanies illness, and it is widely believed that stress may play a part in conditions such as chronic headache, ulcers and asthma. However, it is often difficult to distinguish cause and effect in this area: a person may experience stress *because* he or she is ill, or some third factor, such as personality, may influence both stress and illness.
- Disruption of attention and performance. The distraction associated with stress may interfere with concentration on demanding activities. Stress has been implicated as a source of pilot error contributing to air crashes, and it has been estimated that recent life stress raises the risk of a motor vehicle accident by two to five times (Selzer and Vinokur, 1975). Less dramatically, stress may also interfere with productivity at work, and with performance on tests and examinations (Sarason, 1988).

The following sections examine in more detail the consequences of stress for health and for attention and performance, as these outcomes have attracted the most systematic research.

Health and illness

Investigating the health consequences of stress

Stress is implicated in a wide variety of medical conditions including ulcers, asthma, headaches and two of the main killer diseases, coronary heart disease (CHD) and cancer.

Popular wisdom has it that thinking positively protects against objective physical illness, but is this true? A basic difficulty is determining whether psychological stress is actually a cause of illness. Illnesses disrupt people's lives so it is not surprising that sick people tend to be distressed. To establish that stress factors influence ill health, some sophistication in methods of investigation is required. Some of the ways in which a causal link may be established are as follows:

* Experimental studies. Animal studies can be used to show that inducing stress under controlled conditions provokes illness. Monkeys and rats are prone to develop ulcers when subjected to uncontrollable painful shock. The incidence of ulcers is reduced by a warning signal, and, even more so, by the option of avoiding shock by making a response (Weiss, 1972). Animal work inspired the view that learned helplessness provides a model for human depression: life experiences may have taught the depressed person that he or she is powerless to control aversive events (Seligman, 1975). Obviously, such studies cannot usually be directly replicated in humans, although we may be able to invent acceptable analogues, and there are always questions about the generalizability of animal findings. For example, current work on depression and helplessness emphasizes the individual's beliefs about controllability, rather than learning per se. As in Selye's classic work, animal studies are also useful for investigating physiological responses to stress that may contribute to illness, such as changes in noradrenergic activity produced in the learned helplessness paradigm (Gold, Goodwin and Chrousos, 1988).
* Longitudinal studies of life stress. In 'cross-sectional' studies, stress and health are assessed on a single occasion, but no conclusive causal inferences can be drawn. In longitudinal studies, measures are taken at two or more points in time, and the researcher can test whether stress precedes illness, or vice versa. Statistical modelling techniques such as path analysis are often used. It is more difficult to infer causality from longitudinal studies than from experimental studies, and there are often methodological problems to tackle, such as the validity of the assessments of stress and health.
* Intervention studies. If stress causes illness, psychological therapy for stress should improve the patient's physical condition. For example, relaxation techniques seem to produce improvements in hypertension, tension headache and insomnia, though not necessarily a complete

cure (Lavey and Taylor, 1985). Again, caution is necessary in making statements about causality. For example, it might be muscle relaxation rather than psychological relaxation, which is medically beneficial.

Even if there does appear to be a causal link, difficulties in interpretation remain. There are a variety of mechanisms through which stress might influence health (for example, Cohen and Williamson, 1991). One possibility is that psychological functioning has some direct effect on physiology, mediated by the ANS or endocrine or immune systems. Alternatively, effects may be indirect, in that stress may influence *health behaviours* (Steptoe and Wardle, 1996), which raise or lower the likelihood of illness. Stress might encourage high-risk behaviours such as drinking, smoking, unsafe sex; and physical risk taking, such as driving too fast. Conversely, stress may depress health-promoting behaviours such as choosing a healthy diet and exercising. Stress may also influence behaviours directly related to medicine, such as approaching a general practitioner with a health problem and compliance with treatment regimes. For these various reasons, research on stress and health is difficult, and it is often difficult to make conclusive statements.

Life events and health

Clearly, there are methodological difficulties in assessing life events. In general, it seems that people suffering from a variety of physical illnesses including heart diseases, cancer, infective diseases and multiple sclerosis report relatively high levels of adverse life events in the years preceding onset of illness (see, for example, Brown and Harris, 1989). However, it may be that illness leads people to exaggerate their life difficulties, or that healthy people downplay their problems. In longitudinal studies, some of the best evidence for effects of stress comes from a somewhat indirect source – studies of how much social support is available to the person. Social support refers to the material help, information and sympathy available to the person from social contacts. It seems to mitigate the psychological effects of life events. Berkman and Syme (1979) assessed the social ties available to a community sample in California. They subsequently followed the sample over a nine-year period, and monitored mortality, and found there was quite a substantial association between having few social ties and risk of dying. Marriage and close contacts with friends and relatives were the strongest predictors of remaining alive. Other studies have obtained similar results, although the mechanisms for the effect remain somewhat unclear.

Conversely, hostility from others may be actively harmful. In the clinical context, *expressed emotion* refers to the level of hostility and criticism shown to a person with psychiatric illness by relatives of that person (Kavanagh, 1992). Expressed emotion seems to relate to a poorer prognosis, although its impact on physical illness is uncertain.

Longitudinal studies may also be directed towards specific diseases. Some have shown evidence suggestive of stress effects although the evidence is somewhat inconsistent. There is rather better evidence that more specific types of psychological maladaptation relate to future illness. Studies of occupational stress suggest that heart disease relates especially to a combination of high work demands and low control over the job (for example, Krantz et al., 1988). Executives and doctors are subjected to high demands, but they also have considerable freedom of action in coping with those demands. Heart rate incidence is lower in such jobs than in occupations such as construction worker, machine operator or waiter/waitress, in which the person has little personal control over work demands. In the case of cancer, it seems to be excessive suppression of emotions that may be a risk factor, rather than life stress *per se*. Dattore, Shontz and Coyne (1980) showed that suppression of emotion predicted cancer 10 years later. Cooper and Watson (1991) conducted a study of women attending a clinic for breast disorders. A psychological assessment was carried out prior to medical diagnosis. Women who subsequently turned out to be suffering from breast cancer reported more life events related to loss at the initial assessment. They also had fewer coping skills and were less assertive. In general, passive acceptance or restraint in the face of stress seems to be implicated in cancer, whereas 'fighting spirit' may be protective. However, the evidence is somewhat inconsistent, and the causal mechanisms are poorly understood.

Stress and the immune system

As previously discussed, stress may have both direct and indirect effects on physiological functioning and health. One of the specific mechanisms through which psychological stress may increase vulnerability to illness is through effects on the immune system. Selye (1976) originally suggested that the efficiency of the immune response might be compromised during the 'resistance' stage of the general adaptation syndrome. However, the systematic study of psychological influences on the immune system (*psychoneuroimmunology*) is relatively recent. Methods used include experimental studies of animals and humans, and field studies of life stress. A variety of indices of immune function are used, including levels of immunoglobulin A (Ig A), which can be assessed from saliva, and counts of lymphocytes (B-cells, T-cells and natural killer cells). Animal studies show that acute stress of various types depresses immune response and disease resistance. As ever, psychological stress factors are critical: inescapable or uncontrollable stress stimuli arc more likely to influence immune response adversely (for example, Laudenslager et al., 1983). Human studies (Steptoe, 1991) provide some confirmation for the animal studies, although there are also inconstancies and complications. There is consid-erable evidence that 'life stress' factors such as bereavement, loneliness and examination stress relate to lower immune system activity. As with stress reactions generally, availability of social support acts to offset these effects (Jemmott and Magloire, 1988).

These data are clearly important in suggesting a possible explanation for empirical findings such as the effects of social support on mortality (Berkman and Syme, 1979), and psychological influences on cancer. There have also been attempts to boost immune system function in cancer and AIDS patients through psychological intervention (Antoni et al., 1990), with promising results. However, the extent of clinical benefits resulting remains uncertain. In addition, the physiological pathways involved are poorly understood, but probably complex. One hypothesis is that stress has an indirect effect on immunosuppression, involving the autonomic nervous system and hormone secretion (Hall and Goldstein, 1981). Sympathetic nervous system activation may be associated with release of several hormones that may impair immune response, including catecholamines (adrenaline and noradrenaline) and ACTH, which releases corticosteroids (for example, cortisol).

Personality, stress and illness

As previously discussed, life events are a relatively poor index of the stress symptoms actually experienced by the individual, because they are so dependent upon appraisal and coping. People differ in how resilient or hardy they are. Some individuals seem generally resilient, even when facing major crises, whereas others crumble under minor pressure. The personality trait most consistently related to hardiness is neuroticism. More neurotic individuals show higher levels of stress symptoms in a variety of stressful circumstances. The association between neuroticism and psychological responses such as negative emotion is straightforward (see above), but the relationship between neuroticism and other person-ality factors to illness as a stress outcome is more controversial. Cross-sectional studies of the personality characteristics of patient groups suggests that neuroticism is elevated in a wide variety of conditions, including CHD, asthma, ulcer, arthritis and headache (Booth-Kewley and Friedman, 1987). Neuroticism also relates to psychosomatic conditions such as chronic fatigue, non-ulcer dyspepsia and irritable bowel syndrome (Kirmayer et al., 1994). However, such studies have several limitations. First, there is a shortage of longitudinal studies demonstrating that neuroticism predates illness. Second, neuroticism relates more strongly to subjective reports than to objective systems. One view is that neurotic individuals are simply 'complaint prone' (Stone and Costa, 1990), although evidence that neuroticism relates to some specific objective conditions is now starting to appear (Matthews and Deary, 1998). Third, causal mechanisms are unclear. As with psychological factors generally, neuroticism effects might be direct or indirect. If there are direct effects, they might reflect either the biological or cognitive factors underpinning neuroticism.

Various other narrow traits associated with stress vulnerability have been investigated as predictors of health (see Friedman, 1990). Consistent with cognitive models of stress, more optimistic individuals seem to adjust better to illness, and to recover more quickly than pessimists. So too do those with beliefs in personal control. It is unclear whether these aspects of personality predict onset of illness. There has been extensive research on the Type A personality and CHD. The aggressive, time-pressured, achievement-oriented Type A personality has been said to be more prone to myocardial infarction and angina pectoris than the more laid-back Type B (Rosenman et al., 1975). However, recent research suggests that Type A is a complex of distinct traits, which are not all related to CHD. It may be especially hostility which is associated with risk of disease (Miller et al., 1996).

Finally, one of the most striking but also most controversial instances of personality and stress research concerns the work of Grossarth-Maticek and Eysenck on predictors of mortality (see Eysenck, 1988). In a large study conducted in former Yugoslavia, Grossarth-Maticek classified people into various types, of which two are particularly relevant. Type I individuals were characterized by dependency, helplessness and emotional suppression. Subsequently, these individuals were highly likely to die of cancer. Type II individuals were easily frustrated and angered, and were prone to die of cardiovascular disease. Another study suggested that mortality might be much reduced by giving people behaviour therapy appropriate to their personality. A study conducted in Heidelberg showed that the combination of stressful life events and high-risk personality type led to a particularly high risk of death. The research findings bear some resemblance to other findings: for example, Type II personality resembles Type A. However, this work has attracted particular interest because the magnitude of the personality and stress effects is very large. Usually, psychological factors in illness have only modest effects. The Grossarth-Maticek and Eysenck research has been severely criticized by Pelosi and Appleby (1992), who point out various methodological difficulties such as limited documentation of research design. It remains to be seen whether these findings will replicate; in the interim, they should be treated with caution.

Attention and performance

Research methods

Studies of attention and performance are important because they allow the psychological expression of stress and emotion to be investigated using objective measures. Methods for investigating stress effects on performance reflect the alternative definitions of stress outlined previously. The stimulus definition lends itself to experimental manipulations of stressors, whose effects may be controlled with appropriate control conditions. These may include physical stressors such as noise and heat, biological agents such as drugs, and cognitive-social stressors such as explicitly evaluating performance. Often, task demands are varied so as to test hypotheses regarding the information-processing mechanisms sensitive to the stressor. For example, compared with performance in a quiet environment, loud noise appears to be particularly damaging to attentionally demanding tasks, implying that noise may reduce the attentional 'capacity' available for processing task stimuli (Fisher, 1986).

The response definition of stress leads to attempts to measure stress symptoms such as anxiety and worry, and to relate them to performance. Often measurement of negative emotion is combined with experimental manipulations intended to heighten emotion. Emotion may be induced directly by suggestive techniques such as hypnosis (Bower, 1981), or indirectly through manipulations such as providing feedback on performance indicating that the person has failed to perform adequately. People differ in their susceptibility to such inductions of emotion, so we must take care to distinguish vulnerability to emotional responses from the actual emotions. Figure 8.2 shows a widely accepted formulation developed by Spielberger (1966) to explain anxiety effects on performance. The person's immediate state of anxiety depends on both trait anxiety (vulnerability) and on external stressors, such as a failure experience. Trait anxious subjects react more strongly than non-trait anxious individuals to experiences of this kind. It is then state anxiety that directly impairs information-processing efficiency, and, consequently, performance.

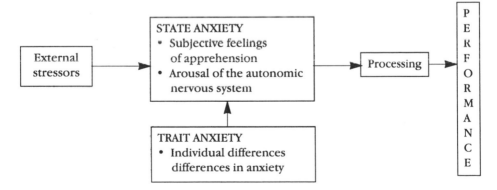

Figure 8.2: A state–trait model for anxiety effects on performance (see Spielberger, 1966).

The transactional definition of stress has inspired not so much particular methods, but awareness of the limitations of conventional laboratory studies. It implies that effects of stress manipulations may, to some extent, depend on the way in which the stressor is evaluated, and the way in which the person chooses to cope with it. For example, Cohen (1980) showed that loud, uncontrollable noise impaired performance even after the noise had been switched off. It may be that people tended to cope with the noise by withdrawing effort from the task, and this passivity carried over to the quiet period that followed.

Theories of stress

Until relatively recently, work on stress and performance was dominated by arousal theory (Duffy, 1962). The psychobiological construct of arousal, previously discussed, was linked to performance by the *Yerkes–Dodson law*, based on animal research conducted by Yerkes and Dodson (1908). This 'law', illustrated in Figure 8.3, has two parts. First, it asserts that states of moderate arousal are optimal for performance. Efficiency of the cerebral cortex, and hence performance, is impaired when arousal is low, in states of sleepiness, and also when arousal is high, in states of strong emotion or agitation. Second, the optimal level of arousal is inversely related to task difficulty; the more difficult the task, the lower the optimum. This application of arousal theory has some common-sense appeal. It is also supported to some degree by studies of interactions between stress manipulations (Broadbent, 1971). Performance is often impaired when the person performs under combinations of two arousing stressors, or two de-arousing stressors. Arousal theory has fallen from favour in performance research for several reasons. These include the difficulties in assessment of arousal previously mentioned, and evidence that, when scrutinized in detail, performance data often fail to conform to the Yerkes–Dodson law (Neiss, 1988).

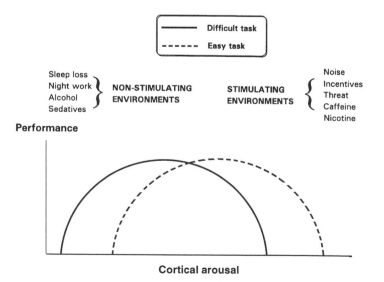

Figure 8.3: Hypothesized inverted-U relationships between cortical arousal and performance (the Yerkes–Dodson law).

However, perhaps the most important shortcoming of arousal theory is the one identified by the *cognitive critique* of arousal theory. Cognitive psychologists (Eysenck, 1982; Hockey, 1984) have pointed out that the effects of stressors on performance tend to vary with the type of information processing required by the task. For example, a stressor might facilitate performance of a demanding attentional task, but impair performance of an equally difficult task requiring short-term memory. Furthermore, this dependence of the stressor effect on the nature of the task varies from stressor to stressor. Hockey (1984) advocates investigating the *cognitive patterning* associated with specific stressors in detail – investigating which tasks it impairs, which it facilitates, and which it has no effect on. Next, we look at some examples of the information-processing functions that seem to be sensitive to stress, bearing in mind that different stressors have different effects on these functions.

Attentional efficiency

Various stressors are prone to impair performance of tasks which require intense concentration, such as performing two tasks simultaneously (dual-task performance). These include noise, heat, anxiety, depression, subjective tiredness and sleep deprivation (see Smith and Jones, 1992). It is often assumed that concentration on a demanding task requires allocation of *attentional resources* to the processing required to perform the task. Attentional resources are a metaphorical 'power supply' for processing, which is impaired when processing calls for more 'power' than is available, which may happen when the task is particularly demanding, or in dual-task performance (Norman and Bobrow, 1975). The stressors listed may reduce availability of resources. However, they may do so for different reasons. Noise diverts attention on to processing the noise stimuli (Fisher, 1986), whereas heat (Hancock, 1986) and subjective tiredness (Matthews, 1992) seem to reduce the total quantity of resources available, perhaps via biological mechanisms.

Negative emotions such as anxiety and depression seem to have a more subtle effect. Strictly speaking, it is not so much the emotion that is damaging to attention, but the distracting worries and intrusive thoughts which tend to accompany negative emotions (Sarason, 1984). Worries divert attention away from the task at hand. The transactional model of stress provides more insight into this process. Worry tends to be associated with emotion-focused coping: it becomes more important to people to deal with their internal thoughts and feelings than to deal with the external task. Successful treatments for test anxiety are directed towards these cognitions, such as training people to direct attention away from the self and on to the task, or exposing them to models who display appropriate cognitions. Anxious individuals may try to compensate for performance impairment through increased task-directed effort (Eysenck and Calvo, 1992) – task-focused coping.

Attentional selectivity

The focus of attention is often compared to a searchlight that illuminates the stimuli to which the person is attending. It seems that arousing stressors often narrow the searchlight beam, so that *attentional selectivity* increases (Hockey, 1984). The person may develop a kind of cognitive 'tunnel vision'. People may handle crises badly because of over-selectivity of attention: a person trapped in a burning building might fail to notice the escape route. One version of this general hypothesis was put forward by Easterbrook (1959), who suggested that arousal reduces the range of cues used by the person. This hypothesis may provide a partial explanation for the Yerkes–Dodson law. Under-aroused people take in information from many sources and so are prone to become distracted from the task at hand. Over-aroused individuals use so few cues that they tend to neglect important aspects of the task, again leading to poor performance. In states of moderate arousal, the person manages to take in all the task cues while ignoring irrelevant cues, leading to optimal performance.

The selectivity hypothesis can be tested in dual-task studies. The person performs two tasks, one of which is designated of primary importance, and the other the secondary task. Of course, people tend to focus more attention on the primary task. However, stressors tend to accentuate this tendency: performance tends to improve on the primary task, and deteriorate on the secondary task. Changes in attentional selectivity seem quite robust empirically (Hockey, 1984), although they are more reliable for arousing stressors (such as loud noise) than for de-arousing ones (for example sleep deprivation). However, stressors may have additional effects on selective attention (see section on cognitive bias below), and selectivity effects may vary somewhat from stressor to stressor. Furthermore, there is some doubt over exactly how selectivity effects operate. Rather than an automatic narrowing of the attentional searchlight, changes in selectivity may reflect a deliberate strategy for coping with stress. For example, the person exposed to noise, which tends to have detrimental effects, may choose to preserve primary task performance at the cost of impaired secondary task performance.

Memory

As with selective attention, stressor effects on memory may partially reflect arousal mechanisms. In some studies arousal enhances *long-term memory* (LTM) but impairs *short-term memory* (STM). Arousal may affect the *consolidation* of information in LTM. The establishment of a strong trace in LTM requires protection of the information from interference during consolidation. Hence arousal impairs STM while the trace is being laid down, but leads to better LTM. This explanation is appealing but somewhat simplistic, as effects of arousal seem to vary from stressor to stressor (Eysenck, 1982). For example, anxiety seems to relate to impairments of both STM and LTM. It is associated especially with impairment of *working memory*, the combination of short-term storage and active processing of information, for instance while doing mental arithmetic. Stressors may also have quite subtle strategic effects. Noise seems to encourage 'parroting back' of material rather than using more active, meaning-based strategies for retention.

Cognitive bias applies to stress-related emotional states rather than to physical stressors such as noise. Everyday observation suggests that people tend to be more pessimistic when upset and more optimistic when happy. Bower (1981) suggested a general principle of *mood congruence*: for example, people in sad moods should be more sensitive to unpleasant or threatening stimuli, they should be prone to remember unpleasant events and their thinking should show a general negative bias. These ideas can be tested experimentally, either by looking at naturally occurring moods, or by inducing moods artificially, typically using suggestive techniques such as hypnosis. The outcomes of these studies are complex, and mood-congruence is confirmed in some studies only. It seems strongest in studies of *judgement*. For example, Forgas and Bower (1987) report that people rate their social functioning more negatively when an unhappy mood is induced. Conversely, people have more positive opinions of themselves (and others) when a happy mood is induced. Depressed patients show similar negative biases in self-assessment, even when they seem to show no objective impairment. Cognitive bias in *memory* is prone to be unreliable, but it can be demonstrated with care in experimental methods (Ucros, 1989). Some of the strongest effects are shown in studies of real-life memory. Depressed patients tend to recall unpleasant events, although, of course, these individuals may actually have experienced more negative personal histories than others.

Studies of bias in *perception* have been influenced by the Freudian idea that people are motivated to defend themselves against unpleasant stimuli by unconsciously suppressing negative stimuli. *Perceptual defence* seems to be a genuine phenomenon, but it does not seem to operate according to Freudian principles. Perceptual thresholds for threatening words are sometimes higher and sometimes lower than thresholds for matched control words, depending on the exact demands placed on information processing (Kitayama, 1997). Perception also seems to be relatively unaffected by mood-related bias, although depressed individuals are sometimes sensitive to negative stimuli (Wells and Matthews, 1994).

Bias in *attention* has been most often investigated in studies of anxiety. There is now a large research literature (see Wells and Matthews, 1994, for a review) which suggests that, given a choice of stimuli, anxious individuals seem to focus on threatening rather than non-threatening stimuli. A variety of techniques are used to demonstrate bias, but the most widely used is the *emotional Stroop test*. The standard Stroop test requires the subject to name the ink colours of a series of words, typically printed on a card. Response is slowed when the meaning of the word conflicts with the ink-colour (e.g. 'BLUE' written in red ink), showing that people involuntarily process word meaning. A typical emotional Stroop test requires subjects to name the colours of threatening words such as 'TORTURE' and 'FAILURE'. Compared with neutral control words, generalized anxiety disorder patients are slow to name the colours of such words, suggesting that selective attention tends to focus on the threatening meaning (MacLeod and Mathews, 1991). Similar, if somewhat less robust, effects are found in studies of non-clinical subjects of anxious personality. Emotional Stroop effects have been demonstrated for a variety of different mood and anxiety disorders. Patients tend to be sensitive to words that match their pathology such as spider words (for example 'COBWEB') for spider phobics, disease or contamination words (for example 'DIRT') for obsessional-compulsive patients, and physical/health threat words (such as 'FAINT') for panickers. There has been some controversy over the interpretation of bias in selective attention. It may reflect either an unconscious sensitivity to threatening stimuli in anxious individuals, or a strategy of monitoring the environment for threat (Wells and Matthews, 1994).

Implications for stress management and therapy

Stress symptoms such as negative emotion are a common source of concern to people, but it can be difficult to identify 'stress' as a clinical problem distinct from, on the one hand, ordinary unhappiness and dissatisfaction, and on the other hand, clinically diagnosed mood and anxiety disorders. To some extent, there is simply a continuum of severity from negative emotion to stress to clinical disorder. However, severe disorder is characterized by major difficulties in daily functioning, whereas the 'stressed' individual may still function effectively. *Stress management* most often refers to treatments for relatively minor symptom levels, in the absence of a diagnosis of mental disorder (see Fontana, 1989, for an introduction). Stress management techniques may also be used as components of the more intensive therapeutic interventions required for clinical patients. However, these techniques are too superficial to provide the main basis for treatment of clinical depression and anxiety conditions. Instead, it is important to restructure the underlying 'self-knowledge' that underpins the person's various cognitive maladapations, through cognitive behaviour therapy.

This section outlines, first, varieties of stress management, and second, the theoretical basis for cognitive behaviour therapy for mood and anxiety disorders. Stress management techniques may be divided into those that address symptoms, and those that address coping skills. This division neglects appraisal, which has previously been identified as a key influence on emotion and stress. Some techniques may influence appraisal indirectly. For example, stress counsellors encourage clients to explore different interpretations of their problems, which may lead to change in appraisal. In general, though, maladaptive appraisals may be difficult to change because of their basis in the person's self-knowledge in long-term memory. Appraisal change is more easily effected by the cognitive behaviour therapy methods, directed towards self-knowledge.

Stress management

Relief of symptoms

Various relaxation techniques have been developed that seem effective in alleviating symptoms such as emotional and physiological disturbance. Drug treatments of course are directed towards symptoms, but the techniques described here focus on psychological methods. *Progressive relaxation therapy* (Jacobson, 1938) involves the person systematically tensing and relaxing the main muscle groups of the body. Decrease in muscle tension tends to be associated with a reduction in other indices of autonomic nervous system activity, such as heart rate and blood pressure, as well as subjective calmness. The mechanisms for these effects are not fully understood. As previously discussed, anxious emotion may, in part, represent a label or inference drawn from perceptions of bodily activity. Hence, reducing bodily symptoms may help the person to appraise himself or herself as calm, especially as recipients of the therapy are encouraged to attribute their psychological tension to physiological tension. The person may also learn to self-regulate physiological functioning through *biofeedback*. Trainees learn awareness of physiological state through feedback provided from monitoring devices. They then learn how to influence physiological responses, first in the laboratory, and then in stressful real-life setttings. Biofeedback may help the person regulate aspects of brain functioning normally inaccessible to conscious awareness and control. Relaxation may also be effected by purely psychological techniques, such as *hypnosis*, *guided imagery* of pleasant scenes, and *meditation*.

All the techniques mentioned have at least some efficacy, although any given technique works better for some people than others. For example, people differ considerably in their hypnotic suggestibility. They are limited in that they do not directly address psychological sources of underlying problems (as cognitive therapy does), or provide the person with better skills for dealing with problems (as coping-oriented techniques do). They may have benefits over and above symptom relief through providing people with beliefs that their symptoms are controllable, and, hence, the confidence to tackle difficult situations themselves.

Training coping skills

In some cases, stress may reflect a genuine lack of skills for dealing with certain problems. In such cases, the missing skills may be trained directly. *Social skills* include managing conversation, observing and listening to others, and non-verbal communication. *Social skills training* aims to identify and correct deficiencies in skills of this kind through verbal instruction, modelling and role-play. Other skills that may be taught in this way include assertiveness and anger control. Nezu, Nezu and Perri (1989) have developed a therapy for depression that focuses on general social problem-solving skills, which are often deficient in depressed individuals. The person learns a positive orientation to problem solving, problem definition, generating alternative solutions, decision making, and implementation of the solution chosen. Training in coping may also be packaged together with other therapeutic techniques. Stress inoculation techniques (Meichenbaum and Cameron, 1983) aim to work like vaccination, in exposing the person to a mild, relatively easily controllable stressor. The person is trained in adaptive appraisal or conceptualization of the stressor, specific coping skills, and application of skills to the problem of real-life.

As with relaxation techniques, the efficacy of coping skills training is well-documented, although, again, there are individual differences in how well it works. It also has applications to clinical patient groups, as the example of training in problem solving shows, but training coping in isolation is unlikely to be a successful therapy for patients. For example, training social skills may be helpful to some social anxiety and social phobia patients, but some socially anxious patients do not show social skills deficits (Edelmann, 1992). Patients' difficulties may more frequently relate to difficulties in using or applying their existing social skills. Training in coping skills also has some of the limitations of relaxation techniques, in that it is relatively superficial and it may make it more difficult for people to confront the underlying psychological problem.

Psychological basis for cognitive behaviour therapy

Clinical depression and anxiety may result from maladaptive schemas for organizing self-knowledge, as described previously, so that therapy requires modification and re-structuring of the self-schema (Beck, 1967). Current theory (for example, Wells and Matthews, 1994) points out that the 'schema' represents not just explicit self-beliefs, such as personal worthlessness, but also dysfunctional internal 'programmes' for appraisal and coping. The content of these programmes may not be consciously accessible. For example, the studies of emotion and attention reviewed in the previous section show how programmes controlling threat detection may be systematically biased.

Beck's (1967) cognitive therapy is based on investigating maladaptive elements of the individual patient's self-schema, such as characteristic negative self-beliefs and thinking errors. Modification of self-belief depends not just on discussion but on behavioural 'experiments' that challenge the patient's beliefs. For example, panic patients are prone to believe that physical symptoms such as their heart racing herald catastrophic outcomes such as heart failure. Having the patient exercise vigorously, under the guidance of the therapist, raises heart rate without the catastrophe resulting and so helps these individuals to learn that their beliefs are inaccurate. The specific techniques used depend on the expertise and ingenuity of the therapist, but, in general, the aim is to introduce more realistic cognitions into the self-schema through collaborative analysis of the patient's beliefs and thoughts.

The recent work on attention and cognitive bias discussed in the previous section, provides a slightly different perspective. Abnormality relates not just to the content of self-beliefs and assumptions, but also to the attentional processes which govern the person's dynamic interaction with the external world, and which, in clinical patients, tend to focus attention on problems rather than solutions. Cognitive biases and disruption of attention and short-term memory give the patient a drastically different set of experiences of everyday life. Wells and Matthews (1994) attribute emotional disorder to prolonged engagement of a *self-referent executive function (S-REF)*. This is a mode of attentional control characterized by active monitoring for threat, self-critical emotion-focused coping and self-focus of attention, which generates perseverative cycles of distress and worry.

The S-REF hypothesis suggests the application of therapeutic distraction techniques, which draw attention away from threat stimuli, and of explicit training designed to give the patient more adaptive control of attention (Wells, 1997). The previous section also described how anxiety and depression tend to be associated with loss of functional attentional resources. Loss of resources and impaired concentration make it harder for the patient to modify dysfunctional self-beliefs (Wells and Matthews, 1994). Hence, relaxation techniques may be an important adjunct to therapy, in that relaxation makes it easier for patients to examine and criticize their faulty beliefs. Wells and Matthews recommend *detached mindfulness* as a therapeutic goal: the patient should be aware of their thought processes without being strongly engaged or disturbed by negative thoughts.

Conclusions

Both stress and emotion are multifaceted concepts, which must be understood at several different levels. Arousal of the peripheral and central nervous system is linked to emotion, but the two traditional theories assign different roles to physiology. The Cannon–Bard theory saw stress and emotion as a direct expression of central brain systems, a function performed by the amygdala and other structures according to contemporary theory. The James–Lange theory claimed that emotion is inferred from perceptions of physiological reactions: crying leads to sadness, smiling to happiness, and so forth. More recently, Schachter and Singer described the process of labelling physiological reactions. Contemporary cognitive theories assign appraisal of events a key role in generating emotion. They also emphasize the importance of active coping with demanding events, including seeking social support: successful coping can prevent or mitigate the harmful impact of stressors. Stable personality traits also seem to bias various aspects of appraisal and coping: the broad trait of neuroticism relates to more negative appraisal and, in many cases, ineffective coping.

When the person fails to cope successfully, stress may have a variety of damaging effects, including subjective discomfort, disruption of social functioning, health problems and impairment of attention and cognition. Stress may have both indirect effects on health, mediated by health behaviours, and direct effects dependent on the immune system and other physiological mechanisms. Behavioural consequences of stress are critically dependent on information processing. Studies of attention and performance suggest that stress-related conditions such as anxiety and depression tend to relate both to impairments on demanding tasks, and to cognitive bias favouring processing of negative stimuli. These consequences of stress should be seen in a dynamic context, within which people's appraisals of their problems feed back into further cycles of cognition and emotion. Stress management techniques operate through various aspects of the stress process, including relief of symptoms, modification of maladaptive appraisal and coping, and modification of the core self-knowledge structures that generate maladaptive cognition.

References

Antoni MH, Schneiderman N, Fletcher MA, Goldstein DA, Ironson G, Laperriere A (1990) Psychoneuroimmunology and HIV-I. Journal of Consulting and Clinical Psychology 58: 38–49.

Beck AT (1967) Depression: Causes and Treatment. Philadelphia: University of Pennsylvania Press.

Beck AT (1987) Cognitive models of depression. Journal of Cognitive Psychotherapy 1: 5–37.

Berkman L, Syme SL (1979) Social networks, host resistance, and mortality: A nine-year follow-up study of Alameda County residents. American Journal of Epidemiology 109: 186–204.

Booth-Kewley S, Friedman HS (1987) Psychological predictors of heart disease: a quantitative review. Psychological Bulletin 101: 343–62.

Bower GH (1981) Mood and memory. American Psychologist 36: 129–48.

Broadbent DE (1971) Decision and Stress. London: Academic.

Brown GW, Harris TO (1978) Social Origins of Depression: A Study of Psychiatric Disorder in Women. London: Tavistock.

Brown GW, Harris TO (eds) (1989) Life Events and Illness. New York: Guilford.

Cannon W (1932) The Wisdom of the Body. New York: Norton.

Chwalisz K, Diener E, Gallagher D (1988) Autonomic arousal feedback and emotional experience: evidence from the spinal cord injured. Journal of Personality and Social Psychology 54: 820–8.

Cohen S (1980) After effects of stress on human performance and social behavior: a review of research and theory. Psychological Bulletin 88: 82–108.

Cohen S, Williamson GM (1991) Stress and infectious disease in humans. Psychological Bulletin 109: 5–24.

Cooper CL, Watson M (1991) Cancer and Stress: Psychological, Biological and Coping Studies. Chichester: Wiley.

Costa PT Jr, McCrae RR (1994). Set like plaster? Evidence for the stability of adult personality. In T Heatherton, J Weinberger (eds) Can Personality Change? Washington DC: American Psychological Association.

Cox T (1978) Stress. London: Macmillan.

Dattore PJ, Shontz FC, Coyne L (1980) Premorbid personality differentiation of cancer and non-cancer groups: a list of the hypotheses of cancer proneness. Journal of Consulting and Clinical Psychology 48: 388–94.

Deary IJ, Blenkin H, Agius RM, Endler NS, Zealley H, Wood R (1996). Models of job-related stress and personal achievement among consultant doctors. British Journal of Psychology 87: 3–29.

Duffy E (1962) Activation and Behavior. New York: Wiley.

Easterbrook, JA (1959) The effect of emotion on cue utilization and the organization of behavior. Psychological Review 66: 183–201.

Edelmann RJ (1992) Anxiety: Theory, Research and Intervention in Clinical and Health Psychology. Chichester: Wiley.

Ellis A (1962) Reason and Emotion in Psychotherapy. New York: Lyle Stuart.

Ekman P, Levenson RW, Friesen WV (1983) Autonomic nervous system activity distinguishes among emotions. Science 221: 1208–10.

Endler N, Parker J (1990) Multi dimensional assessment of coping: a critical review. Journal of Personality and Social Psychology 58: 844–54.

Eysenck HJ (1988) The respective importance of personality, cigarette smoking and interaction effects for the genesis of cancer and coronary heart disease. Personality and Individual Differences 9: 453–64.

Eysenck MW (1982) Attention and Arousal: Cognition and Performance. New York: Springer.

Eysenck MW (1992) Anxiety: The Cognitive Perspective. Hillsdale NJ: Erlbaum.

Eysenck MW, Calvo MG (1992) Anxiety and performance: the processing efficiency theory. Cognition and Emotion 6: 409–34.

Fahrenberg J, Walschburger P, Foerster F, Myrtek M, Müller W (1983) An evaluation of trait, state, and reaction aspects of activation processes. Psychophysiology 20: 188–95.

Fisher S (1986) Stress and Strategy. Hillsdale NJ: Erlbaum.

Fontana D (1989) Managing Stress. Leicester: British Psychological Society.

Forgas JP, Bower GH (1987) Affect in social and personal judgements. In K Fiedler, J Forgas (eds) Affect, Cognition and Social Behavior: New Evidence and Integrative Attempts. Lewiston NY: Hogrefe, pp. 183–208.

Friedman HS (ed.) (1990) Personality and Disease. New York: Wiley.

Gold PW, Goodwin FK, Chrousos GP (1988) Clinical and biochemical manifestations of depression: relation to the neurobiology of stress (part 1). New England Journal of Medicine 314: 1329–35.

Gray JA (1987) The psychology of fear and stress (2 edn). Cambridge UK: Cambridge University Press.

Hall NR, Goldstein AL (1981) Neurotransmitters and the immune system. In R Ader (ed.) Psychoneuroimmunology. New York: Academic Press.

Hancock PA (1986) Sustained attention under thermal stress. Psychological Bulletin 99: 263–81.

Hockey GRJ (1984) Varieties of attentional state: The effects of the environment. In R Parasuraman, DR Davies (eds) Varieties of Attention. New York: Academic.

Holmes TH, Rahe RH (1967) The social readjustment rating scale. Journal of Psychomatic Research 11: 213–18.

Hurrell JJ Jr, Murphy LR (1991) Locus of control, job demands, and health. In CL Cooper, R Payne (eds) Personality and Stress: Individual Differences in the Stress Process. Chichester: Wiley.

Jacobson E (1938) Progressive Relaxation: A Physiological and Clinical Ivestigation of Muscle States and their Significance in Psychology and Medical Practice (2 edn). Chicago: University of Chicago Press.

James W (1890) The Principles of Psychology. New York: Henry Holt.

Jemmott JB III, Magloire K (1988) Academic stress, social support, and secretory immunoglobulin A. Journal of Personality and Social Psychology 55: 803–10.

Kavanagh DJ (1992) Recent developments in expressed emotion and schizophrenia. British Journal of Psychiatry 160: 601–20.

Kemp-Wheeler SM, Hill AB (1987) Anxiety responses to subliminal experience of mild stress. British Journal of Psychology 78: 365–74.

Kirmayer LJ, Robbins JM, Paris J (1994) Somatoform disorders: personality and the social matrix of somatic distress. Journal of Abnormal Psychology 103: 125–36.

Kitayama S (1997) Affective influence in perception: Some implications of the amplification model. In G Matthews (ed.) Cognitive Science Perspectives on Personality and Emotion. Amsterdam: Elsevier Science.

Kohn PM (1996) On coping adaptively with daily hassles. In M Zeidner and NS Endler (eds) Handbook of Coping: Theory, Research, Application. New York: Wiley.

Krantz DS, Contrada RJ, Hill DR, Friedler E (1988) Environmental stress and biobehavioral antecedents of coronary heart disease. Journal of Consulting and Clinical Psychology 56: 333–41.

Laudenslager ML, Ryan SM, Drugan RC, Hyson RL, Maier SF (1983) Coping and immunosuppression: inescapable but not escapable shock suppresses lymphocyte proliferation. Science 221: 568–70.

Lavey RS, Taylor CG (1985) The nature of relaxation therapy. In SR Burchfield (ed.). Stress: Psychological and Physiological Interventions. Washington DC: Hemisphere.

Lazarus RS (1966) Psychological Stress and the Coping Process. New York: McGraw-Hill.

Lazarus RS (1984) On the primacy of cognition. American Psychologist 37: 1019–24.

Lazarus RS (1991) Emotion and Adaptation. Oxford: OUP.

Lazarus RS, Folkman S (1984) Stress, Appraisal and Coping. New York: Springer.

LeDoux JE (1994) Emotion, memory, and the brain. Scientific American (June): 32–9.

Leventhal H, Scherer KR (1987) The relationship of emotion to cognition: A functional approach to a semantic controversy. Cognition and Emotion 1: 3–28.

Loehlin JC (1992) Genes and Environment in Personality Development. Newbury Park CA: Sage.

MacLeod C, Mathews A (1991) Cognitive-experimental approaches to the emotional disorders. In PR Martin (ed.) Handbook of Behaviour Therapy and Psychological Science: An Integrative Approach. Oxford: Pergamon.

Maslach C (1982) Burnout: The Cost of Caring. Englewood Cliffs NJ: Prentice-Hall.

Matthews G (1992) Mood. In AP Smith DM Jones (eds) Handbook of Human Performance. Vol. 3. State and Trait. London: Academic.

Matthews G, Deary I (1998) Personality Traits. Cambridge: Cambridge University Press.

Matthews G, Gilliland K (1998) The personality theories of HJ Eysenck and JA Gray: a comparative review. Personality and Individual Differences.

Matthews G, Saklofske DH, Costa PT Jr, Deary IJ, Zeidner M (1998) Dimensional models of personality: a framework for systematic clinical assessment. European Journal of Psychological Assessment 14: 35–48.

Mauro R, Sato K, Tucker J (1992) The role of appraisal in human emotions: a cross-cultural study. Journal of Personality and Social Psychology 62: 301–17.

Meichenbaum D, Cameron R (1983) Stress inoculation training: toward a general paradigm for training coping skills. In D Meichenbaum, ME Jeremko (eds) Stress Reduction and Prevention. New York: Plenum.

Miller TQ, Smith TW, Turner CW, Guijarro ML, Hallet AJ (1996) A meta-analytic review of research on hostility and physical health. Psychological Bulletin 119: 322–48.

Mughal S, Walsh J, Wilding J (1996) Stress and work performance: the role of trait anxiety. Personality and Individual Differences 20: 685–91.

Neiss R (1988) Reconceptualizing arousal: psychobiological states in motor performance. Psychological Bulletin 103: 345–66.

Nezu AM, Nezu CM, Perri MG (1989) Problem-Solving Therapy for Depression: Theory, Research and Clinical Guidelines. New York: Wiley.

Norman DA, Bobrow DB (1975) On data-limited and resource-limited processes. Cognitive Psychology 7: 44–64.

O'Connor K (1985) A model of situational preference amongst smokers. Personality and Individual Differences 6: 151–60.

Pelosi AJ, Appleby L (1992) Psychological influences on cancer and ischaemic heart disease. British Medical Journal 303: 1295–8.

Rosenman RH, Brand R, Jenkins D, Friedman M, Straus R, Wurm M (1975). Coronary heart disease in the Western Collaborative Group Study: final follow-up of 8.5 years. Journal of the American Medical Association 233: 872–7.

Sarason IG (1984) Stress, anxiety, and cognitive interference: reactions to tests. Journal of Personality and Social Psychology 46: 929–38.

Sarason IG (1988) Anxiety, self-preoccupation and attention. Anxiety Research 1: 3–7.

Schachter S, Singer JE (1962) Cognitive, social and physiological determinants of emotional state. Psychological Review 69: 379–99.

Seligman MEP (1975) Helplessness: On Development, Depression and Death. San Francisco: Freeman.

Selye H (1976) The Stress of Life. New York: McGraw-Hill.

Selzer ML, Vinokur A (1975) Role of life events in accident causation. Mental Health and Society 2: 36–54.

Smith AP, Jones DM (eds) (1992) Handbook of Human Performance (3 vols). London: Academic.

Spielberger CD (1966) The effects of anxiety on complex learning and academic achievement. In CD Spielberger (ed.) Anxiety and Behavior. London: Academic Press.

Steptoe A (1991) Psychological coping, individual differences and physiological stress responses. In CL Cooper, R Payne (eds) Personality and Stress: Individual

Differences in the Coping Process. Chichester: Wiley.

Steptoe A, Wardle J (1996) The European Health and Behaviour Survey: The development of an international study in health psychology. Psychology and Health 11: 49–73.

Stone SV, Costa PT Jr (1990). Disease-prone personality or distress-prone personality? In HS Friedman (ed.) Personality and Disease. New York: Wiley.

Thayer RE (1978) Toward a psychological theory of multidimensional activation (arousal). Motivation and Emotion 2: 1–34.

Thayer RE (1996). The Origin of Everyday Moods. New York: Oxford University Press.

Ucros CG (1989) Mood state-dependent memory: a meta-analysis. Cognition and Emotion 3: 139–67.

Weiss JM (1972) Psychological factors in stress and disease. Scientific American 226: 104–13.

Wells A (1997) Cognitive Therapy of Anxiety Disorders: A Practice Manual and Conceptual Guide. Chichester: Wiley.

Wells A, Matthews G (1994) Attention and Emotion: A Clinical Perspective. Hove: Lawrence Erlbaum.

Yerkes RM, Dodson JD (1908) The relation of strength of stimulus to rapidity of habit-formation. Journal of Comparative Neurology and Psychology 18: 459–82.

Zajonc RB (1984) On the primacy of emotion. American Psychologist 39: 117–23.

Zajonc RB, Murphy ST, Inglehart M (1989) Feeling and facial efference: implications of the vascular theory of emotion. Psychological Review 96: 395–416.

Zeidner M, Saklofske D (1996) Adaptive and maladaptive coping. In M Zeidner, NS Endler (eds) Handbook of Coping: Theory, Research, Applications. New York: Wiley.

Chapter 9
Hypnosis and hypnotherapy

PETER DAVIES

Key concepts	Key names
Mesmerism	Mesmer
Hypnotism	Braid
Suggestibility theory	
Dissociation theory	
Reality testing	
Sleep theory	
Conditioning theory	
Role-play theory	
Altered states of consciousness theory	
Stages of hypnosis	
catalepsy	
amnesia	
hypermnesia	
forensic memory	
regression	
time distortion	
ideo-motor activity	
self hypnosis	
Uncovering and 'discovery' technique	
Regression and revivification techniques	
Behaviour therapy and progressive desensitization techniques	
Suggestion therapy	
Creative imagery techniques	
Cognitive therapy and neurolinguistic programming	

Introduction

Many people, from time immemorial, have practised hypnosis under many labels. It is often assumed to have originated with the work of Mesmer in the late eighteenth century – work that was based on underlying assumptions of 'animal magnetism' and the influence of the heavenly bodies. However, 'Mesmerism' was primarily non-verbal with 'suggestion' based upon patients' expectations and Mesmer's personal reputation.

The father of modern hypnotism is generally assumed to be the Scottish physician James Braid who became interested in mesmerism in 1841 when he attended a demonstration in Manchester. Braid rejected the mysterious and occult elements, and based his views on clinical observation and experiment. It was he who coined the word 'hypnotism' from the Greek word *hypnos* and thus inadvertently originated the misconception that hypnosis is somehow connected to sleep.

It is the author's contention that hypnosis is not therapeutic in or of itself. It is a vehicle for therapies, and it is the therapeutic content that makes hypnotherapy a powerful intervention technique. Any therapy that can be used with a hypnotized patient can be used without hypnotizing the patient. The hypnotized patient is extraordinarily open to suggestion and therapeutic suggestions are usually readily accepted and acted upon. However, most modern hypnosis involves profound relaxation, and the relaxation alone may have therapeutic benefit for some patients.

Theories of hypnosis

There are a number of theories of hypnosis. They cannot all be correct, but it has proved to be virtually impossible for any experiment to be performed that would conclusively evaluate them. Each theory has its origin in the explanation of a particular type of hypnosis and the phenomena associated with it.

Fortunately it is possible to practise hypnosis from a pragmatic viewpoint without total adherence to any one theoretical stance. Nevertheless, most practitioners have some implicit theoretical assumptions, often of an eclectic nature, which inform their approach.

Suggestibility theory

According to the proponents of suggestibility theory, the subject's attention is focused upon the words of the hypnotist, thereby narrowing the subject's span of attention. The subject suspends 'reality testing' and uncritically accepts the voice of the hypnotist in place of his or her own inner voice.

It should be appreciated that this is not an explanation – more a description of what it is like to be hypnotized. Suggestibility does not explain the spontaneous occurrence of hypnotic phenomena such as amnesia or hallucinations. It would, of course, explain such phenomena when the hypnotist suggests them.

Perhaps the greatest weakness of this theory is that it implies that only 'the suggestible', or the weak and gullible, should be capable of being hypnotized. This is not the case. It would also imply that the hypnotist ought to be able to make any suggestion to the subject and expect it to be accepted. This also is not the case, and any suggestions contrary to the subject's own ethical or moral code will not be accepted and often lead to the abrupt cessation of the hypnotic state.

Sleep theory

As stated above, the choice of the word 'hypnosis' derived from the Greek word for sleep, is partially responsible for the belief that hypnosis is in some way allied to sleep. Some practitioners refer to hypnosis as 'the sleep of the nervous system'. Most inductions involve eye closure, and the hypnotized person is often immobile. However, even casual observation of any stage performance shows that hypnosis may be maintained in mobile, active, walking, talking subjects with their eyes open.

There are numerous studies that show that the physiological indices of the hypnotized subject such as blood pressure, reflexes, and electroencephalogram (EEG) recordings more closely resemble those of a person who is awake than one who is asleep. The EEG closely resembles that of an awake person actively involved in problem solving. (The waking EEG is characterized by beta waves, and is a very dense trace with moderate amplitude. Sleeping EEGs vary with the stage of sleep, but in all cases individual peaks and troughs can be detected, and during deep sleep the EEG is characterized by delta waves of considerable amplitude.)

When people sleep they become less attentive, not more. Moreover, people who are asleep do not usually respond to, nor retain, suggestions. Sleep learning is just not effective as it lacks the active involvement of the learner's brain. However, hypnotized subjects are very aware of their environment, especially those parts to which the hypnotist draws attention. Hypnosis, apart from some superficial similarities such as eye closure and low mobility, has no relation to sleep.

Dissociation theory

The fundamental assumption of dissociation theory is that hypnosis abolishes volitional control and certain areas of behaviour are split off from the normal stream of awareness. As a consequence, the individual responds with autonomic behaviour at the reflex level.

Dissociation is not unique to hypnosis. It occurs in other states of consciousness such as dreaming and reverie as well as in some of the more intense forms of religious worship.

Conditioning theory

Classical conditioning is a process whereby the response elicited by a particular stimulus is transferred by a process of association to a different stimulus. According to the conditioning theory of hypnosis, the various phenomena of hypnosis are responses not originally elicited by words, but which, by training, come to be elicited by them.

The key to this process is to be found in Pavlov's notion of 'the second signalling system', whereby words take on the role of acting as symbols for primary environmental events that, otherwise, provide the stimuli for conditioned responses. Thus human beings have the unique ability to form conditioned responses to both external stimuli (first signalling system) and their verbal referents (second signalling system). A word, acting as signal or cue, could come to act as the stimulus for a conditioned response that would become involuntary for life.

This view serves as an explanation for many re-inductions of hypnosis through post-hypnotic suggestion. The words cues, or signals certainly appear to act as conditioned stimuli to re-establish a state of hypnosis in a previously hypnotized individual, and such suggestions certainly retain their effectiveness for more than a decade.

The major weakness of the conditioning theory of hypnosis is that in order to establish the necessary associations between the words and the hypnotic behaviour, it would be necessary to induce hypnosis first. Thus, although conditioning probably plays a role in maintaining and re-inducing hypnosis, it cannot have any role in the initial induction process.

Role-play theory

Reduced to its essentials, this theory would suggest that there is no such thing as hypnosis, and that the subject enters into a role to play the part of hypnotized subject 'as if hypnotized'. It reduces hypnosis to a particularly complex form of social interaction in which the social expectations of both hypnotist and subject can be played out; the subject simulates hypnosis.

It cannot be doubted that there are elements of role playing in hypnosis, especially when dealing with voluntary behaviour. In many situations the simulating person is indistinguishable from one who is hypnotized. However, it is difficult to see that role playing and simulation offer any explanation for hypnotically induced anaesthesia. There are many reports of major surgery, including amputations, being conducted with the patient reporting no pain.

Altered state of consciousness theory

A number of hypnotists attempt to explain hypnosis in terms of an altered state of consciousness. Much the same 'explanation' could be given for meditation or yoga. This theory is more descriptive than explanatory.

Hypnosis as a state

The central tenet is that of the 'trance' state, or the hypnotic trance. This is no explanation of how such a state is reached, but is a powerful description of the way in which many hypnotized subjects behave.

Summary

There is no single satisfactory theory of hypnosis. The majority of such theories are descriptive. Moreover, no single theory accounts for all types of hypnosis or the full range of hypnotic phenomena. Typically each theory has been a product of its time, with each theory being more or less congruent with its *zeitgeist*. Conditioning and physiological explanations came early, the altered state and trance theories were contemporaneous with the Western interest in Eastern meditation, and role play echoes the rise of social psychology as psychology in general has shifted its centre of gravity away from its psychophysical origins.

Depth of hypnosis

At one level it is scientifically meaningless to talk of 'the depth of hypnosis'. There is no unique physiological or behavioural index that such a state exists.

However, whatever our difficulties in explaining the nature of hypnosis, both the good hypnotic subject and observers would agree that hypnosis exists, and that different levels of hypnosis are attainable.

Terminology varies but generally five or six depths of hypnosis have been identified, with three of these being of clinical significance:

- insusceptible;
- hypnoidal (a precursor to the hypnotic state);
- light hypnosis;
- medium hypnosis;
- deep hypnosis;
- somnambulism.

Of the above only light, medium and deep hypnosis levels have clinical implications as the somnambulistic level necessarily implies a very deep level of hypnosis. This is of more relevance in the context of stage hypnosis and entertainment.

The various depths of hypnosis can be approached in two ways. Firstly, there are various tests of hypnotic susceptibility that purport to identify the susceptibility (or suggestibility) of individual subjects. A number of test items are administered, and the scores for the individual items are summated to arrive at an overall score, which indicates the 'hypnotizability' of the individual subject. Secondly, the depth of hypnotizability actually achieved by any individual can be deduced from observable behaviours.

Note 1: The author has identified a problem with the susceptibility scale approach. Such scales tend to serve as self-fulfilling prophecies and subjects who achieve only a low score tend to achieve only the lightest levels of hypnosis. If the overall test score is ignored, and the induction process is centred on only the item, or items, where the subject scored highly then such subjects go on to reach deeper levels of hypnosis than the summated score would indicate.

Note 2: The utility of susceptibility scales in clinical practice is also questionable. Apart from the fact that they may become self-fulfilling prophecies, the clinician faced with a single client is more concerned with utilizing whatever level of hypnosis is available than making a comparative judgement about the client's potential for hypnosis. It is not possible to select only the most susceptible as clients!

Nevertheless, the administration of a test of hypnotic suggestibility can have advantages for the relatively inexperienced therapist. If while administering the test it is noticed that the subject is becoming hypnotized then it is possible to abandon the test and move into a full induction. If this is successful the therapist can then say, 'I was testing you, but it was so obvious that you were an excellent subject that I abandoned the test', and if the induction fails he can claim, 'I am only testing'. This can be a marvellous face saver!

Light hypnosis

The subject is likely to exhibit eye closure following suitable suggestions as part of an induction process conducted by an experienced hypnotist. The hypnotist may go on to suggest that the eyes are locked tightly shut, and that the subject cannot open them. This is known as the 'eye catalepsy challenge'; typical wording might be, 'your eyes are locking tightly shut, and even if you were to try to open them, you will find them locking even more tightly shut. Now try to open your eyes'. The subject in a state of light hypnosis is likely to be able to open their eyes when challenged to do so.

The general appearance of the subject is likely to be that of a relaxed person, and no hypnotic phenomena are likely to be elicited.

Medium hypnosis

Subjects will accept an eye catalepsy challenge and be unable to open their eyes within the two or three seconds usually allowed for this test. Some hypnotic phenomena are likely to be elicited, such as time distortion, ideo-motor activity, waxy flexibility of the limbs, and suggestions of limb catalepsy.

Deep hypnosis

Virtually all of the hypnotic phenomena are available in a deeply hypnotized subject, although not all subjects are equally likely to demonstrate all the phenomena to an equal extent. The subject appears to be profoundly relaxed, and responsive only to the suggestions of the hypnotist.

Depth and therapy

It is not essential that the subject should be in a deep level of hypnosis in order to conduct therapy. Even the lightest level of hypnosis is sufficient for therapeutic suggestions to be given. In the author's opinion it is questionable as to whether the prognosis for successful therapy is dependent upon the level of hypnosis attainable. Assuming that the subject's attention is focused, there is much to be said for making therapeutic suggestions when the subject is in a relatively light state of hypnosis and more likely to engage normal cognitive processes. The deeper stages of hypnosis can then be used to reduce interference (a well-known process inhibiting memory) and to reward the subject by going to a deep level of hypnosis that is usually experienced as being extremely pleasant and totally relaxing. However, therapeutic suggestions given to a subject in a very deep stage of hypnosis (if attainable) are usually very effective. Depth is not a prerequisite for effective therapy; do not give up merely because the subject can only achieve a light stage of hypnosis.

Hypnotic phenomena

Catalepsy

The subject will accept suggestions that designated muscle groups will not work and they will find it impossible to open the eyes or move a limb if this is suggested to them. An allied phenomenon is the waxy flexibility that a subject in medium to deep hypnosis will demonstrate. If a limb is moved into some other position it will move without resistance, and upon release either fall back to its original position without any obvious signs of control, or stay in the position in which it is placed according to the suggestions of the hypnotist.

The eye catalepsy test is especially useful as a means of convincing the subject that they are hypnotized. If they are instructed to try to open their eyes and then fail to do so, they are likely to accept that they have been hypnotized. This test is also useful for reassuring the hypnotist that the subject is hypnotized.

Amnesia

If a deep state of hypnosis is achieved, this may occur spontaneously. Normally it will not, but if a medium/deep, or deep, state of hypnosis has been achieved it can be suggested to the subject. The amnesia may be for selected information, such as 'you will forget your date of birth', or all or part of the hypnotic session. Profound amnesia has little or no clinical relevance, though it may be useful to induce it if the session has uncovered repressed material that might disturb the patient.

The deliberate induction of amnesia may be a part of various thera-peutic interventions involving repressing or forgetting anxiety-provoking material. A typical suggestion would be something like, 'lock all these anxieties in this box, and put the box under one of the large stones on the beach. You can even forget which stone you put it under. You will never be troubled by these thoughts again'. If given at the appropriate stage of therapy, such a suggestion can be surprisingly effective.

Hypermnesia and forensic memory

Hypnosis may help in recalling events that have been repressed. It may also help with the recall of material that has been forgotten; however, the hypnotized subject is, by definition, in a highly suggestible state and no forensic reliability should be attached to material recalled in this way. Hypnosis may aid the learning of material, and the recall of material learned under hypnosis. However, there is little reliable evidence that hypnosis actually improves the memory for normally encountered events.

Analgesia

Hypnosis has a long history in the realms of analgesia and anaesthesia. In 1842 W.S. Ward amputated a leg of a patient who was in a mesmeric trance. The patient reported that he felt no pain, and Ward reported the case to the Royal Medical and Chirurgical Society.

Elliotson was involved in the opening of a mesmeric infirmary in London in 1849 and subsequently reported over 200 painless operations under hypnosis.

Esdaile (1808–59) was practising in India and reported about 300 major operations and innumerable minor ones performed with the patients in a mesmeric trance.

The induction of *glove anaesthesia* is often used as indicative of deep hypnosis. The entire hand can be made numb, 'wooden-like', and as insensitive to pain as if an anaesthetic had been injected. The technique not only serves as a test of the depth of hypnosis but it also has a wide range of applications in clinical hypnosis. Often the technique is to induce glove anaesthesia and demonstrate this to the subject before transferring the insensitivity to some other part of the body that is of interest.

Regression

Two forms of regression may be achieved under hypnosis. Firstly there is regression to an earlier period in life when, for example, the subject may have felt happier and more in control of his or her life. Secondly, there is age regression when the subject is regressed to some specified age.

Age-regressed subjects will typically talk and write like a child of the age suggested to them, however, it would be imprudent to assume that such regressions are accurate reconstructions of the subject at that age. It is quite likely that subjects role play on the basis of their adult knowledge of childrens' behaviour.

It is probably unwise to rely upon any regression that involves the subject regressing below the age of two years, and even then it is wise to be sceptical. However, if the subject genuinely believes in the regressed material then this is their subjective reality, and subjective reality is reality as far as the subject is concerned. It is for this reason that age regression can be a useful tool for examining the origins of behavioural problems.

Past and previous life regressions should be eschewed. They almost certainly have no basis in fact. Subjects can also be progressed to future lives when they will also give apparently convincing demonstrations of lives yet to be lived. To accept these as genuine involves accepting some advanced conceptions as to the nature of space/time itself.

False memory syndrome has been a topic of concern. Hypnosis is not essential for the creation of false memories, or 'recovered memories' as they as sometimes called. However, hypnotized subjects are, almost by definition, in a highly suggestible state and are very likely to accept most suggestions put to them. Scotford (1995) notes, 'false accusations arising out of recovered memory therapy are primarily the product of questionable techniques used by over-zealous, and frequently poorly trained, "therapists", including those employing hypnosis'. McCann and Sheehan (1989) anticipate much of the debate surrounding false memory syndrome. Perhaps the most significant words in their paper are, 'hypnotic subjects . . . invested their most distorted responses with the strongest confidence reports'.

The only possible conclusion is that no reliance should be put upon hypnosis when investigating a client's history. Certainly, any information gleaned with the client under hypnosis is likely to be tainted by responses to implicit or explicit suggestions arising from the procedure itself.

Much of the false memory syndrome saga has revolved around alleged sexual assault. We have seen that hypnosis can be employed to create false memories. A related question is whether it can be used to further sexual assault.

Unfortunately, no unequivocal answer can be given. Allegations of sexual assault, up to and including rape, under hypnosis are common. It is a wise precaution to remember this when using hypnosis with a patient and to ensure that there is some independent witness or record of each session.

However, there is no absolute test to demonstrate that a person is in a state of hypnosis; moreover, complainants may have complex motives. Heap (1995) considers a case of indecent assault by a lay hypnotherapist. His analysis is complex and comprehensive and outlines five possibilities ranging from the complainant being hypnotized to the complainant indulging in fantasy.

Time distortion

Time distortion is a common and easily demonstrated hypnotic phenomenon. Subjective estimates of elapsed time can be either lengthened or contracted according to the suggestions given. In the absence of suggestions, subjects are likely to underestimate the time spent in hypnosis.

Ideo-motor activity

It is perfectly possible for a hypnotized subject to walk, talk, and write just like a normally conscious person. However, some schools of thought would suggest that there are advantages in communicating with the hypnotized subject while bypassing cognitive involvement. Such communications involve ideo-motor activity.

A common method is to suggest that one of the subject's fingers will move to indicate agreement, and that a different finger will move to indicate disagreement. When the first suggestion is made the subject is observed carefully and when a finger moves this act is commented upon and confirmed as signifying agreement. The same is done to identify the disagreement signal.

Once these signals have been established it is possible to ask questions requiring 'yes/no' answers of the subject. The subject will move his or her fingers in reply. However, on the termination of the hypnosis session subjects will typically have no recollection of having done so, or even of which fingers they were using to signal.

An alternative approach uses Chevreul's pendulum, typically a piece of cut rock crystal on a fine chain, which the subject holds. The suggestions are that it will swing in one direction to indicate agreement, at right angles to this direction to signify disagreement, and swing in a circular path to indicate uncertainty. This approach introduces rather more flexibility because of the range of answers available, however it has no other advantages.

Hallucinations

Hallucinations may be either positive or negative. A positive hallucination is when the subject reports or responds to the presence of something that is not present, whereas a negative hallucination results in the subject not reporting or responding to something that is actually present. Hallucinations may be induced in most modalities but are commonly visual, auditory, or gustatory. The feeling of alcohol intoxication following the ingestion of water is one of the easiest hallucinations to induce. Visually the subject may hallucinate people who are not present, or 'see through' people or objects that are present. Most stage shows make considerable use of hallucinations, often providing the subject with special spectacles that make other participants or members of the audience appear naked.

On the whole there are relatively few clinical applications for the hallu-cinations although feeling of premature repletion may help with food intake problems, and the induced alcohol intoxication may help in the reduction of actual alcohol intake when treating alcohol-dependent subjects, or those people who drink in order to acquire the confidence to face social situations. A smaller intake can be made to produce the required effect. This intervention is far more likely to succeed, and is far less threatening to the confirmed alcoholic, than any attempt to actually eliminate all drinking. It is the author's opinion that Alcoholics Anonymous would attract far more people if it offered a programme to control drinking rather than only one to terminate it.

Preparing the patient for hypnosis

Before any hypnosis or hypnotherapy is commenced it is essential to carry out the normal case evaluation that would be done prior to any therapy. If hypnosis is going to be used then further procedures must be adopted.

Pre-induction preparation

Most people are anxious about the idea of hypnosis and fear loss of control. If a person has been hypnotized before these fears will be greatly reduced but it would be unwise to assume that they are absent. A good starting point is to ask whether the patient has been hypnotized before, and how he or she found the experience. If the subject had a good experi-ence the rest of this section is of limited relevance. Asking how they were hypnotized, and then using the same method, can save much time. After all, they know that this method works for them.

If patients have not been hypnotized before, then it is a good idea to ask them what they believe hypnosis to be like. Listen carefully to their account and make a note of any misconceptions that can be corrected later.

If they have no specific expectations, or their only experience is of having seen a stage show, then hypnosis must be explained in some detail. The following checklist of points indicates the more important topics to be covered:

- Being hypnotized is not surrendering complete control to the hypnotist.
- The subject is in control. If the hypnotist suggests anything that is contrary to their moral or ethical beliefs they can come out of hypnosis at any time.
- Being hypnotized feels rather like being in a daydream. It is usually described as being a pleasant and relaxing experience. Most people enjoy it.
- In a state of hypnosis you are fully aware of everything going on around you. You can hear quite normally, and you will find that you think quite

normally. However, you may find that although you know exactly what is going on, it all seems rather too much trouble to do anything about it.

- However, despite these feelings, the hypnotist cannot make you do anything against your will.
- The hypnotist cannot force you to be hypnotized. It should be stressed that only you have the ability to hypnotize yourself. The hypnotist will help you to do this.
- You should not try to make anything happen; equally do not stop anything happening. All you have to do is to listen to the hypnotist and concentrate on what is said.
- Is there anything else that you would like me to explain to you? Have you any other questions?

Misconceptions

If your subject has any misconceptions about the nature of hypnosis they must be dealt with before an induction is attempted. This is imperative if the session is to be successful. Even if you think that you have dealt with all the possible misconceptions before starting an induction, it is possible that the patient's behaviour will indicate that at least one remains. Stop the induction process immediately, and deal with the problem.

Perhaps the most common misconception (after the fear of loss of control) is for subjects to expect hypnosis to be a totally novel experience, unlike anything they have experienced before. Subjects who expect too much are the subjects who are later going to claim that they were not hypnotized.

It should be made clear to the patient that hypnosis is rather similar to a state of deep reverie, or total absorption in a book, film or play. The outside world is still available to consciousness, especially if some unexpected event or emergency arises. However, under normal circumstances it is easy to disregard distracting influences. If their expectations are correct then there is a much greater likelihood of a successful hypnosis session.

Resistance

Resistance is most likely to be encountered during the induction phase. It most often arises as a consequence of some misconception regarding either the type of person who is susceptible to hypnosis, or the nature of hypnosis.

Many people equate hypnotizability with gullibility, a lack of will, or imbecility. To combat such resistance it is necessary to address these misconceptions and to point out that highly intelligent, self-motivating, people are usually excellent subjects. They generally have the ability to concentrate and focus their attention in the way required to induce hypnosis in themselves.

Another common form of resistance arises when the subject chooses to challenge or defy the hypnotist, a sort of 'go on then, hypnotize me'.

This attitude can be triggered by the hypnotist using a direct and authoritarian approach. It is usually better to frame all suggestions in an indirect and permissive manner that offers the subject fewer opportunities to challenge them.

To say 'you will close your eyes' is to invite the subject to resist; to say 'you may find that you wish to close your eyes' is far less threatening and allows for the possibility that the subject may choose not to close his or her eyes at that time. If you regard the eye closure as important, you can always come back to it later with a suggestion such as, 'by now, your eyes are probably feeling tired. You would possibly find that they would feel more comfortable if you were to close them'.

Much resistance can often be overcome by reminding subjects that only they can induce their own hypnosis; nobody else can force them to be hypnotized. It is a reasonable assumption that any patient seeking treatment has the motivation to be hypnotized and any resistance to hypnosis can usually be overcome. Where the hypnosis is being undertaken for reasons other than treatment – such as research – this motivation cannot be assumed to exist, and resistance may be harder to overcome.

When handling resistance it is of paramount importance that the hypnotist does not become either angry or impatient. The problem almost certainly lies with some failure of communication rather than with the patient *per se.*

When the communication problems have been sorted out, it is often a good idea to change the method. There are many ways of inducing hypnosis. For example, it is possible that the method first selected involved visual imagery and that the subject is a poor visualizer. Changing to a method involving no imagery may be all that it takes to bring about a satisfactory induction.

Even if the original method did not involve a mismatch with the subject's abilities, it is still a good idea to change the method so that the points where resistance was encountered initially do not recur. Otherwise renewed resistance may be triggered by the process of conditioning. Ideally the new method will be totally different and the subject will progress to a hypnotic state without further problems.

Conditions for hypnotherapeutic work

Hypnosis can be carried out anywhere, but if the purpose is routine therapy (rather than some emergency intervention) it is best to select some quiet and formal environment. It is important that there are no idle onlookers as they will only serve to make the person feel self-conscious. The presence of another person in some formal role such as nurse or secretary will normally not have this effect and can actually be beneficial.

The therapist may also feel more confident when treating a person of the opposite gender if another person is present as an impartial observer (see the later section on the dangers of hypnosis).

Whenever possible a chair offering good support for the patient and the patient's head should be provided. A couch can be used, but the prone position tends to emphasize the power asymmetry between patient and therapist and thus inhibit the establishment of good rapport.

The presence of such a chair in addition to alternative seating arrangements can be an aid to successful induction. If all the pre-induction conversation, the initial discussion with the patient, the taking of the case notes, the explanation of hypnosis, and dealing with misconceptions, takes place in another chair the subject can be told, 'when you are ready to be hypnotized, go and sit in that chair'. An alternative approach is to introduce the idea of a special chair for hypnosis early in the discussion with the words 'you will not be hypnotized until you sit in that chair'. Both techniques can be combined.

When subjects go to sit in the designated chair they have an expectation of hypnosis and are signifying that they are ready to be hypnotized.

It is preferable for the chosen environment to be quiet and undisturbed. However, this cannot always be achieved and some externally originating noise may have to be tolerated. If this is the case then such noise can be built into the procedure. The subject can be told that the noise will not bother them and, because it does not concern them, they can ignore it. Some external noise can even be turned to advantage: 'whenever you hear the telephone next door ring, you will go deeper into hypnosis, even deeper than before'.

Ethical considerations

The dangers of hypnosis: dangers to the subject

Many people exaggerate the dangers of hypnosis. Hypnosis itself is not dangerous – there is no chance that anybody can 'get stuck' in hypnosis, nor can any physical or mental harm become them. The dangers lie in what is done in hypnosis with the principal dangers being the use of badly or carelessly worded post-hypnotic suggestions. Post-hypnotic suggestions are suggestions given to the subject during hypnosis with the intention that they should be acted upon at a later date when the subject is no longer in hypnosis. A necessary consequence is that the therapist will not usually be present when such suggestions are acted upon.

All post-hypnotic suggestions should be worded carefully to ensure that they will not expose the recipient to unintentional harm. They should contain constraints as to time, place, and circumstance. For example, one patient was given a cassette tape to help combat the desire to smoke. No constraint was put upon where this tape should be used, and the patient put the tape into his car's cassette player while driving. He then complained that he had had to pull off the road because he found his eyes closing!

Clearly he should have been told not to use the tape in his car whilst driving. However, even more importantly, the original suggestion that this tape would help re-create the calm relaxation of the therapeutic session and remove his desire to smoke should have contained a rider that the tape would not do this when played in his car.

Another danger is to use post-hypnotic suggestions that are over inclusive. The suggestion that 'the smell of tobacco smoke will be nauseous' may be an effective way of putting somebody off smoking, but if such a suggestion were to be effective it would expose the unfortunate individual to feelings of nausea whenever he or she encountered any other person's tobacco smoke.

All post-hypnotic suggestions for the re-induction of hypnosis need constraints as to when and where they should be employed, and who should employ them. Ideally they should also incorporate an element of personal control. A safe and ethical suggestion would be something like, 'when we are working together in this room, and only when you wish to do so, you will go into a deeply relaxed state when I say . . .'. Worded in this way the situation the suggestion is limited to therapeutic sessions in a given room and to the person giving the chosen signal, and the suggestion will only be effective if the subject wants to go into hypnosis at that time.

Dangers to the therapist

Probably the greatest danger to the therapist is to his or her own ego. It is easy to forget that the hypnotist only possesses skills and not powers. It is not possible to say that you will induce hypnosis any more than it is possible to claim that the therapy will be effective. It does not matter how effective the induction procedure normally is, nor how effective the therapy has normally been, some people are not susceptible to hypnosis and some of those who are do not benefit from the therapy that you associate with it.

Such failures can be dangerous if therapists have foolishly come to believe in their own infallibility. The failure undermines their confidence, and as subjects take their confidence from the therapist's confidence this makes future failures even more likely. The author knew one quite competent hypnotist who entered such a downward spiral after guaranteeing to hypnotize a person who had failed to achieve hypnosis with other people. The resulting failure so undermined his confidence that he finally gave up using hypnosis altogether.

If you accept that it is the subject who is responsible for his or her own hypnosis this danger is circumvented. The occasional failure is of little consequence. All you have to do is to review your choice and use of techniques. Provided these were appropriate, any failure is the responsibility of the subject and you live to fight another day.

Another very real danger is the occasional person who wants to use the hypnosis session for their own purposes, to use 'being hypnotized' as an excuse or justification for antisocial or exhibitionist behaviour. No specific method can be recommended for dealing with these cases as they are so varied. As a general rule, it can be assumed that as you talked the person into a state of hypnosis, you can equally quickly talk them out of hypnosis again and thus terminate the session. After appropriate discussion it should be possible to resume the session, but probably with a considerable shift of emphasis to incorporate the aberrant behaviour.

Possibly the greatest danger to the hypnotherapist is that of suggestions of indecent assault or sexual harassment. Working with an impartial observer present or within call is one safeguard. An alternative is to tape record the session but note that the subject's permission should be obtained prior to any recording.

Contraindications for the use of hypnosis

Hypnotherapy should not be offered where a patient rejects hypnosis for reasons of prejudice or on religious grounds.

Hypnotherapy is not appropriate where the patient exhibits florid psychosis or other severe disturbance of personality.

Hypnotherapy is probably unwise where the person has a tendency to blame others for his or her problems. The patient is likely to merely transfer responsibility to the hypnotherapist!

Some people are not susceptible to hypnosis. This group would include very young children, people of any age of unusually low intelligence, anybody with an attention deficit disorder, and the elderly who show signs of senility. There is also a type of person who is highly intelligent and introspective who analyses his or her own feelings. Each time they detect any change from their normal state of mind, any new physical sensation, such people shift their attention away from the hypnotist to analyse themselves. There is no way to detect these people in advance, but so long as they persist in this type of behaviour they remain intractable.

A pragmatic contraindication for the use of hypnotherapy might well be where the subject is only able to achieve hypnosis with considerable difficulty and takes a long time to induce. With such a subject it is unlikely that it will be possible to establish a post-hypnotic suggestion for reinduction, in which case too large a proportion of the therapeutic time allotted will have to be devoted to establishing hypnosis. As the hypnosis is not, in itself, therapeutic it may be sensible to eschew hypnosis and deliver the therapy in some other way.

Duration of therapy

It is impossible to be dogmatic as to how long therapy should be for any given patient. There is a danger of therapy becoming open-ended unless the likely duration is established at the outset. Many people find hypnosis exceedingly pleasant and will return as often as they can.

In general, most conditions can be treated in five to seven sessions with the spacing of those sessions relating to the nature of the condition; however, many therapists choose to use more sessions. There cannot be any hard-and-fast rule as much depends upon the chosen therapeutic strategy and the needs of the individual patient.

Problems of long standing, such as obesity and changing eating habits, which can only improve slowly, may best be approached with fairly widely spaced treatment sessions. However, many problems such as anxieties and phobias may respond better to short but intensive treatment with goals set between each session.

It is important to guard against the therapy becoming a crutch for the patient, who then becomes reliant on regular and continuing therapeutic sessions. Any such open-ended commitment is not therapeutically valid. If patients actively enjoy the hypnosis sessions they have no real motivation to address the original problem. A possible solution is to set a target for the number of sessions to be given, and to teach the patient self-hypnosis.

Self-hypnosis as a means of reducing the number of therapeutic sessions

It is hard to learn to hypnotize oneself. There are a number of reasons for this, but a major one is that it is extremely difficult to know that hypnosis has been achieved. However, it is very easy to teach people to hypnotize themselves. Once they have been hypnotized, and thus know what the end state feels like, all that needs to be done is to give them a post-hypnotic suggestion that when they carry out some act (such as closing their eyes and counting backwards from 10) they will re-establish a hypnotic state similar to that experienced in the therapeutic sessions. A few practice sessions are needed, and patients need to be reassured that they can set an appropriate time limit for their hypnosis. They must also be given the suggestion that they will come out of hypnosis at any time if any emergency should arise, or if anything else demands their immediate attention.

Supplementing therapeutic sessions with tape recordings

Using self-hypnosis is an effective way of shortening the therapeutic programme. An alternative is to record the penultimate therapeutic session and to give the patient the tape so that the patient can try it out before the final session. Patients may find some problem with the tape, something not quite right for them, and then the tape can be remade during the final session.

If a tape is used in this way, it is wise to suggest that it will diminish in effectiveness each time that it is used. The idea that the patient can ultimately do without the tape has to be implanted. Otherwise the day will come when the tape is lost or wears out and the patient will return for further therapy.

The use of pre-prepared, or general hypnosis tapes is not recommended. Despite their commercial success and wide availability there is little reason to believe that they are of genuine therapeutic value. Recording patients' own sessions, with their own therapists, provides many more cues for evoking the ambience of the original sessions.

Patient discharge

Patient discharge should be the goal from the first session. Typically a programme should be planned so that the first session establishes a post-hypnotic suggestion for future inductions thus freeing up the remaining sessions for therapy rather than hypnosis. During the first session the patient should be given some minor goal to achieve. The easier this is, the more effective it will be. If patients can see that they have responded in a positive way to the suggestions given under hypnosis then their confidence in the effectiveness of the treatment will be increased. It is far better to achieve a very small gain than to have an ambitious programme that is not working. For maximum effectiveness the patient needs to feel successful and in charge of their therapy. Moreover, at all times the patient needs to know how far they have progressed in their therapeutic programme. This knowledge can be motivating in that they are aware of progress having been made. Patients should be able to anticipate a time when they will be free of therapy and responsible for their own behaviour.

Some clinical applications of hypnotherapy

It should be stressed that there is no right way to approach any problem. Therapists are limited only by their own ingenuity and the needs of the patient. Perusal of journals such as the *European Journal of Clinical Hypnosis*, *American Journal of Clinical Hypnosis*, or *Contemporary Hypnosis* (the journal of the British Society of Experimental and Clinical Hypnosis) will reveal numerous accounts and case reports of individual therapies. A selection of different approaches is given below. The coverage of topics in these journals is very extensive and extended sampling will probably reveal a therapy for most conditions. The sample below merely seeks to illustrate the types of material to be found. Unfortunately, constraints of space prevent more than very brief outlines.

Agoraphobia

Hypnosis is ideal for developing scenarios in the imagination of the subjects. Agoraphobia has been treated successfully using the classic desensitization paradigm with a hierarchy of anxiety-provoking journeys being created in the patient's imagination. Anxiety ratings were noted, and no *in vivo* journeys were attempted until those for the imagined journeys were very low (Collins, 1996).

Anorexia

In a case where fear of growing up was identified as significant in the causation of the anorexia, an age regression technique was employed. An acceptable target weight was achieved in 11 weeks (Brooke and Garrett, 1996).

The treatment was behavioural/cognitive therapy with three distinct strands: 'symptom objectification' techniques (to attain control over symptoms), 'resourced maturation' (to achieve a 'grown-up' self-image); and restored awareness of homeostatic 'messaging' (to enhance personal autonomy). A significant part of the treatment was 'to dissociate and separate out the anorectic behaviour and mind-set from the client's sense of identity'. Put more simply, the client was encouraged to let the part of her mind that wanted to be normal 'talk' to the part of her mind that was maintaining the anorectic behaviour.

Bulimia nervosa

Bulimics are highly hypnotizable. Hypnosis has been used as part of a larger group therapy programme for cognitive rehearsal and imagery of dealing with difficult situations, as well as for forward projection to visualize the goal state (Degun-Mather, 1995).

Bruxism

Eight patients were treated using suggestions such as 'lips together, teeth apart' and with hot towels applied to the face. They were encouraged to visualize themselves as being in a dream. Objective measures such as EMG recording and audiotaping were also employed. The conclusions were that hypnosis can be an effective method for treating bruxism, and that the method is not very time consuming (Clarke and Reynolds, 1991).

Chemotherapy

Hypnosis has been employed to combat the side effects of chemotherapy (Alden, 1997; Bejenke, 1996). Many patients, prior to receiving chemotherapy, become anxious as a result of commonly circulating 'horror stories' of side effects.

There is no single therapeutic approach. Alden outlined the methods she adopted to treat needle phobia, nausea and vomiting, anxiety, the experience of chemotherapy itself, and beliefs about chemotherapy. Among the techniques mentioned are cognitive challenges, distraction techniques, hypnotic analgesia, dissociation, reframing and the restructuring of early trauma, and hypnotic desensitization.

However, in her abstract Alden notes, 'one should not lose sight of the need to prevent, rather than treat, psychological problems'. From knowledge of a previous study by Leslie Walker in Aberdeen, which sought to establish the effectiveness of hypnosis for treating chemotherapy side effects, the author can only conclude that what she is referring to is the importance of providing patients with very full information prior to treatment. In Walker's study none of the chemotherapy group reported nausea or vomiting, but neither did any of the control group who had only had the information without any hypnosis. This result does not invalidate the use of hypnosis; rather it emphasizes the role of careful and complete patient preparation.

Claustrophobia

This condition is almost certainly amenable to 'hypno-desensitization' in a manner similar to that given above for agoraphobia.

Claustrophobic patients are, in my experience, quite specific about the situations in which this affects them. A hierarchy of fear-producing situations should be produced, and work commenced by imagining the least fear provoking of these. When these situations can be imagined without overt anxiety it is time to progress up the hierarchy.

Impotence and frigidity

These conditions are frequently assumed to have a psychological origin, though this statement is more likely to be true of frigidity. Assuming that, following appropriate tests and clinical investigation, no underlying physiological nor hormonal problem has been identified, treatment for a psychological condition may be justified.

In both cases a plausible line of approach would be to utilize visualization techniques having first established an ideo-motor signalling system whereby the patient may communicate any feelings of anxiety. Essentially the treatment would be of the generic 'hypno-desensitization' variety with patients indicating when they felt the onset of anxiety.

The ultimate goal would be to visualize the complete sexual act without anxiety. A useful adjunct would be to establish some small physical act such as rubbing the thumb and forefinger together as an anchor for feelings of relaxation thereby providing patients with a means of reducing their anxiety at any time.

Not all cases have similar aetiologies. McGhie (1993) describes a case of impotence arising from childhood trauma, which appears to have centred around hearing, and then later seeing, his mother engaged in a sexual act. The therapy adopted focused on regression and a dream diary. Although the outcome is reported as being successful, there is inadequate therapeutic detail to describe the method, even in outline.

Nail biting

Although this is common in children, who normally outgrow the habit, it is also found in adults as a psychogenic disorder. Treatment is often simple, requiring only the visualization of the hands with strong and beautiful nails. Patients must also be made very aware of the contact of the fingers with the lips or teeth so that they do not bite their nails without being aware of doing so.

Wagstaff and Royce (1994) report a trial with 17 subjects who were either given suggestions alone, or the same suggestions under hypnosis. Their suggestions were prescriptive, such as 'I will not bite my nails today or tomorrow'. The subgoals after each suggestion related to whether the nails had been bitten, rather than the end state of beautiful nails. Only the suggestions given under hypnosis were effective.

Common approaches to therapy

The therapeutic approach adopted is more likely to be determined by the therapist's theoretical stance and preferences than by the constraints of hypnosis. Hypnosis can be allied with most therapeutic approaches. However, the most commonly used approaches are:

- Uncovering and 'discovery' techniques. These may often take the form of questioning the patient under hypnosis, and the use of regression.
- Regression and revivification techniques. Here the patient will be encouraged to regress to some specific time or event and asked to 'relive' the event. Sometimes this is just a device for learning otherwise repressed material; sometimes the opportunity is taken to 'reframe' the events and assign them a new meaning.
- Behavioural therapy and progressive desensitization. Hypnosis is an ideal way of carrying out these classic therapies entirely in the consulting room and in the imagination of the patient. Anxiety-provoking scenes can be created in the imagination, and the patient can be asked to imagine the proximity of anxiety-provoking stimuli. On conclusion of the hypnotherapy part of the programme, the patient may proceed to *in vivo* exposure.
- Suggestion therapy. Suggestions may be given to the patient who is in a highly receptive state during hypnosis. The suggestions may be prescriptive, 'do this, do that', or they may focus on ego strengthening or the achievement of some end goal.
- Creative imagery techniques. These encourage subjects to create scenarios in their imagination and to imagine themselves participating in the events they are visualizing. This is commonly a part of many other approaches, such as desensitization as described above. However, it can also be used for problems with relationships, work situations, sports performances, or excessive shyness.

- Cognitive therapy and neurolinguistic programming (NLP). Much of this can be described as the reassignment of meaning. Many problems arise as a consequence of inappropriate construing of events, and many are quickly and easily dealt with if an appropriate interpretation is provided. The NLP practitioner would describe this process as 'reframing', but it is perfectly feasible to achieve similar results without reference to NLP or its jargon. Much of what they claim to have made their own consists of variants of standard cognitive therapy.

Conditions amenable to hypnotherapy

The following list is not be exhaustive. It should be regarded as indicative:

Psychogenic disorders	*Somatic disorders*
Anorexia	Asthma
Bereavement	Allergies
Bulimia nervosa	Dermatology
Childhood anxieties	Excessive drinking
Claustrophobia	Excessive eating
Generalized anxiety disorders	Glaucoma
Impotence	Headaches
Nail biting	Hypertension
Neurotic depression	Insomnia
Neurotic paranoia	Irritable bowel syndrome
Nightmares	Nocturnal enuresis
Obsessive compulsive disorders	Obstetrics
Panic attacks	Pain control
Phobias	Post myocardial infarction
Performance anxiety	Tinnitus
Stuttering	Warts

In addition to the above conditions, which are commonly thought to be amenable to hypnotherapy, there are some reports of even more surprising cases.

In his book *If This be Magic*, Playfair cites the case of Dr Mason who successfully treated a case of congenital ichthyosiform erythrodermia of Brocq in the mistaken belief that he was dealing with multiple warts. He had cured the incurable. The case is more formally documented in Mason (1952). It would be unwise to expect miracles of hypnosis, although in this case it seems that something like one happened.

References

Alden PA (1997) Using hypnosis with patients undergoing chemotherapy. Contemporary Hypnosis 14(2): 87–93.

Bejenke C (1996) The use of hypnosis and waking suggestions with cancer patients. Symposium presentation and Workshop given at the Meeting of the European Society of Hypnosis and Psychosomatic Medicine, Budapest, August.

Brooke D, Garrett M (1996) Frightened to 'grow up'. European Journal of Clinical Hypnosis 3(3): 20–6.

Clarke JH, Reynolds PJ (1991). Suggestive hypnotherapy for nocturnal bruxism; a pilot study. American Journal of Clinical Hypnosis 33(4): 248–53.

Collins M (1996) On the road to freedom. European Journal of Clinical Hypnosis 3(3): 17–19.

Degun-Mather M (1995) Group therapy and hypnosis for the treatment of bulimia nervosa. Contemporary Hypnosis 12(2): 69–73.

Heap M (1995) Another case of indecent assault by a lay hypnotherapist. Contemporary Hypnosis 12(2): 92–8.

McCann T, Sheehan PW (1989) Pseudomemory creation and confidence in the experimental hypnosis context. British Journal of Experimental and Clinical Hypnosis 6(3): 151–9.

McGhie P (1993) Impotence Caused by Childhood Trauma. The Journal (Winter): 40–2.

Mason AA (1952) British Medical Journal 23: 442–3.

Scotford R (1995) Myth, memories and reality. Contemporary Hypnosis 12(2): 137–42.

Wagstaff GF, Royce C (1994) Hypnosis and the treatment of nail biting; a preliminary trial. Contemporary Hypnosis 2(1): 9–13.

Further reading

Boring EG (1950) A History of Experimental Psychology. New York: Appleton Century Crofts, Ch. 7.

Heap M (ed.) (1988) Hypnosis: Current Clinical, Experimental and Forensic Practices. London: Croom Helm.

Kroger WS (1977) Clinical and Experimental Hypnosis. Philadelphia: JB Lippincott Co.

Marcuse FL (1959) Hypnosis; Fact and Fiction. Harmondsworth: Penguin Books.

Morgan D (1996) The Principles of Hypnotherapy. Bradford: Eildon Press.

Playfair GL (1985) If This be Magic. London: Jonathan Cape.

Weitzenhoffer AM (1989) The Practice of Hypnotism. New York: John Wiley & Sons.

Chapter 10
Sleep, sleep deprivation, sleepiness, circadian rhythms, sleep neurophysiology, sleep disorders, and dreaming

MARK BLAGROVE

Key concepts	Key names
EEG EOG EMG Stages of sleep Circadian rhythm Sleep disorders Dreaming	Rechtschaffen and Kales

The electroencephalograph (EEG), electrooculogram (EOG) and electromyogram (EMG)

Sleep can be defined in terms of brain activity, behavioural responsiveness, or subjective experience. The spontaneous activity of the *EEG* is monitored in the sleep laboratory. Currents in the cortex, which arise at synapses, cause the EEG trace. Many nerve cells and their axons run in parallel, so their electrical potentials summate. The approximately 200 microvolts EEG is amplified to work the galvanometer pens, which can spot fast changes in potential difference. Electrodes are placed on the scalp, and next to the eyes, with reference electrodes behind the ears. The *EOG* uses the corneo-retinal potential to record eye movements. Like EEG changes, these are of the order of 150 microvolts. The EOG does not record eye muscle movement, and does not give information about the direction of gaze – only about its changes.

The *EMG* is recorded under the chin. It shows the lowered muscle tone of light sleep (stages one and two), the further lowering of muscle tone in deep sleep (stages three and four). It identifies movements that may interfere with EEG and EOG, and discriminates rapid eye-movement (REM) sleep, which has muscle atonia.

In the 1920s Berger recorded the alpha rhythm (8–12 Hz), and found that it disappeared if the eyes opened, or if mental effort such as arithmetic was done with the eyes closed, or when loud or painful stimuli occurred. As one falls asleep there is a decrease in fast, low voltage activity (the waking beta waves), decreases in regularity and frequency of alpha, and increases in slow waves activities (delta and theta). The greater the amplitude and the slower the frequency of the EEG, the deeper the sleep. However, the EEG during REM sleep has similarities to the waking EEG, because of the predominance of low amplitude high frequency waves, hence REM sleep has been termed paradoxical sleep.

Sleep stages

The definitions of sleep stages as used in sleep clinics were standardized by Rechtschaffen and Kales (1968). In the nineteenth century it was first noted that sleep is deepest in the first few hours, and becomes more superficial later in the night. When going to sleep alpha drops from 10 Hz to 8.5 Hz, its amplitude decreases, and the waves then disappear. Low voltage slow activity occurs (2–7 Hz), with slow eye movements. This is *stage one*, in which there are also vertex sharp waves, and alternation with wakefulness may occur. This makes stage one difficult to ascertain, especially as amounts of alpha are very idiosyncratic.

Stage two has three main features:

- theta waves;
- sleep spindle bursts (13–15 Hz) which last about 2 s (amplitude increases to 50 microvolts), and
- K-complexes, which are a sudden increase in scalp negativity, followed by a positive wave, lasting 0.5–2 s, 250 microvolts peak to trough.

There is currently dispute about whether K-complexes occur due to brief arousals, or whether they have a function of preserving sleep (Wauquier et al., 1995). During stage two, larger slow waves appear with frequency less than 2 Hz, and the eyes still have low muscle tension. This stage takes up about half of the sleep period.

Stage three typically begins within 20 minutes of sleep onset. In this stage there are high-amplitude slow waves that occupy 20%–50% of the EEG. These can even be picked up by the EOG. *Stage four* sleep is defined as having over 50% slow waves in the EEG. Stages three and four are termed *slow-wave sleep (SWS)*.

The first REM sleep period then occurs after about 1 hour, lasts about 5 minutes, and then recurs at a periodicity of 90 minutes. Each time the length of REMS increases in duration, such that the final REM period of the night can be up to 45 minutes long. Periods of SWS shorten over the night, subjects thus alternate between SWS and REMS, using stage two for the transition. Subjects are unlikely to move during stages three or four, but at the start and end of REM periods movements are common.

Computer analysis of brain waves is now increasing, whereas previously paper printouts were classified into the different sleep stages by eye. Spectral analysis has shown changes to occur within stages. The EEG has both slow and rapid waves, spectral analysis dissociates the signal into its components. For all the components the heights of the peaks decreases over the night, and onset of sleep has an increase in low-frequency bands.

Comparing sleep stages

Horne (1988) reviews the following characteristics of sleep stages: If sleep is lost, only about 30% is made up when recovery sleep is allowed. Most lost stage four sleep is made up, and about half of the lost REMS – other stages are not recovered. At very large amounts of sleep loss, when recovery sleep is allowed, REM sleep is almost entirely pushed out by SWS. The amount of SWS during sleep is more related to hours of prior wakefulness than is REMS. The time of day during which sleep occurs does not affect SWS amount, whereas there is a circadian rhythm in REMS propensity, peaking at 11:00, with a trough at midnight. If we nap during the day, the amount of SWS obtained reduces the next night's total, but REMS in the next night's total remains the same. Afternoon naps have more SWS than morning naps. The amount of SWS in each 90-minute cycle is about half that of the previous cycle. Horne (1988) hypothesizes that this may indicate an exponential decay of sleepiness built up over the period of wakefulness. Waking up time and ability to go to sleep are linked to the circadian body temperature rhythm.

Rapid eye-movement sleep is fragile in the face of stresses such as temperature change and general threats. Rats, rabbits and rhesus monkeys have a tendency to terminate REMS with a brief arousal, whereas humans may move position without awakening. However, note that there is no evidence that these arousals are used for the scanning of the environment, although Horne (1988) suggests that the arousals may have the function of checking if one is cold, wet, or hungry, which is especially needed for small mammals and the newborn, which cannot go for long without food. Human infants may thus check at the end of each cycle, and they need feeding after a few. During non-REM sleep (NREMS) there is a controlled lowering of metabolism and temperature, whereas during REMS breathing becomes irregular, and pulse and blood pressure fluctuate. Among males there are penile erections, and assessment of these can be used to differentiate physiological from psychological impotence. There is twitching of the extremities (such as paws or hands), and in cows and sheep rumination stops in REMS.

Meddis (1977) argues that REMS is evolutionarily the older part of sleep. His evidence is that neonates have a lot of REMS, that warm-blooded thermoregulation is lost during REM sleep, and that reptiles have wakefulness-type brain rhythms during sleep. As reptiles don't need to regulate their body temperature, Meddis claims that the cyclical process of sleep, with its REMS–SWS alternation, evolved to allow long continuous sleep. Meddis claims that this theory explains the fetal predominance of REMS, in that thermoregulation is not needed in the uterus. He says that the small amounts present in adults are not deleterious enough for evolution to remove them, and that the controls for quiet sleep/NREMS may be so entangled with those for active sleep/REMS that it cannot be removed.

The experience of being asleep

Campbell and Webb (1981) review work showing that people tend to verbally report being definitely asleep only if they are in stage two, and possibly not even then if they are poor sleepers. They also review work showing that some subjects in stages three and four claim to have been awake, but that using a push-button device to signal wakefulness they found that only 10% of signals occurred with no EEG sign of wakefulness, or with wakefulness following (such as alpha). The time of EEG arousal would be very close to the signals, so awareness of wakefulness is not gradual. Still, there were many periods of wakefulness that were not signalled, so sometimes we are not aware of being awake, or even asleep. This is relevant to the treatment of insomnia. Exercise may increase depth and continuity of sleep, but there is dispute about whether heating of the body before sleep also has this effect (Youngstedt et al., 1997). Finger-tapping has been used to indicate the moment of falling asleep because it interferes little with sleep onset (Casagrande et al., 1997)

Wrist actigraphs are devices, worn on the wrist, which detect movement. This is summed to give a measure of movement every epoch of one or two minutes. In normal subjects they are accurate in detecting periods of sleep, because most epochs during sleep have zero movement, but they can result in overestimation of sleep length in insomniacs, because quiet wakefulness is judged to be sleep by the device, and they can falsely register the movements of some patients with parasomnias as wakefulness. Software is now available that aims to remove some of these artefacts by algorithmic analysis of groups of epochs, and a major use of the devices is within- rather than between-subject analysis, that is, treatment effects rather than diagnosis (Chambers, 1994). *Quality of sleep* has been shown by Åkerstedt et al. (1994) to correlate with sleep efficiency, that is, the proportion of time from falling asleep to waking up actually spent asleep, and self-reported poor sleepers have a greater proportion of stage two (light) sleep when they are asleep (Monroe, 1967).

The development of sleep

Roffwarg et al. (1966) review the development of the human sleep cycle, hypothesizing that REM sleep has a developmental function in the newborn. The human *neonate* at one month sleeps on a 4-hour cycle. By two months they may go through the night without feeding but won't have been asleep all the time. They wake periodically, even if they remain quiet. Uninterrupted night sleep is uncommon before three months. The normal one year old has the same pattern of sleep as an adult, only in different proportions, and with a different EEG. The neonate's EEG quiet sleep has few slow waves, and no sleep spindles. The slow waves appear in bursts – in the first month these increase in length. Sleep spindles in stage two develop at two to four months. In the first three months sleep stages are very idiosyncratic, unlike in the case of adults. Full-term infants sleep for 17 hours per day, of which 10–13 hours are REM sleep (60–80%). Normal infants will have REM sleep onset for the first 12 months. Period of alternation between active (REM-like) and quiet sleep (SWS-like) is 1 hour. Mature deep slow wave sleep develops during the first year; daytime sleep is displaced by wakefulness, so by the age of three years, REM sleep has dropped from 12 hours to 3 or 4 per night, and stages three and four occupy 3 hours. From 30 years old the amount of SWS starts to decrease, dropping to 13% by the mid-30s, 5% by the 60s, with stage four by this time virtually disappearing, but in old age it is difficult to assess stages three and four, as the slow waves become smaller with age. Older people have more interrupted sleep, and more stage one, possibly due to attenuation of the circadian rhythms such as temperature.

Sleep in other animals

REM-like sleep is present in two types of monotreme (egg-laying mammals), indicating that a REM sleep precursor state was present in the reptiles ancestral to birds and mammals (Huitron-Resendiz, 1997; Siegel, 1997). Horne (1988) argues that because animals such as the Indus dolphin sleep with one hemisphere at a time, in order to avoid stopping swimming, this indicates that sleep has an essential function. However animals that are normally vulnerable to predators but which are kept safe, sleep longer, indicating that part of sleep can be optional. He has thus developed the *theory of core and optional sleep*. Sleep is also the occasion for huddling in small mammals, and hence saves energy, and allows metabolism to fall.

Effects of sleep deprivation

Blagrove, Alexander and Horne (1995) show that the restriction of sleep to five hours per night mainly has effects on mood rather than cognitive performance, whereas deprivation of all sleep for only one night results in cognitive deficits. Horne (1988) reviews work showing that deleterious and sometimes lethal effects of sleep loss in animals may be an inadequate model for humans, because animals are under greater stress. His theory of core and optional sleep holds that the first three cycles of sleep, in which SWS predominates, are core sleep, which allows the brain to recuperate. Evidence for this is that the proportion of SWS increases with increased time spent awake, and that naps early in the day, when sleep is not necessary, are mainly (optional) REM sleep. When humans have less than five hours sleep per night there are cognitive deficits, because core sleep is then reduced. Motivation, for example with payment (Horne and Pettitt, 1985) or knowledge of results (Wilkinson, 1961) can alleviate the effects of sleep loss.

However, some argue that REM sleep is important for *learning*, and is not just 'optional'. Smith and Lapp (1991) have shown that when students learn for examinations, the number of REMs per unit of time of REM sleep increases. Others have shown that REM deprivation leads to memory deficiencies, but this may be due to the stress of the sleep deprivation, and due to the hyperarousal and distractibility that REM sleep deprivation induces. REM sleep deprivation, either by some anti-depressants or by repeated awakening, has been related to the alleviation of depression.

Sleepiness

Subjective measurements

Here patients' goodwill is needed, to avoid inaccurate or hasty answers. One measure is the *Stanford Sleepiness Scale* (Hoddes et al., 1973). The patient states which of the following points describes their present state of alertness:

- Feeling active, vital, alert, wide awake.
- Functioning at a high level but not at peak, able to concentrate.
- Relaxed, awake but not fully alert, responsive.
- A little foggy, let down.
- Foggy, beginning to lose track, difficulty in staying awake.
- Sleepy, prefer to lie down, woozy.
- Almost in reverie, cannot stay awake, sleep onset appears imminent.

Herscovitch and Broughton (1981) showed that the Stanford Sleepiness Scale (SSS) is sensitive to the effects of cumulative partial sleep deprivation and recovery oversleeping, and scores return to baseline after one night's recovery sleep, but there is dispute about whether scores correlate within individuals with cognitive performance. The *Epworth Sleepiness Scale* (Johns, 1991) assesses trait sleepiness by asking patients to rate their likelihood of falling asleep in situations such as watching TV, sitting quietly after lunch, or in a car stopped at traffic.

Sleep onset latency

This is the standardized and arguably objective assessment of sleepiness, and uses the EEG-assessed time to fall asleep at various times of day as the measure of sleepiness. Caskadon and Dement (1979) found the longest sleep onset latencies (and thus lowest sleepiness) at 10:00, 12:00, and 22:00, and for sleep-deprived subjects found a correlation between sleep onset latencies and performance on an addition task and between sleep onset latencies and Stanford Sleepiness Scores. There are two versions:

* Multiple Sleep Latency Test – the patient lies on a bed and tries to fall asleep (Richardson et al., 1978).
* Maintenance of Wakefulness Test – the patient sits in a comfortable chair and resists sleep (Mitler et al., 1982).

There are large individual differences in alpha – both in its amounts, and also in its appearance. This means that for some people its appearance signals sleepiness whereas for others its disappearance signals sleepiness.

Are we chronically sleepy? Prepubescent children are maximally alert throughout the day. Daytime sleepiness develops as maturation occurs, post-puberty it is between 13:30 and 15:30, the 'post-lunch dip'. In Levine et al. (1988) young college students had a mean sleep onset time of 9.9 minutes, significantly less than the older subjects (12.5 minutes), indicating that they are chronically sleep restricted. Webb and Agnew (1975) found subjects sleep 126 minutes longer if allowed to stay in bed, and the authors noted a 1910 study finding that young adults sleep for 9 hours. They noted that we need alarm clocks to wake up, and wake up sleepy, but Horne (1988) points out that sudden sleep extension results in worse performance on memory and vigilance, supporting Globus's description of the 'worn-out syndrome', when sleep is taken to excess. Sleepiness after waking from sleep is termed *sleep inertia*, and is partly dependent upon the pre-arousal sleep stage.

Circadian rhythms

These derive their name from the Latin words *circa* (about) and *dies* (day). Monk (1991) has suggested that subjective feelings of sleepiness are a 'messenger' to the conscious mind, 'leading the individual towards behaviour that represents an orderly, natural and timely transition between the states of wakefulness and sleep'. The best proof that we have of such an endogenous clock is that the pattern is still present even when external ones for sleep and wakefulness are absent. Such rhythms include body temperature, heart rate, and blood pressure.

Monk (1991) reviews how in order to study decisions to go to sleep we must use subjects who

- don't know what time it is, and
- have no pressure on their time.

When these conditions are met humans usually free-run with a period of 24 to 25.5 hours – that is, the time of going to sleep is delayed by about one hour each day. The body can maintain these rhythms despite being in long-term isolation for months. Although the rhythms usually stay integrated, the sleep/wake cycle can become very irregular, with 12 to 15 hour sleep periods mixed with sleep periods of normal length: this is 'spontaneous internal desynchronization', in which the sleep/wake cycle differs markedly from the 25-hour circadian temperature. Some humans shift to very long days, such as 22 hours asleep followed by 28 hours awake, and not all the cyclical functions shift at the same time. When free-running, or under desynchronization, and when the temperature at sleep onset is high and falling, long sleeps are experienced. When the temperature at sleep onset is low and rising, short sleeps occur. The older the subject, the shorter the free-running periods are, producing the earlier bedtimes and waking times characteristic of this group. Note, however, that although in many societies naps occur mid-afternoon, body temperature is high at this time, although sleep latency is low. The influence of circadian rhythms can explain why traffic accidents are highest between 13:00 and 14:00 and between 01:00 and 04:00. Accidents and mistakes in industrial settings also have these two peaks, and are very costly on a national basis (Webb, 1995).

Monk (1991) shows how the persistence of the circadian rhythm is a cause of jet lag. After a flight of five hours it takes several days to adjust the sleep–wake cycle but more than eight days before the cycle of cortisol secretion adjusts. Light is a powerful stimulus to lock the internal clock to the natural day. Light is said to entrain the cycle and is called a *zeitgeber* (German – time giver). Although light is the most important *zeitgeber* for circadian rhythms, it is not the only one. Others are meal times and social cues. For example, congenitally blind humans maintain a rough 24 hour cycle if they are isolated but have social cues. In total isolation they develop a clear 25-hour cycle.

Physiological basis of biological clocks

The master clock is located in the *suprachiasmatic nucleus of the hypothalamus*. This is a small nucleus, containing about 10 000 cells, located in the medial hypothalamus just above the optic chiasm, and receives a direct projection from the retina. Lesions of the SCN abolish the periodicity of behaviour. For example, rats with lesioned SCN still sleep but the sleep periods are randomly distributed throughout the day.

Neurophysiology of sleep

Over the centuries there have been theories that sleep is due to thickened blood, fumes from the blood or stomach, or lack of oxygen. These were based on sleep being a lack of wakefulness. In the 1920s the viral infection encephalitis lethargica spread through Europe. In the first stages there were fever and agitation, after a few weeks lethargy and drowsiness, and then prolonged sleep. Patients who had died were found to have an infected diencephalon. This did not stop the argument, though, as to whether sleep is an active or passive process. The proponent of the active view was Hess, who saw sleep as a replenishing process. He stimulated the thalamus of waking cats with low-frequency pulses; they went to sleep and their EEGs shifted to the high voltage, slow pattern. Sleep was thus shown to be caused by a change in the pattern of neural firing, not by a cessation of that activity. When stimulated, the mid-brain reticular formation arouses the EEG, and muscle tone increases. The generator for REM sleep is in the pons, with muscle tone inhibited by the locus coeruleus, and there are various centres for sleep and wakefulness.

Sleep substances

Horne (1988) reviews work on sleep substances. This shows that sleep has been studied in terms of sleep substances since the discovery of enkephalins and endorphins. Pieron, in 1913, had proposed that during wakefulness a hypnotoxin builds up (sleep poison), and found that the cerebrospinal fluid (CSF) of sleep-deprived dogs can induce sleep in alert dogs. Factor S (S for sleep) was found in the early 1980s to be a small peptide, five amino acids long. Sleep-promoting substance has effects lasting for up to 24 hours, influenced by the phase of the light/dark cycle. Delta sleep-inducing peptide is nine amino acids long. The function of the pineal gland is unknown, but it releases melatonin, particularly during the night, which has been shown to cause sleepiness in humans and to alter their circadian rhythms.

Disorders of sleep

These are reviewed in Williams, Karacan and Moore (1988), and Bonnet (1990), from which some of the following is taken. Note that in investigating patients in the sleep clinic there is a *first-night effect* in which sleep onset time is increased, as is amount of light sleep before SWS and before the first REM period. Hence one acclimatization night is allowed in which data are not collected.

Disorders of initiating and maintaining sleep (DIMS)

Insomnia

This is the major DIMS and is aggravated by depression, by alcohol or drug withdrawal, and by pre-sleep worries. Edinger and Fins (1995) show that although some insomniacs (such as those with depression or psychophysiological insomnia, or subjective insomnia) underestimate their total sleep time, and overestimate the time it takes for them to fall asleep, 20% of insomniac patients (especially those with periodic limb movements) overestimated their length of sleep, so that the condition is worse than suspected. State misperception and sleep onset time misperception occur because behavioural, experiential and EEG definitions of sleep onset can define different moments of sleep onset, and because patients may mistake dreaming for thinking. Furthermore, individuals differ in the amount of sleep they need, and in the amounts that they think they need. Insomnia can be treated by reducing sleep length so as to improve sleep efficiency, and by having strict wake up times, so as to reset zeitgebers. In some cases insomnia can be caused by nocturnal myoclonus, or periodic movements in sleep (PMS) – the frequent jerking of the lower extremities during sleep that increases with age – and by restless leg syndrome, which worsens in the evening and refers to heavy and tired legs with a deep itchiness.

Disorders of excessive somnolence (DOES)

Apnoea

Apnoea involves the frequent stopping of breathing (hypopnea) during sleep for periods of over 10 seconds. Three hundred attacks may occur in a few hours and the skin can turn blue. Fatigue, headaches and sleepiness result during the day, but because individuals wake only very briefly to gasp and to halt the apoxia they have no knowledge that the cause of their sleepiness is frequent awakenings, which are usually only spotted by a partner or in the sleep laboratory. Sufferers are typically male, over 40, and obese; in contrast, premenopausal women have the stimulating effect of progesterone on breathing. Obstructive sleep apnoea results from obstruction of the windpipe, due to the fattened airways and lowered muscle tone during sleep, whereas central apnoea results from a lack of central nervous system (CNS) or brainstem instructions to breathe. In a model of sleep apnoea, Bonnet (1985) found that briefly awakening subjects after each minute of EEG-defined sleep for two consecutive nights almost eliminated SWS and REMS, and resulted in subjective daytime sleepiness and performance decrement, although total sleep time was only reduced by one hour each night. Treatment is by *continuous positive airway pressure* (CPAP), in which a mask and air pump present pressurized air to the sleeping patient throughout the night. Tracheotomy is performed in serious cases, and patients should refrain from sedatives such as alcohol.

Hypersomnia

This refers to an excessive amount of sleep within 24 hours, accompanied sometimes by drowsiness and the confusion, disorientation and automatisms of sleep drunkenness. It can result from the prolonged use of alcohol and anxiolytics.

Narcolepsy

This usually results from brain lesions or disorders of neurochemistry, and there are reports of a genetic component. Disease onset is usually before age 25. It occurs in about 0.5% of the adult population, and has up to four components:

- Sleep attacks: the patient can suddenly, without control, fall asleep, with sleep lasting up to 15 minutes.
- Episodes of cataplexy (muscular weakness): these last up to two minutes and result from intense emotion.
- Sleep paralysis: this can occur on waking, or when about to fall asleep, and can last up to 30 seconds, with the patient conscious throughout.
- Vivid hypnogogic hallucinations: these occur when falling asleep.

Only one in seven patients have all four components. Rapid eye-movement sleep often occurs at the start of a sleep period, and the disorder is theorized as being due to failure of REM sleep control. During sleep the patient may change sleep stages frequently. Hood and Bruck (1997) show that narcoleptics have deficient confidence in their memory, although there is no evidence that their memory is worse than normal subjects.

Disorders of sleep–wake schedules

Delayed sleep phase syndrome occurs in young adults who retire to bed late. *Advanced sleep phase syndrome* occurs in the elderly. Lowered performance and mood, vascular illness, and difficulty sleeping, can occur due to shiftwork, especially in the advanced phase condition.

The DIMS, DOES and disorders of sleep–wake schedules are also referred to as dyssomnias.

Parasomnias

These are disorders that occur during sleep.

Somnambulism

This is sleep walking. It occurs in stages three or four of sleep, because during REM sleep muscle tone is lost. The condition is more prevalent in males, and possibly has a genetic component.

Night terrors

These are also known as sleep terrors. They are a disorder of sudden arousal, usually preceded by sleep stages three or four, which occur early in the night without an accompanying dream, and so can be differentiated from nightmares. They most commonly occur in three to five year olds.

Nightmares

Nightmares (dreams with anxiety) usually occur late in the night during REM sleep; 10–25% of the general population experiences one or more nightmares per month and the incidence decreases with age. The correlation of nightmare frequency with trait anxiety indicates either that such individuals have more nightmares, or that they are just more likely to report them. Belicki (1992) has shown that nightmare distress is related to psychopathology and waking emotional adjustment, whereas nightmare frequency is separate from this and is related to vividness of dreams. Using a retrospective questionnaire to measure nightmare frequency can greatly underestimate, by a factor of 2 to 10, the number of nightmares reported by a contemporaneous sleep log.

Other parasomnias

Other parasomnias include nocturnal enuresis (bedwetting – the majority of sufferers are boys aged five to seven); bruxism (teeth grinding); and automatisms resulting in violence and amnesia.

Dreaming

Psychophysiology

Aserinsky and Kleitman (1953) and Dement and Kleitman (1957) showed that REM sleep is associated with high frequency of dream recall, with longer REM sleep periods and dreams occurring later in the night. Subjects were considered to have been dreaming only if they could relate a coherent, fairly detailed description of dream content, which we now know biased the study against finding NREM sleep dreams. Some subjects were better than others, and there was no practice effect. Subjects were more emphatic about not dreaming if they were wakened from stage two than from stage four. There was a connection between dream length and REM sleep period length, and they concluded that dreams progress at a rate comparable to a real experience of the same sort, and are not therefore instantaneously upon awakening. However, dreams recalled after 30 minutes of REM, or after as much as 50 minutes, weren't much longer than those at 15 minutes REM, showing an inability to remember all the details of very long dreams, although subjects would have the impression they'd been dreaming for a long time. The work of Antrobus (1983) and Foulkes (1962) shows that dreams do occur in non-REM sleep, and may just be shorter and less vivid than REM sleep dreams.

The activation-synthesis model of dreaming (Hobson and McCarley, 1977)

This major psychophysiological theory of dreaming holds that neurophysiological activation of memories during sleep by the pontine brain stem is followed by cognitive synthesis of the dream plot as an attempt to make sense of the random assortment of activated memories. The EEG shows ponto-geniculo-occipital spikes during REMs, which are hypothesized to cause the almost random activation of memories. Bizarreness in dreams is thus held to be due to this random activation of memories.

These authors hold that the brain cannot organize information in a coherent manner and achieve full self-awareness during sleep. The brain and mind are active, but external and internal realities cannot be tested, and attention is lacking. This theory accounts for the following characteristics of dreams:

- Hallucination – we hallucinate because there is no sensory input and motor output. The brain assumes it is awake.
- Delusion – the dream is taken as reality.
- Discontinuities – due to the barrage of internally generated information, with attempts made to synthesize the memories into a single plot.
- Intensification of emotion, both cognitively and autonomically, because the limbic system is activated, as well as the brain-stem startle networks, for example heartbeats and breathing speed up.
- Amnesia – synthesis occurs, but not remembering, the dream just stays as short-term memory.

Reinsel et al. (1986) oppose this theory by claiming that dreamlike mentation can occur during the waking state, and during NREM sleep, and they find that discontinuous mentation is more prevalent in daydreaming than in night dreams. Solms (1997) shows the importance of parietal and frontal cortex to dream production.

Other work on dreaming

In the activation-synthesis theory dreams are not obscure but transparent, containing meaningful, undisguised impulses and memories. Freud's (1900) theory, by contrast, holds that initial latent thoughts, usually unconscious, are translated into more acceptable symbols, with secondary revision then making the final manifest dream more coherent and even more disguised. The unconscious thoughts, the most important of which are wishes, gain expression by the use of symbols and also occurrences from recent days (day residues). Freud held that the dream is decoded by the process of free-association in which individual components of the manifest dream are thought about in a non-judgmental manner, collecting the patient's uncensored reactions to each such component, and achieving a 'royal road to the unconscious'. Dreams, for Freud, were thus akin, in their evidential value, to neurotic symptoms and slips of the tongue. The use of free-association to access and categorize the sources of the dream is now used by Cavallero (1993).

Foulkes and Rechtschaffen (1964) found that a pre-sleep showing of a violent film led to REMS dreams that were more imaginative, more vivid, more emotional, and longer than were dreams following a neutral film. External stimuli applied during sleep, especially sound, can become incorporated into dreams (Arkin and Antrobus, 1991). Blagrove (1992) reviews work showing that stresses can affect dreams, which can thus be held to be meaningful. For example, Kramer showed that judges can assign a set of randomized waking concerns to their corresponding dream series reports, Breger found that individuals undergoing vascular surgery and psychotherapy had dreams that depicted these experiences, and Cartwright (1986, 1991) has shown that length of recovery from divorce is indicated by aspects of dream content, which has resulted in the view that dreams aid the adaptation to stressful events (De Koninck and Koulack, 1975). Hill et al. (1993) have shown that psychotherapy using the studying of one's own dreams leads to greater depth and insight than the studying of events or, as a control, the dreams of other people, but Blagrove (1996) reviews the conflicting claims of whether dream cognition is deficient – the view that dreams tell us no more than we already know in waking life – versus the views that hold that dreams are insightful and adaptive, aiding in problem-solving, memory-searching or the metaphorical expression of current concerns. The latter view of the adaptive function of dreams is supported by claims of the function of REM sleep in aiding memory consolidation, and by instances of creativity provoked by dreams, such as in Kekulé's account of the discovery of the structure of the benzene ring (Strunz, 1993).

Summary

Going to sleep is controlled by many factors, such as how long one has been awake, and one's circadian rhythm. Sleep is composed of five stages:

stages three and four (slow wave sleep) and REM are concerned with brain recuperation and memory consolidation respectively. Dreams can occur in any sleep stage, but are more vivid in REM sleep, and the function and meaningfulness of dreams is currently a matter of dispute.

References

Åkerstedt T, Hume K, Minors D, Waterhouse J (1994) The meaning of good sleep: a longitudinal study of polysomnography and subjective sleep quality. Journal of Sleep Research 3: 152–8.

Antrobus JS (1983) REM and NREM sleep reports: comparison of word frequencies by cognitive classes. Psychophysiology 20: 562–8.

Arkin A, Antrobus J (1991) The effects of external stimuli applied prior to and during sleep on sleep experience. In S Ellman, J Antrobus (eds) (1978) The Mind in Sleep. New Jersey: Leonard Erlbaum.

Aserinsky E, Kleitman N (1953) Regularly occurring periods of ocular motility and concomitant phenomena during sleep. Science 118: 361–75.

Belicki K (1992) Nightmare frequency versus nightmare distress: relations to psychopathology and cognitive style. Journal of Abnormal Psychology 101: 592–7.

Blagrove M (1992) Dreams as the reflection of our waking concerns and abilities: a critique of the problem-solving paradigm in dream research. Dreaming 2: 205–20.

Blagrove M (1996) Problems with the cognitive psychological modeling of dreaming. Journal of Mind and Behavior 17: 99–134.

Blagrove M, Alexander C, Horne J (1995) The effects of sleep reduction on the performance of cognitive tasks sensitive to sleep deprivation. Applied Cognitive Psychology 9: 21–40.

Bonnet M (1985) Effects of sleep disruption on sleep, performance, and mood. Sleep 8: 11–19.

Bonnet M (1990). The perception of sleep onset in insomniacs and normal sleepers. In RR Bootzin, JF Kihlstrom, DL Schacter (eds) Sleep and Cognition. Washington DC: American Psychological Association.

Campbell SS, Webb WB (1981) The perception of wakefulness within sleep. Sleep 4: 177–83.

Cartwright RD (1986) Affect and dream-work from an information processing point of view. Journal of Mind and Behavior 7: 411–28.

Cartwright RD (1991) Dreams that work: The relation of dream incorporation to adaptation to stressful events. Dreaming, 1: 3–9.

Casagrande M, Gennaro LD, Violani C, Braibanti P, Bertini M (1997) A finger-tapping task and a reaction time task as behavioral measures of the transition from wakefulness to sleep. Sleep 20: 301–12.

Caskadon M, Dement W (1979) Effects of total sleep loss on sleep tendency. Perceptual and Motor Skills 48: 495–506.

Cavallero C (1993) The quest for dream sources. Journal of Sleep Research 2: 13–16.

Chambers MJ (1994) Actigraphy and insomnia: a closer look. Part 1. Sleep 17: 405–8.

De Koninck J, Koulack D (1975) Dream content and adaptation to a stressful situation. Journal of Abnormal Psychology 84: 250–60.

Dement W, Kleitman N (1957) The relation of eye movements during sleep to dream activity: an objective method for the study of dreaming. Journal of Experimental Psychology 53: 339–46.

Edinger JD, Fins AI (1995) The distribution and clinical significance of sleep time mis-perceptions among insomniacs. Sleep 18: 232–9.

Foulkes D (1962) Dream reports from different stages of sleep. Journal of Abnormal and Social Psychology 65: 14–25.

Foulkes D, Rechtschaffen A (1964) Presleep determinants of dream content: effects of two films. Perceptual and Motor Skills 19: 983–1005.

Freud S (1900) The Interpretation of Dreams. Translated by J Strachey. Penguin Freud Library Volume 4, 1976 edition. Harmondsworth: Pelican.

Herscovitch J, Broughton R (1981) Sensitivity of the Stanford Sleepiness Scale to the effects of cumulative partial sleep deprivation and recovery oversleeping. Sleep 4: 83–92.

Hill CE, Diemer R, Hess S, Hillyer A, Seeman R (1993) Are the effects of dream interpre-tation on session quality, insight, and emotions due to the dream itself, to projec-tion, or to the interpretation process? Dreaming 3: 269–80.

Hobson JA, McCarley RW (1977) The brain as a dream state generator: an activation syn-thesis hypothesis of the dream process. American Journal of Psychiatry 134: 1335–48.

Hoddes E, Zarcone V, Smythe H, Phillips R, Dement WC (1973) Quantification of sleepi-ness: a new approach. Psychophysiology 10: 431–6.

Hood B, Bruck D (1997) Metamemory in narcolepsy. Journal of Sleep Research, 6, 205–10.

Horne JA (1988) Why We Sleep: The functions of sleep in humans and other mammals. Oxford: Oxford University Press.

Horne JA, Pettitt AN (1985) High incentive effects on vigilance performance during 72 hours of total sleep deprivation. Acta Psychologica 58: 123–39.

Huitron-Resendiz S (1997). Sleep in reptiles. Sleep Research Society Bulletin 4: 32–7.

Johns MW (1991) A new method for measuring daytime sleepiness: the Epworth Sleepiness Scale. Sleep 14: 540–5.

Levine B, Roehrs T, Zorick F, Roth T (1988). Daytime sleepiness in young adults. Sleep 11: 39–46.

Meddis R (1977) The Sleep Instinct. London: Routledge & Kegan Paul.

Mitler MM, Gujavarty KS, Browman CP (1982) Maintenance of wakefulness test. a polysomnographic technique for evaluating treatment efficacy in patients with excessive somnolence. Electroencephalography and Clinical Neurophysiology 53: 658–61.

Monk T (1991) Circadian aspects of subjective sleepiness: a behavioural messenger? In T Monk (ed.) Sleep, Sleepiness and Performance. Chichester: John Wiley.

Monroe LJ (1967) Psychological and physiological differences between good and poor sleepers. Journal of Abnormal Psychology 72: 255–64.

Rechtschaffen A, Kales AA (1968) A Manual of Standardized Terminology, Techniques and Scoring System for Sleep Stages of Human Subjects. Bethesda MD: National Institute of Neurological Diseases and Blindness.

Reinsel R, Wollman M, Antrobus JS (1986) Effects of environmental context and cortical activation on thought. Journal of Mind and Behavior 7: 259–76.

Richardson GS, Caskadon MA, Flagg W, Van Den Hoed J, Dement WC, Mitler MM (1978) Excessive daytime sleepiness in man: multiple sleep latency measurement in narcoleptic and control subjects. Electroencephalography and Clinical Neuro-physiology 45: 621–7.

Roffwarg HP, Muzio JN, Dement WC (1966) The ontogenetic development of the human sleep dream cycle. Science 152: 604–18.

Siegel JM (1997) Monotremes and the evolution of REM sleep. Sleep Research Society Bulletin 4: 31–2.

Smith C, Lapp L (1991) Increases in number of REMS and REM density in humans following an intensive learning period. Sleep 14–330.

Solms M (1997) The Neuropsychology of Dreams. Mahwah, NJ: Lawrence Erlbaum Associates.

Strunz F (1993) Preconscious mental activity and scientific problem-solving: a critique of the Kekulé dream controversy. Dreaming 3: 281–294.

Wauquier A, Aloe L, Declerck A (1995) K-complexes: are they signs of arousal or sleep protective? Journal of Sleep Research 4: 138–43.

Webb WB (1995) The cost of sleep-related accidents: a reanalysis. Sleep 18: 276–80.

Webb WB, Agnew Jr HW (1975) Are we chronically sleep deprived? Bulletin of the Psychonomic Society 6: 47–8.

Wilkinson R (1961) Interaction of lack of sleep with knowledge of results. Journal of Experimental Psychology 62: 263–71.

Williams RL, Karacan I, Moore CA (1988) Sleep Disorders: Diagnosis and Treatment. Chichester: John Wiley.

Youngstedt SD, O'Connor PJ, Dishman RK (1997) The effects of acute exercise on sleep: a quantitative synthesis. Sleep 20: 203–14.

Chapter 11
Neuropsychology – studying behaviour following brain damage

M. EACOTT

Key concepts	Key names
Modules	
Neurological specificity	
Isomorphism	
Equipotentiality	Lashley
Achromatopsia	
Hemianopia	
Scotoma	
Macular sparing	
Akinotopsia	
Visual object agnosia	Lissauer
Tactile agnosia	
Auditory agnosia	
Apperceptive agnosia	
Associative agnosia	
Prosopagnosia	
Double dissociation	
Visual disorientation	
Neglect	
Short-term store	
Long-term store	
Declarative	
Procedural	
Engram	Lashley
Mass action	
Korsakoff's amnesia	
Wernicke's encephalopathy	
Amnesic syndrome	
Broca's area	
Wernicke's area	
Aphasia	
Expressive/non-fluent/motor	
Receptive/fluent/sensory	(contd)

(contd)

Key concepts	Key names
Prosody	
Executive dysfunction	
Wisconsin card-sorting test	
Perseveration	
Thurstone word fluency test	
Pseudodepression	
Pseudopsychopathy	
Contention scheduling	Norman and Shollice
Supervisory activating system	
Anosognosia	
WAIS-R	
National adult reading test	
Warrington's graded naming test	

Neuropsychology can be defined as the study of the relation between brain function and behaviour. It combines insights from anatomy, physiology and psychology and involves studying the effects that brain damage has on behaviour in an attempt to determine the relationship between the brain and behaviour. The term itself is relatively recent, being first used in the subtitle to Hebb's 1949 book *The Organisation of Behaviour: A Neuropsychological Theory*. Since then the discipline of neuropsychology has flourished.

Neuropsychological investigation relies on several underlying assumptions. The first is that the brain is the organ of behaviour. This may be accepted as commonplace today, but it was not always so – Aristotle (384–322 BC), for example, believed that the heart controlled behaviour. The second assumption is that behaviour is controlled by *modules.* Modules are relatively independent cognitive processing systems that control different aspects of behaviour. The modularity principle would, for example, suggest that memory and visual perception are controlled by different modules, which engage in processing in isolation from each other (Fodor, 1983). Neuropsychology aims to study the organization of these processing modules by examining the effect that damage to modules has on behaviour. This requires one further key assumption – that modules physically exist in the brain and so can be affected by brain damage. This assumption that the organization of the brain and the organization of the mind bear some relation to each other is called *neurological specificity* or *isomorphism*. If one accepts these assumptions, damage to different parts of the brain may be expected to result in different patterns of behavioural impairment. For example, one could damage the parts of the brain controlling memory but leave those controlling visual functions relatively intact. Conversely, one could damage the visual parts of the brain but leave memory intact. However, this view has not always been widely accepted.

In 1929, Lashley published an influential paper that suggested that the brain showed *equipotentiality* – that is, all parts of the brain had equal potential for controlling all types of behaviour. If the brain is indeed equipotential, it would not be possible for a patient to have specific problems in memory, but none in visual perception, because both are controlled from one unitary, damaged brain system. Instead, equipotentiality suggests that brain damage should result in a *graceful degradation*, that is a gradual decrease in all mental functions as increasing amounts of brain tissue become damaged. As we shall see over the subsequent parts of this chapter, brain damage to different regions can result in very specific and differing patterns of impairments in behaviour. These impairments suggest that the brain is modular in its organization and that it is not equipotential.

Deficits in visual perception

In humans, vision is the dominant sense. As a reflection of its importance to us, it has been claimed that 55% of the total surface area of the human brain is devoted to processing visual information. Not surprisingly, therefore, damage to this cortex has repercussions on our visual abilities and the nature of the disabilities reveals something of the organization of this mass of cortex.

Visual field defects

Damage to the primary visual cortex within the occipital cortex (see Figure 11.1) affects the cortex, which receives visual information from the eye via the midbrain. Not surprisingly, therefore, such damage has a profound effect on the ability to see. Within the visual system, the principle of division of labour applies, so that different parts of the visual cortex process information that originated in different parts of the visual field. In fact, one can think of the primary visual cortex as having a map of visual space overlaid on it, so that each part of the visual cortex will receive visual information which came exclusively from one part of the visual field. This is achieved via the *optic chiasm*, where nerve fibres that originated in either eye are recombined and sent to each hemisphere according to the part of visual space in which they collected the visual information (Figure 11.2). As a result, unilateral damage to the primary visual cortex will result in a blind region for the corresponding part of the visual field. A small blind region caused by such damage is called a *scotoma*. Strangely, if the scotoma is small, a patient may be unaware of the blind region because constant movement of the eyes and a psychological process of filling in missing information means that the absent visual information rarely has any real-life implications. If more cortex is damaged, the scotoma will become correspondingly bigger. In some cases the primary visual cortex of an entire hemisphere will be damaged. In this case, the patient will be unable to see anything that occurs in the visual field opposite (contralateral) to the brain damage. Such a blind region is called a *hemianopia*. Although it is true that each hemisphere receives visual information from the opposite side, both hemispheres receive information about the central few degrees of visual space. For this reason, a hemianopia often has intact vision for the very centre of the visual field, while all other portions of the visual field are lost. As the centre of the visual field is known as the *macula*, this sparing is called *macular* sparing.

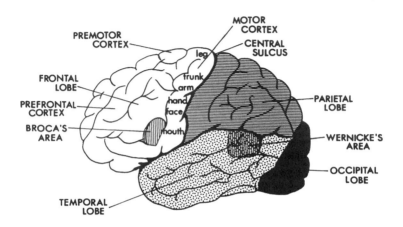

Figure 11.1: The left hemisphere of a human brain.

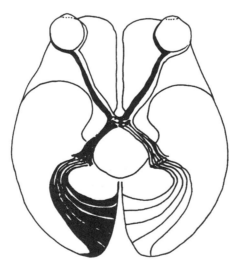

Figure 11.2: The optic chiasm shown within the human brain as viewed from below. The eyes can be seen at the top of the figure and the primary visual cortex at the bottom. It can be seen that light falling on the left-hand side of each eye (and thus originating from the right-hand side of space) will be channelled into the primary visual cortex of the left hemisphere.

Selective loss of visual abilities

It has already been noted that a great deal of cortex is devoted to processing visual information. However, equipotentiality does not exist within this cortex because different regions of the cortex process different aspects of visual information. As discussed above, primary visual cortex contains a map of the visual field, but Fellman and Van Essen (1991) found that there are as many as 32 maps of the visual field within the visual system of a monkey. A similar picture is beginning to emerge of the human brain. Why does the brain contain so many maps of the visual world? One possible answer to this question is that each of the visual areas is processing different aspects of the visual scene. For example, one of these areas may be primarily extracting information about the colours present, whereas other areas are extracting information about the relative distances between objects, or their positions, or whether they are moving. If this were the case, one might expect that brain damage would sometimes, by chance, damage just some of these visual areas, leaving others intact. One might expect, therefore, occasionally to find patients who are able to see, but who have lost the ability to process colour, depth or movement in their visual world. Although they are rare, such patients do occur. For example, following brain damage, patients may have a difficulty seeing colours, complaining that their world looks drained of colour, like a black-and-white photograph (for reviews see Meadows, 1974; Cowey and Heywood, 1997). An impairment of colour perception following brain damage is called *achromatopsia*. A similar impairment in the ability to extract movement information from vision has also been reported (Zihl, Von Cramon and Mai, 1983) and is termed *akinotopsia*.

Impairments of object recognition

Patients with achromatopsia will not necessarily have any problem recognizing objects unless recognition is critically dependent on the colour of the object (for example a picture of a tomato and an apple might be confused by an achromatopsic patient). However, there is a group of patients who appear to have complete visual information, and yet nevertheless show a puzzling failure to recognize objects. This can be seen in the clinic, but also in their own homes. A failure to recognize everyday objects that is not due to a general intellectual deterioration, language loss, or basic sensory dysfunction (such as hemianopia) is called *visual object agnosia*. The term agnosia comes from the Greek and means 'without knowledge'. Although it is rare, the existence of visual object agnosia has been recognized for over 100 years. Lissauer (1890) described a classic case. An elderly gentleman, known as GL, hit his head in a fall during a snowstorm. Apparently unharmed, he retired to bed. However, he later complained that he was not able to see as well as before. On testing GL's visual acuity was found to be normal for his age and he was able to draw reasonable copies of things he could see. In many ways, therefore, his vision was intact. However, he was unable to recognize many common objects. As his vision seemed superficially intact, one might suppose that GL had lost knowledge about the objects he failed to recognize – that is, he had forgotten about common objects. However, one can test a patient's knowledge about objects by asking simple questions. For example, if a patient has failed to recognize a fork, one could test whether he has lost all knowledge about forks by asking 'what implements might you use to eat your dinner?' GL, however, like many agnosic patients, showed normal knowledge about objects that he could not recognize visually. Indeed GL was also able to identify the objects by touch or if they made a characteristic sound. Visual object agnosia is therefore a specific inability to recognize objects from vision. Although less thoroughly investigated, equivalent problems in recognizing objects from touch (*tactile agnosia*) or from their characteristic sounds (*auditory agnosia*) also exist.

Lissauer (1890) realized that visual object agnosia could theoretically arise for several different reasons. He distinguished and named two of these: *apperceptive agnosia* and *associative agnosia*. He proposed that apperceptive agnosia arose when there was a breakdown of the final stage of perceptual processing of visual information. According to Lissauer, an apperceptive agnosic patient was able to process basic visual information and so could describe many aspects of the object (for example 'round', 'shiny', 'golden') but could not put all the information together to gain a full mental representation of the object. A representation of the object is known as a *percept*, hence the name apperceptive agnosia. One way of determining whether patients have an adequate percept is to ask them to draw an object. A patient with apperceptive agnosia will fail to draw an object and may even have difficulty copying a line drawing of an object. Apperceptive agnosia is therefore a deficit that arises as a failure to form an adequate percept of an object and will usually result in a failure to draw or copy objects, as well as a failure to recognize them.

However, some patients, like Lissauer's patient GL, will make perfectly adequate drawings of objects that they nevertheless fail to recognize. These patients are called *associative agnosics*. The ability to draw accurately suggests that the percept is complete. Why then do patients fail to recognize the object? When I recognize the pen that I have before me, what I am really doing is matching the percept of the pen that my visual system has assembled (containing full information about its shape, colour, texture, and so forth) and knowledge in memory about similar classes of objects that I have seen before. Once I have compared my percept of my pen and matched it with the concept of pen in my memory, I can confidently produce a name ('pen') and some characteristics of my pen (it will write, and it will probably soon be lost). Recognition is demonstrated by the ability to produce this information. If I claimed to recognize an object, but was unable to produce any relevant information about it, you may doubt that I had truly recognized it. Note that my recognition need not involve naming the object, or indeed any ability to speak. Correct recognition of a pen could be demonstrated by miming a writing action, or by choosing 'pencil' as the associated object given a choice of visually similar objects such as pencil, knife and knitting needle. Associative agnosia can therefore be seen as a failure to match a percept with previous experience.

Some patients have agnosic deficits for a limited range of objects. For example, two patients of Warrington and Shallice (1984) were relatively good at recognizing man-made objects but very poor at recognizing animals and other living things. Other bizarre selective agnosias (agnosias that affect some classes of objects more than others) have also been found. For example, Warrington reported that a patient was able to recognize pictures representing abstract concepts such as enticement, but failed to recognize a picture of a carrot (Warrington, 1981). The interpretation of such cases is still controversial, but they do suggest that visual agnosia should always be tested with a range of objects or pictures to ensure that testing does not cover only a small range of pictures with which the patient is relatively good, only to ignore a large class of objects with which the patient has great difficulty.

Prosopagnosia

One particular selective agnosia has a long history and has been much studied. In 1947, Bodamer described a series of patients who had difficulties in recognizing people visually. For example, one of his cases, who sustained a head injury during the Second World War, could no longer recognize people – not even those who were well known to him. He could see the faces adequately as he could point to the individual features (eyes, nose, mouth), but even well-known faces produced no feeling of familiarity in him. When he unexpectedly met his own mother, he failed to recognize her. This selective failure to recognize people from their faces is called *prosopagnosia* (from the Greek 'prosop' meaning face). The deficit often co-occurs with visual object agnosia. However, prosopagnosia and visual object agnosia can each also occur by themselves. This pattern of occurrence is called a *double dissociation* as each impairment can occur independently of the other, although many patients have both problems. When there is a double dissociation between two cognitive processes (such that deficits in each may occur without the other), there is reason to believe that the two rely on different underlying mechanisms in the normal brain, each of which can be separately damaged. The double dissociation between impairments in object recognition and face recognition has been held as evidence that faces represent a special class of objects in the brain and are not processed as other visual objects.

Like visual object agnosia, prosopagnosia is probably not a single entity and there may be several different reasons for face recognition impairments. For example, some prosopagnosic patients report that the faces look strange and distorted, while for others the faces appear normal, although unfamiliar. Some also have problems making judgements about the age or even gender of people based on their facial characteristics. Equally, some prosopagnosics are unable to interpret people's emotional state on the basis of their facial expression, so that smiling or frowning no longer has any meaning to them (Bornstein, 1963). However, note that the problem lies in the faces of the people, as many prosopagnosics report that they can learn to recognize people from the sound of their voices, or from non-facial visual characteristics, such as their walk, clothes or hairstyle. As a result, a prosopagnosic patient may be duped by the simplest of disguises (a moustache or a limp), because, unlike most people, they do not recognize the invariant facial characteristics. The ability of many prosopagnosic patients to function in everyday life by relying on voice recognition or other visual characteristics reveals that the underlying problem is not that the patient has all lost memory for the person concerned. The problem may be a failure to access stored knowledge about the person from the visual information contained within the face.

Deficits in visual-spatial processing

Patients with visual agnosia (whether for objects or for faces) have an impairment in knowing what (or who) something is, but they have no problem in knowing where it is. Indeed, if allowed, patients with visual object agnosia will often reach out to grasp an unknown object and touching the object may be sufficient to allow them to identify it. However, there are other patients who have a specific problem in dealing with the spatial aspects of their visual world, despite the fact that they may have no problem in recognizing objects. Thus there is a double dissociation between knowing what an object is and knowing where it is, and either of these abilities may be separately impaired by brain damage.

Visual disorientation

The most complete, early description of patients who suffered from problems in visual localization following brain damage comes from Holmes (Holmes, 1918). Holmes studied a group of soldiers who had suffered from head injuries during the First World War. He described eight patients who had difficulties determining the location of objects that they could see. The first and most famous of these patients is Private M, who was wounded by shrapnel. He was considered to have recovered well and had no lasting problems with language, paralysis or intellectual functioning. His acuity was normal for the central part of his visual fields and he could recognize objects well. However, Private M had a problem determining the location of objects that he saw and could recognize. As a result, he could not reach out and pick up objects, often groping for them as though he were in the dark, despite his obvious ability to see the desired object. This was not just a problem in controlling the muscles involved in reaching, as Private M could also not say which of two objects was closer to him on the basis of vision alone, although he was accurate if he was allowed to feel the relative positions of the objects. Thus Private M's problem was making judgements about the location of objects from vision. This condition is known as *visual disorientation*.

Visual disorientation can result in difficulties over and above those that seem superficially concerned with the localization of objects. Private M, like other patients with similar problems, could read single words or short sentences but could not read longer pieces. These patients have problems controlling their eye movements as nothing seems fixed in space. Therefore the controlled eye movements required for reading are beyond them. They report that the words appear to jump around the page and they quickly lose their place in the text.

Holmes' (1918) report of eight patients with this problem noted that all had bilateral lesion of the parietal lobes (see Figure 11.1). However, since then, unilateral parietal lobe lesions have been reported to result in similar problems, which are confined to localization within the opposite side of space (Brain, 1941). The involvement of the parietal cortex contrasts with the lesion causing the visual agnosic deficits discussed above. Agnosic deficits are associated with damage to the temporal lobe or at the junction of the occipital and temporal lobes. This accords with an idea that has emerged from consideration of the anatomy and physiology of the region that has been determined mainly using the brains of animals, including monkeys. This has suggested that visual information is channelled into at least two major streams in the brain (Ungerleider and Mishkin, 1982). The first stream courses ventrally to the temporal lobes and processes information primarily concerned with an object's identity ('what'). The second courses dorsally to the parietal lobe and primarily processes the object's localization ('where'). These two streams have become known as the *ventral* and *dorsal* processing stream respectively (see Figure 11.3).

Unilateral neglect

Damage to the parietal lobe can also cause a related but different problem. Following damage to the right parietal cortex, patients may have an impairment in responding to events that happen to the left side of their bodies. Similar problems after damage to the left parietal cortex are much less commonly seen. This condition is known as *unilateral (or contralateral or hemispatial) neglect* and can be defined as a failure to report, respond, or orient to stimuli presented to the side contralateral to a brain lesion in the absence of elementary motor or sensory deficits. This failure to respond to events on the side contralateral to a lesion can be simply

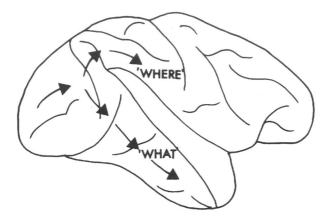

Figure 11.3: The brain of a monkey showing the route of the proposed dorsal ('where') and ventral ('what') processing streams.

demonstrated. For example, in the *line bisection task* a patient is simply asked to mark the centre of a horizontal line drawn on a piece of paper. A patient with contralateral neglect will bisect it towards the right, reflecting a failure to take sufficient account of the left-hand side of the line. Equally, a patient can be presented with a random array of ticks on a page and asked to cross out each tick. A patient with unilateral neglect will typically conscientiously cross out all the ticks on the right of the page but show a conspicuous failure to cancel those on the left. Their partial compliance with the task instructions demonstrates that they have understood what is required, but ignored ticks on the left. Failure on the line bisection and cancellation task might be thought to reflect a hemianopia, that is a sensory loss that hides half of each page. However, we can rule out this simple explanation for two reasons. First, patients who have hemianopia often complete these tasks well, as simply moving the eyes over the page will compensate for the hemianopia. Second, patients with contralateral neglect also fail to respond to non-visual stimuli in the neglected field. For example, a patient may fail to report a touch to the left shoulder while reporting touches to the right side of the body. If asked to raise their arms patients may raise only the right arm, even when reminded that both arms should be raised. Thus, unlike hemianopia, which is specifically a visual problem, contralateral neglect affects all modalities. It may also affect a patient's drawing. Asked to draw a clock, for example, a patient may draw a distorted circle, much less full on the left than the right hand side, and will then complete only the numbers on the right side of the clock face, failing to fill in those numbers that should fall on the left. Contralateral neglect may extend to all aspects of the patient's life – a patient may fail to eat from the left of the plate or neglect to shave the left of the face. In fact, contralateral neglect has also been shown to affect the imagination. In a famous study, Bisiach asked an Italian patient with neglect to describe the central square in Milan (with which he was very familiar) from a particular viewpoint (Bisiach and Luzzatti, 1978). The patient accurately described the right-hand side of the square from his imagined viewpoint and neglected to describe the left. Bisiach then asked him to imagine the square from a different and opposite viewpoint. Now the patient described buildings which had been neglected in his first account and failed to report buildings now to the left, but which he had previously mentioned. Thus the patient neglected whatever was on the left of his imaginary representation of the square. This and other evidence has led to the view that neglect is a failure to attend to positions on the contralateral side of space and is therefore a deficit in spatial attention. The fact that contralateral neglect is much more common after right-hemisphere lesions than left suggests a special role for the right hemisphere in the spatial control of attention that is not shared by the left hemisphere.

Memory

The above discussion of visual functions within the brain suggested that perception is not a single entity within the brain but can be subdivided into perception of specific attributes such as colour and movement, and the recognition and localization of objects. Similarly, memory cannot be viewed as a single entity that can be impaired by brain damage. Modern psychologists recognize that memory should be subdivided into a temporary, short-term, store (STS) and a memory store for long-term or permanent storage (LTS). Equally within LTS, psychologists subdivide memory into declarative and procedural memories.

The physical representation of a memory within the brain is called an *engram*. Lashley attempted to determine the brain structures that contain the engram (Lashley, 1929, 1950). His repeated failure to find the engram located in a single region resulted in him supporting the idea of *equipotentiality*, or *mass action*, as discussed above. Specifically, he suggested that all areas of the brain contributed equally to memory functions. However, the principle of equipotentiality proved to be as inappropriate for memory processes as it was found to be for visual functions.

An early clue to the localization of engrams came in the 1950 when Penfield investigated the brain function of patients about to undergo brain surgery. The patients had only local anaesthetic and so were fully conscious while Penfield passed a small electrical current through the brain to stimulate neurons. Some of these stimulations resulted in the patients reporting feelings or perceptions (Penfield and Perot, 1963). For example, if their visual cortexes were stimulated, patients would report flashes of light. When Penfield stimulated the cortex of the temporal lobes, patients reported experiences that seemed like memories. Thus it appeared that Penfield had discovered the location of the engram, and by stimulating the cortex was eliciting playback of these memories. The areas that Penfield was stimulating, the lateral and medial surfaces of the temporal lobe, were suggested to be the storehouse of memory. However, since then it has become apparent that Penfield's finding were not quite what they at first appeared. It is probable that his stimulations caused electrical after-discharges that spread to brain areas other than those Penfield thought he was stimulating. More recent studies have found that memory-like responses are most commonly found after stimulating a group of structures that comprise the *limbic system* (Halgren et al., 1978). The limbic system is composed of the hippocampus and amygdala (which lie within the temporal lobes and are therefore known as *medial temporal structures*) and parts of the thalamus and hypothalamus (see Figure 11.4).

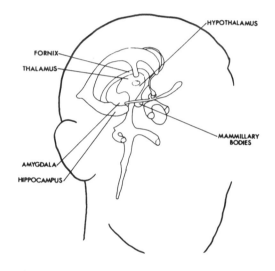

Figure 11.4: Structures involved in memory processes in the human brain.

Further evidence implicating some of these regions in memory came from the case of a young man known as HM. HM underwent bilateral removal of portions of his temporal lobe in an attempt to relieve intractable epilepsy. As a result of his surgery he became densely amnesic. He had lost some memories for events that had occurred prior to his brain surgery (*retrograde amnesia*) and was unable to add any new memories of events that occurred after his operation (*anterograde amnesia*) (Scoville and Milner, 1957). Thus the case of HM points to the structures within the medial temporal lobes that were removed in his surgery as being crucial to memory functions. Specifically, HM had substantial damage to the hippocampus, the amygdala and the cortex of the temporal lobe, which surround these structures. Further study of patients and animals with either hippocampal or amygdala damage has suggested that the damage to the hippocampus was primarily responsible for HM's amnesia.

However, amnesia is a relatively common consequence of brain injury and some of these cases have verified damage to the brain that is far removed from the hippocampus. This evidence has suggested to some that there may be at least two different causes of the symptoms of memory loss that we label as amnesia. For example, one of the more common forms of amnesia is *Korsakoff's amnesia*. Korsakoff's amnesia follows an acute neurological condition named *Wernicke's encephalopathy*. The symptoms of Wernicke's encephalopathy include ataxia, optic abnormalities and gross confusion, and it is usually associated with prolonged alcohol abuse. On recovery from the acute stage, these patients are left with profound anterograde amnesia (Victor, Adams and Collins, 1971). Studies of the brains of these patients have suggested that the locus of the brain damage is in the mammillary bodies at the base of the brain and also in the thalamus. Both of these locations are far removed geographically from the medial temporal lobe (see Figure 11.4). Moreover, a patient known as NA suffered a bizarre accident in which a minature fencing foil entered his brain though his right nostril, through the cribiform plate and into the left forebrain. NA recovered from this unfortunate accident, suffering only from a mild paresis of upward gaze and severe memory impairment for verbal material. Computerized tomography (CT) scans have revealed that NA has damage to the medial dorsal nucleus of the thalamus (Squire and Moore, 1979). Thus again, as in Korsakoff's amnesia, we see damage within the thalamus causing amnesia. The fact that amnesia can follow damage to two geographically distant brain regions has led some to suggest that there may be more than one type of amnesia. A more parsimonious account is provided by the idea that the hippocampus and central regions of the thalamus form a tightly linked memory circuit that includes the hippocampus, fornix, thalamus and mammillary bodies. In this case, damage anywhere within this circuit will result in amnesia (see Figure 11.4).

The introduction to this section emphasized that memory is not a unitary entity and amnesic patients have many memory abilities still intact. For example, their short-term memory (STS) and semantic memory remain unimpaired and their skill learning may be intact. This implies that these abilities are subserved by other brain circuits that remain unaffected by the brain damage usually seen in amnesic patients and discussed above. The STS system may be interrupted by damage to other brain regions. For example, Warrington and Shallice (1969) report the case of KF who suffered damage to the left cerebral hemisphere. As a result he had an auditory digit span of only one digit. Digit span is seen as a measure of STS capacity and a span of around seven is considered normal. KF's digit span was therefore grossly abnormal and reflects a severe deficit in STS. Other work has implicated the prefrontal cortex (see Figure 11.1), or connections to it, as being the critical regions for causing deficits in STS.

Interestingly, KF's digit span was much improved if the digits were presented to him visually, rather than spoken. This suggests that there may be a dissociation within STS for auditory information and for visual information. A similar pattern may exist in LTS. NA, the patient with damage to his thalamus following a fencing accident mentioned above, in fact had damage confined to his left thalamus. NA's amnesia was most marked for verbal information and was better (although far from perfect) for visual information. In general, it seems that, at both the level of short-term memory and long-term memory, the left hemisphere plays a much greater role in verbal information whereas the right hemisphere contributes more fully to retention of visual information.

Language functions

The association between the left hemisphere and memory for verbal information accords with a long-known association between the left hemisphere and language functions. The first documented association between a brain area and a behavioural impairment was published by Paul Broca (Broca, 1861). Broca's celebrated case, known as 'Tan', had a profound *aphasia*, that is an impairment in language (from the Greek for 'lack of speech'). In fact, Tan's impairment was so severe that he could utter only the single sound, 'Tan'. On his death, Tan was found to have damage to a region in the third frontal convolution of the left hemisphere, which subsequently became known as *Broca's area* (see Figure 11.1). Patients who have language impairments similar to Broca's patient, Tan, are called *Broca's aphasics*. Clearly Broca's area plays an important role in language functions.

Around the same time, Wernicke had noticed a different group of patients with language impairments following brain damage (Wernicke, 1874). However, the pattern of their impairment differed from that noted by Broca and the region damaged was also different. While Broca's patient could produce almost no language, aphasics of Broca's type typically have some comprehension of language, although it may not be entirely normal. In contrast, aphasics of Wernicke's type typically produce fluent speech, although it may contain many errors, but their comprehension is very poor. In addition, Wernicke's aphasics do not have damage in the frontal lobe, but more posteriorly in the superior portions of the temporal lobe (see Figure 11.1). Thus there are at least two regions that can produce deficits in language, although they produce different types of language impairments. Broca's aphasics have most difficulty in producing speech and for this reason are sometimes known as *expressive, non-fluent* or *motor aphasics*. Note that Broca's region lies very close to the frontal regions, which control the speech musculature and that Broca's aphasia is a disorder relating to the production of language. Conversely, Wernicke's aphasics have most difficulty with the comprehension of speech and are therefore sometimes known as *receptive*, *fluent* or *sensory aphasics*. Again, it may be of interest to note that Wernicke's area lies close to the auditory projection zone, an area of the brain concerned with processing auditory input. Wernicke's aphasia is a disorder relating to the processing of incoming speech.

However, the picture of Wernicke's area processing incoming speech and Broca's area processing outgoing speech is probably too simplistic. It has been noted that aphasia may also follow damage to regions far removed from both Broca's and Wernicke's areas. Even in the nineteenth century it had been suggested that aphasia may follow damage to subcortical structures. However, this view was not given much credence until Penfield and Roberts (1959) suggested that the thalamus, especially the pulvinar, played an important role in language functions. The studies involved placing electrodes in the pulvinar as part of a surgical treatment for movement disorders. Stimulation of the pulvinar during this procedure caused speech difficulties, including an inability to name objects, slowed or arrested speech, and a tendency to repeat previous words (Ojemann, 1975). However, the roles that the thalamus and pulvinar play in language functions are not yet clear.

Language functions are usually associated with the left hemisphere (although the situation may be different in some left-handers). Nevertheless, the right hemisphere does have a role in language that should not be underestimated. Language does not just consist of words strung together in a grammatical sequence. Normal verbal interaction requires that appropriate intonation and expression are added to those words in order to add emphasis and emotion and occasionally to change the meaning. For example, the words 'green house' may mean a glass shed for raising plants or a green-coloured abode, depending on the stress given to the word 'green'. Equally, the phrase 'you are not going out tonight' could express a command, astonishment or merely a question depending on the pattern of pitch and stress used. These aspects of language, known as *prosody*, rely on the right hemisphere. Patients with damage to the right hemisphere may be unable to use prosody to understand language (Heilman, Scholes and Watson, 1975). This may lead them to misunderstand conversations despite intact language comprehension as measured in standard clinical tests. They may also have difficulty using prosody effectively and therefore their speech will appear to be monotonous and dull (Ross and Mesulam, 1979).

In summary, we have seen that language is not a single function in the brain, any more than is memory or perception. Language functions may break down in a number of ways following damage to a number of brain regions. The left hemisphere plays a major role in most language functions in most people, but the right hemisphere plays an important role in prosody.

The frontal lobes

The area at the front of the brain has long been recognized as being important to normal human functioning. The special emphasis comes from the fact that it is a vast amount of cortex, representing about 20% of all cortex in the human (see Figure 11.1). In addition, it is clear that over the process of evolution from lower animals to humans, it is the prefrontal cortex that has expanded more than other parts of cortex. This has given rise to the idea that it is the prefrontal cortex that gives us the essential qualities of humans, as contrasted with the animals. Indeed, until the 1930s, the frontal lobes were considered as the seat of the highest intellect.

The frontal lobes themselves consist of three distinct regions: the motor cortex, premotor cortex and prefrontal cortex (see Figure 11.1). The motor and premotor cortex can be considered as part of the motor control system. Damage to motor cortex results in paralysis. However, because each part of the motor cortex controls one muscle group, partial damage can result in paralysis of just some of the body. The motor cortex can be seen as containing a map of the body, with the upper body towards the bottom of the strip, the lower body at the top, and the representation of the legs continuing on to the medial surface of the brain (see Figure 11.1). However, it is a slightly strange map of the body because the amount of cortex devoted to each part of the body is not proportional to the size of the body part. Instead, it is proportional to the amount of control we have over movements of that part of the body. For example, we have exquisitely fine control of the mouth, lips and tongue, which allows chewing and swallowing, as well as all our speech. A relatively large amount of motor cortex is devoted to controlling the fine movements required for these functions. In comparison, fine control of movements of the hips and legs is limited, perhaps because relatively little cortex is controlling these movements.

The premotor cortex is intimately connected with the motor cortex and can be seen as an executive control area for the motor cortex. If the motor cortex controls the execution of movements, the premotor cortex selects the appropriate movements to be executed. However, the premotor cortex receives a large amount of information from the prefrontal cortex. The prefrontal cortex has been described as a region that is involved in collecting information from the sensory regions about the world, collecting relevant information from the memory systems and combining this in order to choose an appropriate plan of action. Thus the entire frontal lobe may be seen as the output system for the brain. The prefrontal cortex assesses the current situation and determines an appropriate course of action. The premotor cortex determines appropriate movements to achieve this and the motor cortex controls this movement plan.

Some evidence for the role of the prefrontal cortex in complex planning of actions comes from patients who have damage to the prefrontal region. The most famous patient to have suffered damage to the prefrontal cortex was a Victorian railway worker named Phineas Gage, first reported by Harlow in 1868. As a result of the accidental ignition of explosives during construction of a railway line, a metal bar was driven through the entire frontal portion of Gage's brain, causing extensive damage to prefrontal regions. Astonishingly, Gage quickly recovered, and had few overt signs of his brain damage. After a few weeks, his perceptual, motor, language and memory functions were all entirely normal. However, Gage suffered a complete change in his personality. Gage had been a foreman on the railways and had been considered a sober and responsible worker. Following his injury he became irresponsible, rash and impatient, with a tendency to profanities. He was unable to continue in his former work and travelled the country with a circus, ever hopeful of making his fortune.

Although it is extreme, Gage's case is not untypical of the results of damage to prefrontal cortex. The patients appear unable to make rational assessments of their situation and make appropriate decisions based upon it. These deficits are known as *executive dysfunction*. In the clinic, these deficiencies can be seen in their performance on standard tests. Although their memory, language and perceptual functions are all intact, patients will fail apparently simple tasks. One classic task is known as the *Wisconsin card-sorting test* (Milner, 1964). It consists of a pack of cards, each of which has on it a number of coloured shapes. However, there are three possible shapes (for example square, circle, and star), three possible colours and either one, two or three exemplars of the shape could appear on each card. For example, a card may show two blue stars or one red circle. The patient has to sort a pack of these cards into three piles but is given no instructions as to the sorting principle. The pack could plausibly be sorted into three piles on the basis of the colour on the card (ignoring differences in shape and number) or could be sorted according to shape or number. The patient has to choose a sorting principle and lay a card at a time on the piles and is given feedback as to whether the card is correct or incorrectly laid according to a predetermined principle. Once the patient has worked out the rule the tester has in mind, the sorting principle can be changed (for example switching from colour to number) without telling the patient. The patient, through trial and error, must determine the current rule. Patients with damage to the prefrontal cortex have enormous difficulties with this task. Many will work out the initial rule, but will fail to switch from this rule to another when the rule changes. This is typical of the behaviour of these patients in many situations. Such rigidity in behaviour or thought is called *perseveration* and can be seen in many tasks. Perseveration may result in repetitive behaviour, so that the patient may repeat an action such as pacing, but may also result in a patient having difficulty changing a from one idea to another, so the patient may become fixed on a single thought or idea. For example, a patient may show perseveration in the *Thurstone word fluency test*. The Thurstone word fluency test requires patients to write or say as many words starting with a given letter as they can think of in five minutes. Prefrontal patients will typically become stuck after a few words, or may perseverate the same few words repeatedly. Perhaps this repetitive behaviour is akin to another sign of frontal lobe damage – an inability to modify behaviour according to subsequent information. Having determined on a rule or strategy, patients will continue with it despite clear evidence that it is, or has become, inappropriate.

These impairments are seen in clinical tests, but patients with prefrontal cortex lesions may also show inappropriate behaviour in everyday situations. Like Phineas Gage, these patients may show inappropriate social or sexual behaviour, perhaps failing to take account of highly complex and sometime subtle rules that govern such behaviour. In addition, damage to the prefrontal cortex, particularly the lower portions (called the *orbitofrontal cortex*) have been associated with *pseudodepression* and *pseudopsychopathy* (Blumer and Benson, 1975). Pseudopsychopathic patients display immature behaviour with a lack of social and behavioural restraint. Phineas Gage is an example of pseudopsychopathy. In contrast, patients showing pseudodepression display outward apathy and indifference, initiating almost no activity, including conversations. It has been suggested that pseudodepression is more commonly seen after left frontal lesions whereas pseudopsychopathy is associated with right hemisphere damage, although bilateral damage may be necessary to cause severe cases. Although pseudopsychopathy and pseudodepression seem such different symptoms, they may be functionally related. It is possible that pseudodepression is a result of no action plan being determined by the prefrontal cortex. In contrast, damage to the system may result in pseudopsychopathy, where any change in the environment triggers a new plan of action, yet none is followed through to its conclusion.

The prefrontal cortex is a large area of cortex and studies in monkeys have shown that it is composed of areas that differ in their connections and cell types. We should therefore expect that they will differ in the behavioural consequences of damage too. It is thus expected that there should be a range of different behavioural consequences of damage to prefrontal regions. They share the underlying principle that the behaviour becomes disorganized. This has led Luria to describe the function of the prefrontal cortex to be for programming and regulating behaviour (Luria, 1966). This idea has been developed by Norman and Shallice (1980, 1986). They proposed that behaviour is controlled in two major ways. First, many behaviours are almost automatic, so we are hardly consciously aware of them. For example, we may be capable of driving a well-known route, responding appropriately to traffic lights and other drivers and yet arrive home with no recollection of the journey. Norman and Shallice suggest that such behaviour is automatically controlled by a process they named *contention scheduling*. However, sometimes contention scheduling is not sufficient as the conditions may call for some behaviour for which we do not already have a set of routine operations, or those routine operations may be inappropriate. For example, if instead of driving your normal route home you have to remember to call in at the dry cleaners, you will have to override the contention scheduling in order to arrive home with the dry cleaning. They call this override system the *supervisory activating system* (SAS). The SAS will operate when automatic, well-known routine behaviours are not working or we have none available for the given situation. However, Norman and Shallice suggested that prefrontal damage disrupts the operation of the SAS. Patients with prefrontal cortex damage therefore rely on contention scheduling. This will allow them to deal with routine situations well. However, in novel situations or when a novel solution to a problem is required, the failure of the SAS will become apparent. The patients are likely to follow well-established routines even though it may be apparent that they are wrong and that a new strategy is required. Such a failure could result in many of the impairments shown by patients with prefrontal cortex damage, both in everyday life and in clinical settings.

Techniques in neuropsychological assessment

There are a great many neuropsychological tests that aim to assess various aspects of the mental functioning of a patient after brain damage. Some of those that are most commonly associated with particular impairments have been mentioned above in the appropriate sections. The choice of test depends to some extent on the nature of the damage suffered by the patient, the subjective reports of the patient and the aim of the assessment. Assessment will ideally pinpoint the nature of the deficit, but it may also help to highlight areas of relatively preserved ability, which may help in the rehabilitation process.

One approach is to ask patients where they are experiencing difficulties. Although this may indeed be helpful, it may not produce a full answer. In many cases patients are not aware of the nature of their difficulties. Patients with achromatopsia, for example, may not spontaneously report problems seeing colour, although they are aware that things do not seem clear. Contralateral neglect is commonly associated with *anosognosia*, a denial of any problem despite sufficient evidence. For example, a patient asked to raise both arms and who only raises the right arm as a result of neglect of the left arm may claim that there is nothing wrong. Patients with pseudodepression also show an absence of appropriate concern about their situation. Spouses or other family members may be a better source of information on the patient's abilities. However, family members cannot be aware of changes in the patient's perceptions or thoughts. Thus one aim of neuropsychological assessment will be to provide a detailed analysis of the patient's abilities and impairments. However, this should of course be balanced by consideration of the impact of these impairments on the patient's lifestyle. For example, assessment may reveal that a patient has a mild prosopagnosia and relatively more severe impairments in visual memory (both deficits associated with right hemisphere damage). However, the prosopagnosia may have a much more severe impact on the patient's life if their job involves meeting people, while for them the memory impairment may be simply bypassed using verbal memory strategies.

There are a variety of tests that specifically test abilities associated with particular neuropsychological deficits. Some of these have been mentioned in the preceding sections. For example, the Wisconsin card-sorting test or the line bisection task might be useful when one suspects prefrontal or parietal damage respectively. Alternatively, one may use standardized test batteries. Test batteries assess a range of abilities and have instructions for administration and scoring so they can be widely used by those who do not necessarily have much experience of neuropsychology. There are many test batteries available and choice depends on availability and personal preferences more than anything else. In assessing a patient's abilities one must bear in mind individual differences in intelligence and educational level that may affect vocabulary or other aspects of the test. For example, Warrington's graded naming test is a test of a patient's ability to name pictures, which starts with common words and proceeds to less common words. One can assess the severity of any naming deficit as increasing severity of the disorder results in more frequent words being lost. However, one must take into account premorbid vocabulary because a word in the midrange of the test may be a very unusual word for someone with little education but could be commonplace for an educated patient. The Wechsler Adult Intelligence Scale Revised (WAIS-R) may help in determining ability, but brain damage may affect this measure itself. Alternatively, the National Adult Reading Test (NART) assesses ability to read and pronounce irregular words (such as 'bouquet') and has been found to be relatively resistant to the effects of brain damage and may again give some indication of premorbid attainment levels.

Summary

This chapter began by introducing the concept of modularity. The subsequent sections have demonstrated that brain damage can differentially affect visual, memory, language and higher-level functions. Even within each of these functions, there may be differential impairment of just one aspect. For example, within the visual modality, deficits in object recognition, object localization and face recognition may be identified. The purpose of neuropsychology is to use this evidence to understand the way these functions are organized in the brain. This knowledge may usefully be applied to rehabilitation so that brain-damaged patients may concentrate their efforts on using those functions which remain relatively intact.

References

Bisiach E, Luzzatti C (1978) Unilateral neglect of representational space. Cortex 14: 129–33.

Blumer D, Benson DF (1975) Personality changes with frontal and temporal lobe lesions. In DF Benson, D Blumer (eds) Psychiatric Aspects of Neurologic Disease. New York: Grune & Stratton.

Bodamer J (1947) Die prosopagnosia. Archiv fur psychiatrie und zeitschrift fur neurologie 179: 6–54.

Bornstein, B (1963) Prosopagnosia. In L Halpern (ed.) Problems of Dynamic Neurology. Jerusalem: Hadasseh Medical Organization, pp. 238–318.

Brain WR (1941) Visual disorientation with special reference to lesions of the right cerebral hemisphere. Brain 64: 244–72.

Broca P (1861) Remarques sur le siege de la faculte du langage articule suivre d'une observation d'aphemie. Bull Soc Anat Paris 6: 330.

Cowcy A, Heywood CA (1997) Cerebral achromatopsia: colour blindness despite wavelength processing. Trends in Cognitive Sciences 1: 133–9.

Fellman DJ, Van Essen DC (1991) Distributed hierarchical processing in the primate cerebral cortex. Cerebral Cortex 1: 1–47.

Fodor JA (1983) The Modularity of Mind. Cambridge MA: MIT Press.

Halgren E, Walter RD, Cherlow AG, Crandall PH (1978) Mental phenomena evoked by electrical stimulation of the hippocampal formation and amygdala. Brain 101: 83–117.

Hebb DO (1949) The Organisation of Behaviour: A Neuropsychological Theory. New York: Wiley.

Heilman KM, Scholes RJ, Watson RT (1975) Auditory affective agnosia. Journal of Neurology, Neurosurgery and Psychiatry 38: 69–72.

Holmes G (1918) Disturbances of visual orientation. British Journal of Opthalmology 2: 449–68.

Lashley KS (1929) Brain Mechanisms and Intelligence: A Quantative Study of Injuries to the Brain. Chicago: Chicago University Press.

Lashley KS (1950) In search of the engram. Symp Soc Exp Biol 4: 454–82.

Lissauer H (1890) Ein fall von seelenblindheit nebst einem beitrage zur theorie derselben. Archiv fur Psychiatrie und Nervekrankheiten 21: 222–70.

Luria AR (1966) Higher Cortical Functions in Man. London: Tavistock.

Meadows JC (1974) Disturbed perception of colours associated with localised cerebral lesions. Brain 97: 615–32.

Milner B (1964) Some effects of frontal lobectomy in man. In JM Warren, K Akert (eds) The Frontal Granular Cortex and Behaviour. New York: McGraw-Hill, pp. 313–31.

Norman DA, Shallice T (1980) Attention to action: willed and automatic control of behavior. Centre for human information processing (report no. 99). Reprinted in revised form in RJ Davison, GE Schwartz and D Shapiro (eds) (1986) Conciousness and Self-Regulation, Vol 4. New York: Plenum Press.

Ojemann GA (1975) The thalamus and language. Brain and Language 2: 1–120.

Penfield W, Perot P (1963) The brain's record of auditory and visual experience. Brain. 86: 595–696.

Penfield W, Roberts L (1959) Speech and Brain Mechanisms. Princeton NJ: Princeton University Press.

Ross EG, Mesulam M-M (1979) Dominent language functions of the right hemisphere? Archives of Neurology. 36: 144–8.

Scoville WB, Milner B (1957) Loss of recent memory after bilateral hippocampal lesions. Journal of Neurology, Neurosurgery and Psychiatry 20: 11–21.

Squire LR, Moore RY (1979) Dorsal thalamic lesion in a noted case of human memory dysfunction. Annuals of Neurology 6: 503–6.

Ungerleider LG, Mishkin M (1982) Two cortical visual systems. In DJ Ingle, MA Goodale, RJW Mansfield (eds) Analysis of Visual Behaviour. Cambridge MA: MIT Press, pp. 549–86.

Victor M, Adams RD, Collins GH (1971) The Wernicke–Korsakoff Syndrome. Philadelphia: Davis.

Warrington EK (1981) Neuropsychological studies of verbal semantic systems. Philosophical Transactions of the Royal Society of London, Series B 295: 411–23.

Warrington EK, Shallice T (1969) The selective impairment of auditory verbal short-term memory. Brain 92: 885–96.

Warrington EK, Shallice T (1984) Category-specific semantic impairments. Brain 107: 829–54.

Wernicke K (1874) Der Aphasishe Symptomenkomplex. Breslau: Cohn & Weigart.

Zihl J, Von Cramon D, Mai N (1983) Selective disturbance of movement vision after bilateral brain damage. Brain 106: 313–40.

Further reading

A more detailed but readable account of many of the disorders discussed in this chapter can be found in:

Ellis AW, Young AW (1988) Human Cognitive Neuropsychology. New Jersey: Erlbaum.

This book does not cover executive dysfunction. An equally good source that does include the deficits that follow damage to prefrontal cortex is:

McCarthy RA, Warrington EK (1990) Cognitive Neuropsychology: A Clinical Introduction. San Diego CA: Academic Press.

Chapter 12
Intelligence and its measurement

JOHN PICKERING

Key concepts	Key names
Metacognition	Metcalfe and Shimamura
Psychophysical approach	Galton
Mental age	Binet
IQ	Stern
Intelligence scales	Stanford-Binet; Wechsler
Factor analysis	Spearman
General and specific factors	Spearman
Independent primary factors	Thurstone
'Fluid' and 'crystallized' abilitites	Cattell
Seven types of intelligence	Gardner
Artificial intelligence	Newell
Triarchic theory	Sternberg
Emotional intelligence	Damasio, Goleman
Cultural assimilation	Vygotsky, Wertsch

There is no generally accepted definition of 'intelligence', nor are there objective units in which to measure it. The history of the area shows that measurement techniques have become, essentially, an exercise in comparing individuals to norms. Most intelligence scales assess performance on a number of different tasks that involve different aspects of intelligence. The overall results give a deviation from a norm, which is usually related to age and gender. The extent of this deviation is now the meaning of the term 'intelligence quotient' or IQ. The pattern of results can also show something about a person's individual strengths and weaknesses. There seem to be both specific and general components to intelligence, although there is some controversy as to what the specific ones are specific to. Recent research has moved in both specific and generalized directions. The specific information processing mechanisms of intelligence have been investigated in neuropsychology, in cognitive psychology and in artificial intelligence. There has also been research into the way in which people's skills and knowledge in general are integrated into the social world and adapted to new situations. Enduring issues in the area remain, such as the balance between hereditary and environmental factors and the issue of whether intelligence scales are culturally fair.

Introduction

The word 'intelligence' is used in general conversation and yet it is rather difficult to define it specifically and to find ways to measure it. It is perhaps not surprising that there remains a contrast between common usage and the devising of rigorous definitions and measurements. What counts as intelligence varies across individuals, cultures and historical periods, and so an explicit and stable definition may be an unrealistic objective. Perhaps the best that can be expected is to find concepts and techniques of measurement that are sufficiently clear and reliable to be useful in given situations.

Indeed, if we look into the history of the idea it is clear that despite the persistent conceptual and practical difficulties, many working definitions and reliable practices have emerged and here we offer a brief historical survey of some of them. The survey will show that this area has always been strongly influenced by the changing social context surrounding psychology so that no single definition or measurement system has prevailed. In fact, it is a sign that psychological science is responsive to the intellectual climate and that the study of intelligence is still actively progressing. We will thus finish the chapter by looking at some enduring questions and some current issues in the area.

The measurement of intelligence

If people tell you what they mean by intelligence, many similar ideas will tend to appear, such as: 'clever', 'smart', 'bright', 'brilliant', 'sharp', 'quick on the uptake', 'on the ball' and so on. These are clearly not terms with objectively grounded meanings on which we might base a system of measurement. It is instructive to compare the terms used in the measurement of intelligence with those used in the natural sciences. There we find a language of well-defined units, like centimetres, grams and seconds and of equally well-defined procedures for measuring those units. Nothing so objective is yet to be found in the measurement of intelligence. Despite almost a century of steady effort, and much progress, the measurement of intelligence remains a matter of approximation and of competing views on what is being measured.

One solution to this problem has been to define intelligence as 'that which is measured by intelligence tests'. Psychologists were well aware of the circularity in taking this line. The point was that it seemed almost impossible to define intelligence and attempts to do so appeared to leave psychology at a theoretical *impasse*. Therefore, this oddly self-referential definition was advocated so that psychologists could get on with the business of deriving and perfecting tests, and, perhaps more importantly from the practical point of view, finding out how well they worked in real world situations like educational and vocational selection.

In fact it has been found possible to reach an adequate consensus on what intelligence is taken to mean, without this rather radical step. What has emerged is a middle ground between the informal language of everyday talk about human intelligence and rigorously objective measurement. Ideally, psychology would want to discover terms, units and measurement techniques that would be as explicit about intelligence as physics is about, say, mass. This ideal is probably an unrealistic goal. In any case, the measurement of intelligence does not have to conform to this image of scientific precision in order to be useful. Accordingly, in what follows, the techniques for measurement and the definitions of 'intelligence' will be approached through a brief historical survey of what psychologists have done to measure intelligence. The reader should bear in mind that this history is still in progress.

A working definition

Aspects of intelligence that are incorporated into most working definitions refer to three linked aspects of human psychology. The first is the cluster of cognitive skills covering *understanding* and *using knowledge*. The second is the ability to *learn* from experience and to *apply* what is learned to *new situations*. These two aspects of intelligence are part of the broader issue of *adaptive action*. To act adaptively is to respond to the problems and situations that constantly confront us in a way that allows us to not just survive but to achieve *goals* effectively. In fact, the developmental psychologist Jean Piaget offered a neat definition of intelligence as: 'Knowing what to do when you don't know what to do'. This captures nicely the adaptive sense of being able to confront new situations and to find from experience an appropriate course of action.

The third aspect of intelligence is the capacity for *reflection and self-monitoring*. This is a relatively recent perspective on intelligence and reflects research into the capacity to think about thought – what has become known as *metacognition* (Metcalfe and Shimamura, 1994; Nelson, 1992). To be self-aware and to be able to think about thought processes, both those of the thinker and those of others, is something that critically distinguishes human from animal intelligence. Therefore what we call intelligence in human beings may well be linked to the ability an individual has to do this. Although it leaves many questions unanswered, this three-aspect view – concerning learning, adaptive action and metacognition – will be adopted here as a working definition of the word 'intelligence'.

This word appears to have arrived in the English language in about the twelfth century. It derives, via old French, from the Latin roots *inter*, meaning coming within or between things, and *legere*, meaning linking or reading. Its origins thus reflect rather well the first of the three linked senses above – that of associative understanding. The contexts in which the word is found in early records show that it referred to the human world of ideas and knowledge. This contrasts somewhat with its contemporary meaning, which has now extended to cover non-human intelligence and the adaptation to the natural environment.

Although intelligence has long been taken as a central aspect of human mental life, it was the emergence of science that gave rise to the idea that it might be measured. Two aspects of scientific work are important here. The first is the technical means to make appropriate measurements. The instrumentation required, for example, to time human actions precisely, simply did not exist prior to the scientific revolution. With the rise of astronomical and medical research, however, particularly during the middle and late nineteenth century, there appeared both the instrumentation and the methods, especially statistical techniques, to go with it.

The second aspect is the theory of *evolution*. The idea that the natural world had changed and that this change had something to do with the ability to survive focused attention on the role of intelligence in adaptive action. It was this second aspect of the late scientific revolution that produced one of the first attempts to systematically measure intelligence in the context of a scientific theory.

Francis Galton approached human intelligence as a matter of *heredity*. As he was a cousin of Charles Darwin and was related to other eminent thinkers of his day, this may have been of particularly personal interest! He investigated the occurrence of *exceptional abilities* and *eminent individuals* in family trees. Some of the methods he used were similar to those used by natural historians like Darwin and the other systematic biologists of his time. Having established to his own satisfaction that genius could be inherited, Galton then went on to use the methods of laboratory science to try to show more specifically what was inherited (Galton, 1914).

Galton believed that intelligence comprised various internal processes such as memory, thought, judgement and reasoning. It was difficult to measure these directly but he reasoned that they must derive from more basic psychological processes like perception, motor skill and sensory discrimination. Therefore, it was possible to measure intelligence by measuring the processes on which it depended. He and colleagues such as James Cattell tested how well people could perform physical tasks requiring speed and judgement. This was called the *psychophysical approach* because of the sorts of techniques they used in their investigations of things like the absolute sensitivity of sight and hearing, the ability to make fine and rapid discriminations and the speed and strength with which people could make particular movements. The expectation was that intelligence would correlate with performance on such tests as these and that this would prove to be the basis of how high intellectual performance was transmitted from one generation to the next.

This research had mixed results. Although sensory capacities could be measured reliably, the expected correlations between sensory function and other measures of intelligence, such as college performance, were neither high nor reliable. It was expected that if intelligence reflected a high level of sensory function this should be detectable in all senses. Thus it was expected that high correlations would be observed between sensory functions in particular individuals but, again, there was little evidence for this. It was also clear that in many of Galton's studies intelligence was being defined by how a particular class and culture at a particular point in history judged people to be 'eminent' and 'subnormal'. This clearly would not do as the basis of a scientific theory that would apply to the whole spectrum of people. However, as we shall see below, the idea that intelligence might be measured by measuring some aspect of how the brain works has reappeared in recent years.

The psychophysical approach declined quite rapidly during the early part of the twentieth century and was replaced by what remains today the principal approach to intelligence, although it has developed into a wide variety of forms. This approach takes intelligence to be less to do with special cases and the workings of the senses and more to do with how the general range of people perform everyday tasks. Genius and mentally deficiency are regarded as extremes on a continuum. The concern of psychologists is less with how eminent individuals appear within families and more with how intelligence is distributed in the population as a whole and hence with how individuals relate to this distribution.

This shift is, in effect, a shift from elitism to popularism. It illustrates how the study of intelligence is particularly sensitive to the political and social currents flowing around psychological science. Around the turn of the twentieth century these currents were, broadly, in the direction of mass communication and of social programmes directed at the majority of large urban populations. Screening and selection of very large numbers of individuals for the educational system and for military service, for example, caused a shift of interest from the capacities of exceptional individuals towards the spread of abilities in the whole population, and especially the young. There was a rapid rise in the power and reliability of testing procedures and with it came a deepening of the theories on which these tests were based. This work laid the foundations of the modern view of intelligence and its measurement.

The work of the French psychologist, Alfred Binet, and his colleagues in Paris between 1890 and 1911 reflects just these influences from the wider political and social sphere. A major impetus for Binet's work, and for work like it elsewhere in Europe and America, was the development of large-scale public educational systems. Tests were needed that would detect abnormally low levels of educational ability or progress. Binet was not convinced by Galton's and Cattell's emphasis on sensory function. Instead he proposed that general knowledge, reason, judgement and the ability to respond adaptively to the demands of new situations were the essentials of intelligence and they could be measured directly.

He devised a wide range of tasks which were then systematically refined and composed into test batteries that discriminated between individuals of the same age and between the performance of the same individual at different ages. A central idea here was *mental age*. This was a level of mental competence that was empirically established as typical of a child at a particular chronological age. This idea was developed by William Stern, a German psychologist, into the notion of IQ or *intelligence quotient*. This is simply the mental age of an individual divided by his or her chronological age and multiplied by 100. This notion was widely used for decades but is gradually being replaced by the idea of a deviation IQ, which will be explained below.

Binet's research, subsequently developed and modified in the early 1930s by Louis Terman at Stanford University, gave rise to the first major system for measuring intelligence, the Stanford-Binet Intelligence Scales. These are still in use today (see, for example, Thorndike et al., 1986) but more widely used still are a set of scales known as the Wechsler scales (Wechsler, 1974). However, the underlying theory and methodology of both scales are fairly similar. They are both referred to as a 'scales' since the fundamental process is one of comparing individuals with a scale of performance on a set of tasks.

Scales like the Stanford-Binet and the Wechsler are administered as a series of tests of different abilities. The Stanford-Binet scales comprise of tests that measure verbal, numerical and spatial reasoning and of various types of short-term memory. The Wechsler scales have two major sections dealing with verbal and performance skills, within these sections there are separate tests of comprehension, information and reasoning.

Each test is presented as a graded series of similar tasks. The series begins with easy items followed by ones that are progressively more diffi-cult. For each test there is a stopping criterion based on the failure to complete a number of successive items in the series, the score on the test being a function of how far along the series the person taking the test was able to get. When this criterion is judged to have occurred, the next series is administered and so on until all tests have been given. The tests probe different aspects of intelligence, and this allows the scale to give more than just a single overall result. It is possible to look at the results of individual tests or groups of tests to see how the overall figure breaks down into strengths and weakness in particular areas. This is especially useful in clinical and educational work.

The scoring of individual tests and of the whole scale is by reference to a scale or set of norms. These norms are the result of giving the tests to a very large number of people selected to be representative of the population as a whole and grouped by age and gender. This provides data with which individuals may then be compared. Stern's original idea of comparing mental and chronological age has changed into the idea of comparison with a norm. Although the term 'IQ' has been retained, it now stands for how an individual deviates from the norm of his or her peer group.

This deviation is expressed in terms of the *normal distribution*, which is illustrated in Figure 12.1. This is a characteristic bell-shaped curve that is found when we plot a frequency distribution of a single measure that is influenced by many different factors. The statistical properties of this curve are very well known – such as what proportion of the whole distribution lies within a given number of *standard deviations* above and below the *mean*. It is usual to assign arbitrary values to the mean and standard deviation, to make calculations easier. In intelligence scales, in order to connect with the idea that an 'average IQ' is 100, the assumption is made that the mean, for both individual tests and for the scale as a whole, is 100. The standard deviation is assumed to be 15.

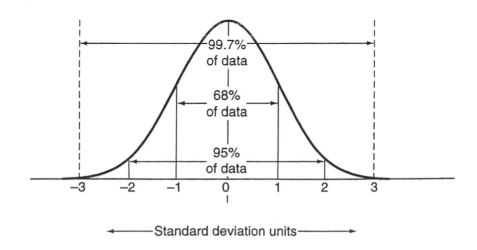

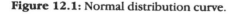

Figure 12.1: Normal distribution curve.

This allows any individual raw score to be converted by referring to tables that show how many standard deviations above or below the mean it is. The deviation scores from all the tests making up the scale are then combined into an overall score that gives what is called a deviation IQ. Strictly a deviation IQ is no longer a quotient, that is, a figure obtained by dividing one number by another as it was in Stern's original idea. Instead it is a measure of how far away an individual is from the most typical level of performance for a relevant comparison group.

An analogy with the height of people at different ages may be useful here. We say of children that they are tall or short 'for their age'. We would be less likely to say this about adults, although we do say that someone is taller or shorter 'than the average'. However, and in a more absolute sense, we can actually measure the height of any individual on a ratio scale like inches or centimetres. Clearly, the Wechsler scales and the many other systems like them for 'measuring' intelligence are not actually measuring anything in this latter sense. There is no ratio scale available – merely norms to which individuals may be compared.

This is now the principal way intelligence is measured. There are scales for different populations and for different aspects of intelligence. A great deal of research has gone into the design, the use and the validation of such scales, which are widely used in education, medicine and in various sorts of selection. The normal distribution is a way of categorizing different levels of performance. An IQ of more than three standard deviations from the mean indicates extreme cases covering less than 1% of the population. At the lower end, such individuals will be expected to have multiple organic disabilities and require permanent special care. At the upper end, special educational provision is strongly indicated. Between two and three standard deviations we find about 5% of the population. Again, special care will probably be necessary at the low end, but at the upper end, individuals will normally be able to fulfil their potential within conventional education and, through performance, receive the attention they need. Between one and two deviations below the mean, remedial attention may be advisable during education and sheltered occupations as adults may occasionally be needed. For the remainder of the range, both educationally and in adult life, we encounter individuals who are able to function well, at their various levels, within normal social surroundings.

The development of scales at present is away from general intelligence and towards specific cognitive abilities, like reading. Some general scales attempt to assess intelligence in a *culturally neutral* way, as far as that is possible. That is, they try to find tests that are independent of what an individual might know because they belong to a particular social or cultural group. One such scale is the Raven's Matrices (Raven et al., 1991), where the completion of a series of increasingly complex visual analogies is the principal task. Figure 12.2 shows an example of a relatively easy analogy, and Figure 12.3 shows a more difficult one. As the series progresses successful performance requires comparing, inferring and the holding in visual memory of increasingly large amounts of information. However, general knowledge or specific skills, like the ability to handle words or numbers, are not involved.

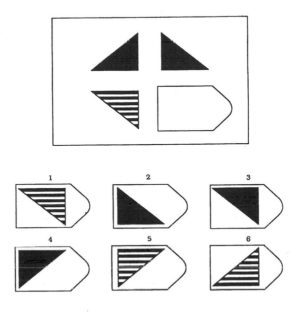

Figure 12.2: An example of an easy analogy from Raven et al., 1991.

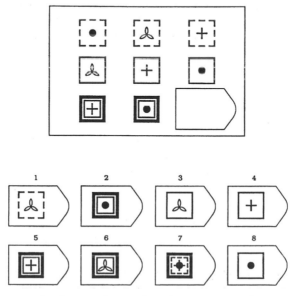

Figure 12.3: An example of a complex analogy from Raven et al., 1991.

Such scales, therefore, are taken to be measuring processing capacity itself, over and above any particular skills or information that an individual may have had the opportunity to learn. From a more general psychological point of view, however, it is well to remember that there is nothing being measured in the absolute sense here. Such scales only indicate where an individual is in relation to some population. They do not aim to show what intelligence actually is – not directly at least. In the next section we will look at some more direct attempts to do so.

The nature of intelligence

Is intelligence one thing or many? This question has been at the heart of a number of attempts to say more explicitly what intelligence actually is. These have generally taken as their starting point the measurement of ability in a wide variety of tasks that seem to require intelligence. This tells us relatively little on its own. As we saw in the previous section, we can establish norms of performance and compare individuals' performance with them, but although this tells us something about the individuals it is not really very informative about what might be determining the ability to perform a task. However, a technique called *factor analysis* does try to get at just that.

Factor analysis is basically an exercise in *multiple correlation*. If we give a wide variety of tasks to a large number of people we are likely to find that performance on groups of them tends to be related. That is, patterns of correlation are likely to appear where performance on tasks within the group will predict performance on other tasks within the group, but not on tasks outside it. There may be a number of such groups with relatively high correlations within them and relatively low correlations between them. Statistical procedures can identify such groups, referred to as factors, and can show how independent they are from each other. By choosing a wide but representative range of tasks it is assumed that all the factors of intelligence will be analysed out, hence the name: factor analysis.

In general, what factor analysis shows is that there are a small number of principal factors to intelligence and a larger number of smaller ones, each with varying degrees of independence from each other. What aspect of intelligence any factor actually is, has to be found by looking at the tests that are associated with it. Over the many factor analytic studies of intelligence, the picture varies. Factors have been identified that seem to cover spatial, numerical, logical and verbal abilities. Just how interrelated these factors are, and what the pattern of relationships is, is a matter of argument.

The principal originator of this method, Charles Spearman, maintained that there was a single *general factor*, which he called 'g', for general ability, and then a number of *specific factors* having to do with specific aspects of intelligence (Spearman, 1927). The general factor was something that appeared in the performance of any task, whereas the specific factors related to abilities in particular areas. As an illustration, consider what we might find if we were to give a set of five visual and five verbal tasks to a large number of people. We might expect that people who do well overall will have higher than average scores on all 10 tests, leading to a correlation between them. This would be evidence, in Spearman's terms, of a 'general' factor that influences performance on any test. We might also find that, independently of overall performance, performance on either the five verbal or the five visual tasks was also correlated. The pattern of results here might be that performance on one, say, verbal test correlated well with that on other four verbal tests, but not with any of the five visual tests. Likewise, visual tests might correlate with each other but not with verbal tests. Both these sub-patterns of correlation might reflect the overall level of performance to some extent, but nonetheless could not be predicted from it. In the language of factor analysis, this would be evidence for a general factor and for two specific factors to do with visual and verbal tasks.

Spearman's pioneering work has been modified considerably by subsequent factor analytic studies. Early revisions tended to challenge the idea of 'g'. For example, the work of Louis Thurstone suggested there were seven relatively *independent primary factors*, which are briefly listed in Table 12.1 (Thurstone, 1938). The most recent studies have returned somewhat to Spearman's original view and seem to show that there is a hierarchy of factors with varying degrees of stability (for example Carroll, 1993). One particularly interesting idea to emerge from factor analysis is the distinction between what Raymond Cattell called *fluid* and *crystallized* abilities (Cattell, 1971). Fluid abilities have to do with manipulation of information and the general dynamics of mental life, such as the speed with which things may be compared or the flexibility of approach to a problem. Crystallized abilities, by contrast, have to do with accumulated knowledge, such as general facts and information about the world, vocabulary and the orderliness and accessibility of what we know.

Table 12.1: Thurstone's seven general factors

Factor	Typical relevant tasks
Number facility	Speed and accuracy in arithmetic tasks.
Word fluency	Finding word meanings, naming things.
Visualization	Image manipulation and visual sorting.
Memory	Speed and accuracy of short-term recall.
Perceptual speed	Finding targets in confusing backgrounds.
Induction	Finding general rules from specific cases.
Verbal reasoning	Solving analogies, interpreting proverbs.

Notice that the question at issue in factor analytic studies of intelligence is not: 'how much has an individual got?' 'what is the structure of intelligence itself?' 'has it got components?' 'how are the different components related to each other?' Such questions might be used to design tests for intelligence, as indeed they are, but this is not the primary aim. The primary aim is to investigate the nature of intelligence itself and the broad conclusion from these studies is that it has components and these are related in a hierarchy.

Although not strictly a factor analytic approach, one of the most radical claims that intelligence is composed of different components is that of Howard Gardner (Gardner, 1983). He suggests there are, in fact, seven separate types of intelligence (not related to Thurstone's seven factors) and that these have relatively independent biological roots in the biological structure of the brain. His types of intelligence cover intellectual abilities such as number and language, social abilities such as knowledge of self and others, and physical abilities to do with space and movement. His claim that these are linked to biological factors is based on evidence from brain damage, developmental profiles of exceptional abilities and on arguments from evolutionary psychology. Although the evidence on which Gardner bases his claims may not be as systematic as that of the factor analytic theorists, it has been convincing enough for it to be used in educational psychology, especially in the education of people with exceptional abilities (Gardner, 1993).

Gardner and the factor analysts ask: 'are there components to intelligence and if so what are they?' In short, it is an inquiry into *structure*. This approach can be complemented by another, which looks at intelligence from the point of view of process. This approach derives from what has been the principal paradigm in psychology since the late 1950s, namely, *cognitive science*. This treats the activity of the brain by analogy with that of a computer and would identify the basis of intelligence as the acquisition, storage, retrieval and *processing of information*. Although it is clear that the brain is not literally like a computer, the analogy is perhaps taken rather more seriously than most scientific analogies used in scientific research because it is possible to programme computers to do things that we would say showed intelligence if human beings did them.

This project, known as *artificial intelligence* or AI, has had some remarkable successes. Programs have been written that have a systematic way of solving any problem. So-called 'expert systems' have been developed that carry out such tasks as medical diagnosis, the analysis of complex chemical data and the tracing of faults in complex machinery to a level that is as good as human experts. Some progress has been made in handling natural language and quite good machine translation is now routine in many areas of human activity. Computer controlled robots are now built that can see, act with a surprising degree of autonomy, and make elementary decisions. Such examples could be multiplied, and the rate at which human intelligence is being supplemented and even replaced by computer intelligence is a clear sign of how practically applicable AI is.

Developments like these have led a number of psychologists to take AI as a general theory of intelligence (Newell, 1991). If we accept this, then perhaps intelligence can be studied in a new way. We can discover the processes that enter into intelligent action and describe them in a particularly explicit and open way by expressing them as computer programs. Armed with this theory of intelligence it may be easier to analyse what human intelligence comprises, possibly with the result that we can improve or amplify it. This approach is thus an effort to see how intelligent computers can become, to compare what they do with what people do, and to bring human and artificial intelligence into a deeper relationship.

This project is treated with enthusiasm by some (Moravec, 1988) and with disdain – even horror – by others (Weitzenbaum, 1984). The fact is that this sort of research has had mixed results. In specific areas – chess would be an obvious example – it has proved possible to create computer intelligence that far exceeds what most people can manage. However, there has been much less success in producing the sort of general intelligence that is used in the mundane business of surviving in a world that is complex and always changing. It is presently quite beyond AI to come up with a system that is anywhere near as good at doing what we do when we move about, interact socially using language, and solve the very general and unpredictable problems of everyday living.

What seems to be the difficulty for AI is capturing the way human intelligence grows out of *interaction* with a highly structured, social environment. Moreover, as this interaction proceeds, human beings are able to monitor their own activities and subject them to critical analysis and development – the issue of *metacognition* mentioned at the beginning of the chapter. Computer programs and robots cannot, yet, interact with their environment in this way. Their intelligence has largely been programmed into them, although some systems can learn. This is quite sufficient when the objective is to produce intelligent actions or decisions in a specific domain, like chess or medical diagnosis. However, when general intelligence that can move from one domain to another is required, AI fails. It is this capacity for generalization that makes human intelligence the formidable thing that it is. It is not just that we can become expert at this or that – it is also that what is learned in specific areas, especially during early development, becomes generalized into the basis for flexible adaptive intelligence that can be applied anywhere and in any context.

Now the human context is a complex social world and intelligence is expressed within it. In what he has called his *triarchic* approach, Robert Sternberg combines three elements: the internal world of mental operations, the external world of social action, and the open-ended world of creative experience (Sternberg, 1985, 1995). The first element covers the internal mental operations that underlie performance on specific tests. Here he adopts the approach of cognitive science in using laboratory tasks to reveal just what these operations are and how they proceed. The second element covers the way we use such operations to respond adaptively in the real world. The third element deals with how we monitor and adapt our skills in order to apply them in new situations. It is clear that Sternberg goes beyond mere assessment to address how intelligence is used in the actual world in which human beings find themselves.

Enduring issues in the psychology of intelligence

This brief survey of the psychology of intelligence needs to be seen in the context of what was said in the introduction. The study of intelligence is an area particularly responsive to the *social context* surrounding psychological science. We find, therefore, that some controversial issues constantly arise, such as whether intelligence is something that can be inherited. The most common attitude encountered at present is that intelligence has a *genetic component*, but that the *interaction* between that and the influence of the *environment* is so profound and complex that making decisions about, say, education or immigration policy on the basis of genetic differences between individuals or ethnic groups is unjustified (Colman, 1987, Chapters 2 and 3).

Intelligence is also clearly a culturally relative matter. The skills, aptitudes and knowledge that are useful in one cultural setting may not be useful in another. Efforts to find culturally neutral or *culture fair* scales for intelligence have generally been regarded as unsuccessful. Here culture need not only mean the rather more obvious differences between, say, people living in urban environments in the developed countries and people living in more traditional ways in the less developed world. It should also be taken to mean the different groups of people within a single culture. The ethnic communities of multi-cultural societies will also differ in language, values, skills and social relations. These, in the sense of Sternberg's theory, provide very different contexts in which cognitive skills need to be used. Even though those skills may be fundamentally similar, the ways in which people learn to apply them will be very different. A scale developed to assess intelligence in one community may therefore not be of much use in another.

In fact, the use of intelligence scales in general, especially those that work by comparison with norms, has always been subject to a great degree of caution. Are these norms stable? Will the measure made of individuals at one stage of their development predict a similar measure made at a later stage? Do the measures reflect the real nature of intelligence, or merely the choice of items of a particular sort – something that is clearly linked to the question of cultural relativism noted above.

Questions like these have led a number of psychologists to return to something like the *psychophysical* approach of Galton. For example, the idea that intelligence depends on the speed with which the brain works is appealing because there are objective ways in which the speed of mental operations can be measured (Matarazzo, 1992). Some research has suggested a correlation exists between IQ scores and speed on simple information processing tasks (for example, Deary and Stough, 1996) whereas other research suggest that recordings of *brain activity* may show how rapidly information is processed and thus, likewise, predict performance on IQ scales (for example, Barratt and Eysenck, 1992).

However, the scope of these objective techniques at present still seems rather limited. It is recognized, for example, that intelligence is not merely a matter of information processing, and a number of psychologists are now suggesting that intelligence is intimately bound up with other aspects of mental life such as emotion. The evolutionary origins of intelligence are likely to have to do with the ability to manage our social relations through language (Dunbar, 1996) and to manage our sexual relations through strategic planning (Badcock, 1994). Now social and sexual behaviour are intrinsically bound up with emotional experience. This, along with the sense that creativity and productivity in thought too are very much emotionally loaded matters has led to important recent works on the idea of *emotional intelligence* (Damasio, 1994; Goleman, 1995).

There are as yet no tests or scales that come from this work, but it needs to be borne in mind that the familiar scales that are so widely used emphasize the rational aspect of intelligence. Important as this aspect is, it is increasingly recognized that it will need to be placed within a more inclusive framework for mental life that treats feelings and experience more explicitly.

Conclusion

What has been presented here is only a small sample of a large and constantly changing area of psychological research. The definition and measurement of intelligence are issues to which psychologists will constantly return. Ideas and techniques that reflect other areas of psychological research and the wider social context will continually be brought to bear. Presently, we see intelligence as a matter of information processing activity in the brain. The speed and the organization of this activity – what might be called processing capacity – is perhaps the most commonly accepted definition of the internal components of intelligence.

Well-developed scales exist against which to compare the processing capacity of an individual to group norms. However, the limits of the scales have always been recognized. The growing points of contemporary research on intelligence have to do with contextualizing and extending what such scales show. There is a growing recognition that other elements of mental life need to be included in the definition of intelligence. These include emotion, self-reflection, and the capacity to apply skills in new situations.

These situations are not to be identified with particular social and cultural conditions. Human cultures value different things and transmit different skills to individuals as they develop. Although he was not directly concerned with intelligence per se, the work of the great Russian psychologist Lev Vygotsky has attracted increasing attention over the past decade or so (see, for instance, Wertsch, 1995). Vygotsky took the view that the psychological development of intelligence was the result of the *assimilation* of skills from the *cultural context.* Individual differences arose not only from the richness or the impoverishment of this context but also from the capacity of individuals to explore it and to learn from it.

Contemporary research into the nature and measurement of intelligence is likewise paying attention once again to the idea that what underlies intelligence is not merely what might be going on inside the head. Intelligence has to be treated as a measure of how well an individual is able to integrate their own mental resources with the cultural and social structures around them. This integration is not a function of internal information processing alone. It also requires flexibility, self-monitoring and the ability creatively to recognize where skills learned in one area may be applied in another.

References

Badcock C (1994) Psychodarwinism. London: Flamingo.

Barratt P, Eysenck H (1992) Brain evoked potential and intelligence. Intelligence 19: 361–81.

Carroll J (1993) Human Cognitive Abilities: A Survey of Factor Analytic Studies. Cambridge: Cambridge University Press.

Cattell J (1971) Abilities: Their Structure, Growth and Action. Boston: Houghton Mifflin.

Colman A (1987) Facts, Fallacies and Frauds in Psychology. London: Hutchinson.

Damasio A (1994) Descartes' Error. London: Macmillan.

Deary I, Stough I. (1996) Intelligence and inspection time: achievements, prospects and problems. American Psychologist 51: 599–608.

Dunbar R (1996) Grooming, Gossip and the Evolution of Language. London: Faber.

Galton F (1914) Hereditary Genius: An Inquiry into Its Laws and Consequences. New York: Macmillan.

Gardner H (1983) Frames of Mind: The Theory of Multiple Intelligences. New York: Basic Books.

Gardner H (1993) Multiple Intelligences: The Theory in Practice. New York: Basic Books.

Goleman D (1995) Emotional Intelligence: Why it can Matter More than IQ. New York: Bantam.

Matarazzo J (1992) Biological and physiological correlates of intelligence. Intelligence 16: 257–8.

Metcalfe J, Shimamura A (1994) Metacognition: Knowing About Knowing. Cambridge MA: MIT Press.

Moravec H (1988) Mind Children: The Future of Robot and Human Intelligence. Cambridge MA: Harvard University Press.

Nelson T (1992) Metacognition: Core Readings. Boston: Allyn & Bacon.

Newell A (1991) Unified Theories of Cognition. Boston: Harvard University Press.

Raven J, Court JH, Raven J (1991) Manual for Raven's Progressive Matrices and Vocabulary Scales. Oxford: Oxford Psychologists Press.

Spearman C (1927) The Abilities of Man. New York: Macmillan.

Sternberg R (1985) Beyond IQ: A Triarchic Theory of Human Intelligence. New York: Cambridge University Press.

Sternberg R (1995) What it means to be intelligent: the triarchic theory of human intelligence. In Tomic W (ed.) Textbook for Undergraduate Intelligence Course. The Netherlands: Open University Press.

Thorndike R, Haya EP, Sattler JM (1986) The Stanford-Binet Intelligence Scale. Chicago: Riverside.

Thurstone L (1938) Primary Mental Abilities. Chicago: Chicago University Press.

Wechsler D (1974) The Measurement and Appraisal of Adult Intelligence. Baltimore: Williams & Wilkins.

Weizenbaum J (1984) Computer Power and Human Reason. Harmondsworth: Penguin.

Wertsch J (1995) Sociocultural Studies of Mind. Cambridge: Cambridge University Press.

Chapter 13
Some empirical approaches to individual differences

MARYLIN J. WILLIAMS

Key concepts	Key names
Dependent and independent variables	
Assessment methods	
observation	
interview	
questionnaire	
Scales	
nominal	
ordinal	
interval (cardinal)	
ratio	
Rating scale	
Subscale	
Reliability	
test–retest	
alternate forms	
inter-rater reliability	
Validity	
concurrent	
criterion	
face	
content	
predictive construct	
Norm-referenced tests	
Criterion-referenced tests	
Semantic differential scales	Osgood
Equal-appearing intervals	Thurstone
Likert-type scale	Likert
Grids	Kelly
Q-sorting	Stephenson
Longitudinal approach	
Cross-sectional approach	
Cohort and individual designs	
Cross-sequential designs	
Microgenetic studies	
Life-course study	

Like other scientists, psychologists depend greatly on fundamental empirical dimensions such as time, quantity, frequency and distance for many of their measurements of behavioural variables (such as response time and movement). However, there are important features of human performance and experience (including intelligence, personality, attitude, feelings) that do not lend themselves to direct measurement. In order to measure such variables, psychologists have developed a number of methods, all aimed at transforming people's judgements of their own subjective experience so that they become 'knowable' and quantifiable.

Use of these methods over time has had the effect of making psychologists' abstract concepts (such as intelligence, attitude) more concrete; hypothetical constructs have become transformed into 'real' entities. These concepts are slippery, but what they represent matters to people in their everyday lives: people's attitudes influence what they consume, how they feel, whom they help or harm. So it is important that we are able to assess these variables as effectively as possible. Furthermore, in order to understand what is meant by references to such concepts as 'intelligence', 'attitude' or 'personality', in a particular research study, we can best do so by attending to how they were measured. Indeed, the way in which a variable is measured provides us with a working or 'operational' definition of that variable.

This chapter summarizes the main measurement techniques that have been developed to harness concepts such as attitude and personality. They are best viewed as tools for use in psychology (and other social science) research studies. Given the variety of research study designs (correlational, experimental and so forth) it is not surprising to find that intelligence, personality or attitude can appear as *dependent* (caused) or *independent* (causes) variables or simply as candidates for association with other variables (in correlational designs). Studies of human development over time involve particular difficulties in research design. Some alternative approaches to research in this area will be discussed in the final part of this chapter.

Techniques for measuring intangible psychological variables have not been developed solely for their use in research studies – measures are needed for the assessment of individuals and the prediction of their behaviour (such as their response to treatment). Methods for assessing an individual's abilities or intelligence, personality, attitudes and feelings, involve assumptions about the relative *stability* of these characteristics. One assumes that the intelligence and skill of healthy people endures over extended time periods, personality somewhat less so, and current state, by definition, is unlikely to remain constant for long.

Assessment methods encompass a variety of scenarios, ranging from observation of task performance, play behaviour or social interaction, to (typically) responses in interviews or completion of questionnaires by the person being assessed. Whether the measurement method is based on the responses of trained observers or on those of the assessed people themselves, the same principles of measurement apply.

Before outlining the principles involved in 'scaling', an example will serve to illustrate the issues addressed.

A group of people may watch a film and then discuss its virtues. Each person may focus on a particular aspect of the film (its visual quality, direction, plot, skills of actors) and use a variety of words to express their evaluation of these features. To achieve a single overall impression of how the group as a whole evaluated the film one would first have to establish a 'common metric'. This would involve at least two steps: firstly, a single dimension would have to be agreed, such as 'good–bad'; secondly, a measure of the degree of goodness/badness of the film as judged by the group as a whole would have to be obtained. This could be done simply by asking each member whether they thought the film good or bad; the number (frequencies) of people judging the film good and the number judging it bad would then provide an impression of the group's overall view. Alternatively, one could ask each group member how good or bad the film was, and provide different levels of goodness/badness for them to choose from when making their judgements. Thus, 'excellent, very good, good, quite/fairly good, average, somewhat bad, bad, pretty awful, terrible', might be alternative descriptions. These alternatives can be seen as points along a continuum/dimension of meaning which could be referred to as a 'nine-point scale', and could be presented as a 'visual analogue scale'.

By assigning numbers (1 to 9) to the scale points, people's evaluations could be summarized to give a total score representing the group's opinion of the film.

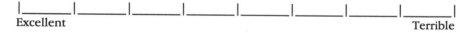

Excellent   Terrible

Figure 13.1: A visual analogue scale.

The same scale could be used by the group to evaluate (or 'rate') different films, or used to compare different groups' judgements of the same film. More subtle measurements could be made by using more than one scale to focus on different qualities of the film ('exciting–boring', 'uplifting–degrading' and so forth) and/or by considering different scenes. Indeed, quite an elaborate measurement tool could be developed for evaluating films (and/or their viewers), based on this simple strategy for representing subjective experience.

Scaling

Possibly the simplest form of measurement is by classification into two or more categories on the basis of one or more characteristics (such as male–female) thus producing a *nominal scale*. It could be argued that 'scale' is a misnomer here because no dimension is represented and there are no gradations of 'level' to which numbers might meaningfully be applied. In contrast, *ordinal scales* do permit the arrangement of people along a dimension in rank order (for example, according to tidiness of appearance). Ordinal scales permit interpretations of relative level (John is tidier than Pam, who is tidier than George), but do not represent distances in tidiness between the scale positions as equal (John cannot be said to be twice as tidy as George). The next step 'up' in measurement level is the *interval (cardinal)* scale. This has equal units of measurement, but no fixed zero, so one can meaningfully add and subtract the numbers representing scale points, but one cannot multiply or divide them by each other. For example, two people with scale positions 1 and 2 on an eight-point interval scale of 'healthiness' could be said to be as far apart from each other in terms of healthiness as two people at scale points 7 and 8, but not that a person at point 8 was eight times as healthy as one at point 1. Most rating scales assume equal intervals. *Ratio scales* are the 'best' level of measurement; having a fixed zero and equal intervals, scale differences and relative magnitude can be compared. Although time and length can be measured on ratio scales, temperature (and psychological variables like attitude) cannot. These principles of scaling are relevant to decisions about the statistical procedures that can meaningfully be applied to data arising from use of the different forms of scale. The higher the measurement 'level', in general, the more powerful the statistical procedures that can be applied.

The examples given above (gender, tidiness) are simple, and might lead one to ignore a further, and major, problem in the scaling of psychological variables – that of dimensionality. A linear scale should be relevant to only one dimension. One would find a single scale purporting to measure both tidiness and outgoingness difficult to use, and any scores arising from its use extremely hard to interpret. The problem of linearity and dimensionality is more complex when a number of scales are used in conjunction in order to achieve finer and more reliable discrimination between people than a single scale permits. If a single dimension (whether assessed by use of one or more scales) is being used to assess people's attitudes, personality or ability, it is important that the scale represents the full range of possible positions on the scale for the population of people being assessed.

Before considering more specific forms of measurement, it is worth noting that a variety of different terms have been used to refer to the tools by which measurements are made – general terms such as a 'measure', a 'technique', an 'instrument', and more specific ones such as 'scale' and 'test'. The term *scale* has been used in a variety of different ways in the psychological literature; its over-use may create confusion. 'Scale' can refer to the examples outlined above, i.e. assessment of a single dimension, sometimes referred to as a 'rating scale'. There are two important ways in which single scales used as, or as elements in, measures of individual difference vary. A scale may be used to report/assess different levels of endorsement with respect to a variable, either by being the vehicle for an 'agree/disagree' or 'prefer/least prefer' or 'very much/not at all' type of response to a statement or question. Thus the statement or question is presented independently of the response scale. Alternatively, the scale itself may embody the variable of interest. For example, bipolar adjective-scales (such as 'very happy/very sad') invite responses signifying level and dimension (pole of adjective). In the first form, the variable is presented separately from the scale measuring direction (+ or −) and intensity of response, whereas, in the second, dimension and intensity and direction of response are all integral to the scale. Examples of the first include Likert-type scales and of the second, semantic differential scales. Both are discussed below.

When rating scales are used by observers in an attempt to arrive at an objective assessment of a person's behaviour, observers may need considerable training so that they agree not only with each other but with researchers/practitioners elsewhere, about what the scales represent and what the different scale points signify. Agreement between different raters is termed *inter-rater reliability* and *intra-rater reliability* refers to the degree to which the same rater uses a scale consistently on different occasions. Published sets of rating scales currently in use in psychiatry include Hamilton's (1967) rating scale for depression (HRSD), which consists of a number of three- and five-point scales, one for each variable. Others involve a series of items, each being rated on two or more scales; for example, Beigel et al.'s (1971) manic-state rating scale (MS) has a number of items, each separately rated for frequency and severity. These two examples also illustrate the variety of ways in which rating scales can be used by professionals: the HRSD was designed to be completed by the interviewer as a summary of an unstructured interview; the MS was intended for use by nurses following observation of a patient's behaviour. Rating scales are discussed further below.

Another usage of the term 'scale' refers to questionnaires designed to assess personality, ability, attitudes/values or other individual differences. As will be described below, such questionnaires are built up from a number of items (questions, problems, statements) all having been shown to be related to a particular trait, aptitude or attitude, so that a total score incorporating scores of responses to the individual items can be taken to indicate the person's position on a hypothetical 'scale' referring to the dimension representing levels of the construct concerned. When an overall total score can be shown to include correlated but distinct subgroups of items referring to components of the trait, aptitude or attitude, these subgroups of items are said to comprise *subscales*.

An alternative term, which is, like 'scale', used in a variety of ways is 'test'. Typically used to refer to methods for assessing intelligence and other abilities, either using paper and pencil (the questionnaire) or other methods, the term is also used to refer to measures of personality (again, usually by means of the ubiquitous questionnaire, but sometimes by other projective techniques).

Development of individual difference measures

Before discussing specific techniques for construction of particular kinds of measure, some general points will be addressed. The development of measures ('tests', 'scales', 'questionnaires' or 'inventories') assumes relatively stable, enduring dispositions underlying and reflected in behaviour. It is through observation of behaviour, or self-reports of behaviour, that the nature and level of these underlying characteristics, or traits, is sought. The task of the test constructor is to formulate questions, or statements ('items') that successfully cover the range of the behaviour (the domain of content) believed to be trait related. Items must be verbally 'framed' (phrased) in such a way that the various biases in responding that have been demonstrated in research are avoided. For example, content that is likely to be responded to in a socially desirable way, in a dishonest way, or which may offend or upset respondents by referring to sensitive topics should be avoided. An important response bias to be avoided is 'acquiescence response set' (a tendency to agree or disagree with items regardless of their content). In order to nullify the effects of this latter bias it is often recommended that positively phrased items (such as 'I find parties very enjoyable') are balanced with negatively worded equivalents (for example, 'parties are very stressful for me') – scoring of one of the 'pairs' of such items must, of course, be reversed.

Stylistic concerns are also important. Ambiguous questions, double questions ('do you buy milk or cream?'), and complex questions are unlikely to be answered effectively by respondents. Other practical issues of design include provision of adequate instructions to respondents and ensuring a comprehensible layout.

Reliability and validity

Another general issue concerns the degree to which a measure can be said to be valid and/or reliable. *Reliability* concerns the degree to which a person's 'true' score on the characteristic being measured is reflected in his or her observed score. One is aware that one's watch is unreliable when the time indicated relates inconsistently to the time shown by other indicators of time (such as a clock). The 'true' score is hypothetical and may be unattainable, but the degree to which a particular instance measuring that characteristic is likely to be reliable can be assessed in various ways (and should be reported in manuals and research reports describing the measure). *Test–retest reliability* refers to the consistency of test results over time. Unless a characteristic being measured (for example, current state) is expected to vary over time, the same test performed on separate occasions should yield the same or similar results in terms of the ordering of people from higher to lower scores. Similarly, alternative forms of the same instrument should provide consistent results. If an instrument is made up of a number of items (problems, questions, scales), all allegedly contributing to the measure of a single attribute or character-istic (such as verbal intelligence, extroversion, or anti-Semitism) then that instrument is only reliable if it is *internally consistent* – that is, if all items consistently contribute to the accuracy of the overall score.

When observers are using a common method to assess the behaviour of one or more individuals, inter-rater reliability (the degree to which they agree) is taken as an indication that they are basing their evaluation on the same criteria. All these forms of reliability are typically evaluated and expressed as correlation coefficients – a level of 70% (0.7) often being the minimum acceptable level for continuing use of the measuring instru-ment. An instrument may be reliable, but not *valid* – it may not be measuring what it is purported to measure.

Validity may be assessed in a variety of ways. *Concurrent validity* concerns how well scores obtained using an instrument correlate with those obtained using one or more other instruments designed to measure the same characteristic, while *criterion validity* requires that people with different scores differ in other, predicted ways; *predictive validity* is achieved if the scores obtained predict future behaviour successfully.

High *content* and *face validity* denote that the content of the instru-ment actually concerns what is being assessed and is 'transparent' in this respect (for example a depression measure asking people how often they feel depressed). Establishing the *content validity* of measures of attain-ment (in education, for example) typically involves consulting experts about the degree to which different items, or tasks, reflect the skill being assessed and to which particular levels of achievement in this skill area cover the full range of experiences relevant to the characteristic.

The *construct validity* of an instrument concerns the nature of the variable being assessed; research studies using the instrument provide further information about what it measures. A variety of statistical techniques (for example factor analysis, principle components analysis) permit detailed study of the dimensionality of the variable and may provide a more fine-grained view – subscales may be developed, for example, where evidence suggests that a variable is composed of a number of relatively distinct component variables. Studies of content and criterion validity can, then, add to information about the nature of the variable under scrutiny, as well as about content and criterion validity per se.

Issues of reliability and validity are relevant to all attempts at measure-ment.

Interpretation of scores

A further concern, which pertains particularly to composite measures of attitude, personality, ability and attainment, is the question of how people's scores on such measures may be interpreted. When a test of personality or ability or attitude is used, the *observed* or *raw* scores (that is, the total scale/subscale scores that are first obtained) may not be immediately meaningful, but require interpretation. Observed scores for a test of personality or ability are typically transformed into *norm scores*, which can then be compared with those shown in norm tables, indicating scores obtained by different proportions of particular populations. For example a score obtained on a test by an undergraduate, after transformation into a norm score, would be compared with known norm scores for an undergraduate population, so that it could be interpreted according to the extent that it was below or above average.

Manuals for such *norm-referenced* tests include norm tables for different populations. Raw scores on *criterion-referenced* tests (typically of attainment or dysfunction) on the other hand, are interpreted in a different way. Rather than permitting comparison of the abilities or personality traits of the person tested with those of other similar people, scores on criterion-referenced tests concern a person's performance in relation to the content of the test: 'The focus is clearly on what test takers can do and what they know, not how they compare with others' (Anastasi, 1998: 102). A test of mathematical attainment, for example, might include groups of problems of different difficulty level. A person's score on such a test indicates the most difficult level of performance he or she is able to achieve, and is best understood by reference to the actual mathematical problems that this level of performance indicates. Criterion-referenced tests may be designed and used so as to predict performance in particular jobs, as well as to evaluate success of training or level of dysfunction.

Development and construction of personality tests and inventories

Individual differences in emotional, cognitive and interpersonal orientation and responsiveness, motivation, values and attitudes have been assessed in a variety of ways, most prominently by means of self-report questionnaires. Some tests of personality focus on one or a few characteristics, such as self-esteem (for example Coopersmith, 1981). Other measures are designed, on the basis of more general theories, to cover as exhaustively as possible the main personality factors that distinguish between individuals, and which, in their distinctive combinations, can confer individuality.

Murphy and Davidshofer (1988) succinctly summarize the main methods of constructing personality measures as rational, empirical and factor-analytic.

Rational methods are theory based; items are designed to reflect the personality typology generated by theory about the mechanisms (biological, cognitive) underlying individual differences in behaviour. The content of items is closely tied to the particular personality theory, so the items tend to have high 'face' and content validity. For the same reason, however, they are easy for respondents to 'see through', and responses are therefore easy to fake if a socially desirable impression is being presented.

An empirical approach is exemplified by the development of the Minnesota Multiphasic Personality Inventory (MMPI). Initially, like some other famous and much-used inventories, the Minnesota Multiphasic Personality Inventory (Hathaway and McKinley, 1943) was designed to assess levels of mental illness, as well as levels of the relevant personality characteristics in the 'normal' population. During development of the MMPI, some items were tested by comparing responses from specific clinical groups with those from normal adult groups, a procedure known as *empirical criterion keying*. Only items successfully discriminating between the groups were retained for the 'clinical scales' in the final version of the inventory. Criterion keying was also used to select items for other MMPI scales, but the criteria were non-clinical in nature. Similar techniques were used to construct the California Personality Inventory (CPI), the 1987 version including 20 scales, and designed for use with normal adult populations. Both inventories involve a certain degree of overlap between the scales; their multidimensionality is valuable in enabling a complex picture of an individual person to be derived, based on the profile of scores on the different scales. Thus the pattern of scores on the different scales is illuminating as a clinical diagnostic tool. Training in interpretation of the score profiles is essential if proper use is to be made of the information they provide.

Construction of inventories by factor analysis involves developing a set of items (on the basis of theory and/or observation), administering them to respondents and then assessing the intercorrelations between scores on the different items. Further statistical manipulations are applied and then the factors accounting for most of the variability in responding are identified. Interpretation of the factors then involves inspection of the items that are highly correlated with a factor and arriving at an intuitive summary of what seem to be the features that these items have in common. Cattell et al. (1970) designed the Sixteen Personality Factor Questionnaire (16PF) on the basis of factor analysis of ratings of people using 171 trait names, for example.

These methods of construction do not preclude each other; inventories designed initially by factor analysis may be validated empirically (by comparing groups of people who would be expected to differ in terms of scores on the different factors). Scores on items in rationally derived tests may be factor-analysed, and so on.

Rating scales

The use of rating scales by 'objective' trained or untrained observers or their use in 'subjective' self-report measures as structures for responses to questions or statements have been discussed. In both contexts rating scales permit summary evaluations of a person's characteristics, behaviour or attitudes. Rating scales may take the form of a visual analogue scale or their 'points' may be represented by numbers or by alternative verbally stated answer categories. The number of response categories may vary (typically between two and nine); both 'objectively' and 'subjectively' completed scales may include greater numbers of points if visually presented (for example, printed) than if presented verbally (in interview, or by telephone) especially if the verbal description of the scale points varies scale-by-scale; respondents find it difficult to hold more than three response alternatives in mind while deciding which is most appropriate. Some rating scales are unipolar – that is they have an extreme point at one end and a zero (or 'don't know') option at the other. Other scales are bipolar ranging from one extreme, having a zero (or 'don't know') point in the centre and an opposite extreme at the other end. Scoring should reflect this polarity.

Summary evaluations are the ultimate aim of many research projects designed to assess services such as those involved in medical care (for example, Jenkinson, 1997). There is debate (see Fitzpatrick, 1997) as to the value of the single, global 'satisfaction' measure obtained by analysis of responses to a single question on a single scale as against a summary score based on responses to a number of questions on a number of scales. The latter permits response to a number of facets of service (some of which a patient may evaluate positively, some not) to be combined. In addition, the combined scale scores permit statistical analysis to assess internal reliability (by assessing, for example, Cronbach's alpha) of the whole questionnaire/collection of scales; the questionnaire may then be enhanced by editing out information provided by scales or items contributing to unreliability. Further analysis (by factor or principal component analysis) will reveal the main factors underlying evaluation (which may well not correspond to the theoretical variables that initially led the researcher to design the items/scales). So, evaluation based on a single scale of 'good' to 'bad' is both limiting from the observer's or respondent's point of view and may give little information to the researcher or practitioner.

Semantic differential scales

Osgood et al. (1957) illustrated the value of combining a series of rating scales, subsequently called *semantic differential (SD) scales*. Such scales are simply bipolar scales representing descriptive dimensions. Their end points are labelled by adjectives with opposite meanings, and they typically have seven points. In studies designed to 'measure meaning', Osgood et al. asked respondents to use a collection of differently labelled visual analogue scales (e.g. 'good–bad', 'true–false', 'hard–soft', 'hot–cold' 'fast–slow', 'sane–insane') to rate a range of concepts, such as 'beauty', 'war', 'nurse', 'physics'. Factor analysis revealed three main factors underlying 'meaning': evaluation, potency and activity. Researchers using such scales to assess narrower ranges of concepts (such as foods) have identified different basic factors underlying the meanings ascribed, as would be expected. A further use made of the scale scores by Osgood et al. was the derivation of 'profiles' for concepts, based on the pattern of relationships between the mean scale values for each dimension provided by a particular group of respondents. Such profiles provide a visually immediate indication of areas in which a new product 'fits' a company's typical product profile, when the technique is used in market research, for example, or of an applicant's 'fit' with the ideal profile for a job, when selection for employment is concerned. Osgood et al. themselves argued that evaluation is akin to attitude, so that bipolar rating scales measuring the evaluative factor can constitute a means of measuring attitudes. Peck (1993: 181) notes that, in psychiatry, 'the SD is flexible, sensitive, reliable and, above all, simple, and is particularly useful in the assessment of change'.

Attitude measurement

Attitude concepts are associated with feelings, affect, evaluation, directed toward objects, persons, groups in the environment. There is an overlap between the concepts of personality and attitude in that certain 'types' of people have been believed to have certain types of attitude. This overlap is exemplified by tests of personality such as the measures of authoritarianism by Adorno et al. (1950) and dogmatism by Rokeach (1960). It is not surprising, therefore, that methods for measuring attitudes share many principles with those for the measurement of personality. The range of possible intensities of attitudes towards an 'object' must be covered, typically by providing statements or questions reflecting this range, and/or alternative responses referring to different levels of endorsement (agreement or approval), which may be represented as visual analogue scales. Remembering that single items or scales are intrinsically unreliable as indicators of attitude and that 'attitude' is regarded as a composite of a number of specific orientations to its elements, numerous different items are needed to reflect this complexity.

The use of semantic differential scales for measuring the evaluation of, or attitudes towards, concepts has already been described. Two techniques specifically designed for the assessment of attitudes are those of Thurstone and Likert.

Thurstone scales

Through his method of 'equal-appearing intervals', Thurstone (1931) hoped to achieve a true interval scale. Although it is arguable whether his method achieves this, the technique illustrates well some scaling principles and is therefore worth discussing in some detail.

The process requires the scale constructor to:

* Collect statements ('items') about object of attitude.
* Reduce the number of items to approximately 100 by removing duplicates, ambiguous items, 'double' statements and those that make questionable assumptions.
* Write each item on a card.
* Give each of approximately 50 'judges' a full set of items.
* Ask each judge to sort items into seven (or nine, or eleven) piles, according to their objective assessment of the items' degrees of favourableness towards the attitude object, in such a way that the items appear to be equally spaced along the 'favourable–unfavourable' continuum, the middle pile representing a 'neutral' point.
* Discard sortings that are evidently deviant (due to such factors as judges misunderstanding instructions).
* Score the piles from 1 to 7 and calculate the median value for each item, such that half the remaining judges give the item a lower position, and half a higher. Also assess the interquartile range, which indicates the scatter of judgements (variability of judgements).
* Reject items with high scatter.
* Select approximately twenty items to cover the range of attitudes and which appear to be about equally spaced along the seven-point scale (as indicated by medians).
* Arrange selected items in a questionnaire in random order, inviting respondents to endorse all items with which they agree.
* The respondent's scale score is the average (mean or median) of the values of all the items he or she endorses.

Note that each item provides only one of two possible scores (zero or the item value).

Thurstone scales are *differential* rather than *cumulative* – if a scale is sound and reliable, a respondent will agree only with items *around* his scale position (rather than only with those *less extreme* than his/her position). If sufficient items 'qualify' for inclusion in the scale, two 'matching' scales may be derived, giving the opportunity for 'alternate-forms' reliability assessment.

Disadvantages of the method are that it is time consuming and may be expensive; if judges come from a population very different from that of the respondents, and the initial judgements of favourability are not truly 'objective', the scale values may be inappropriate. However Moser and Kalton (1971) argue that research evidence indicates that: '... there are some fairly reassuring indications of the independence of scale values from the judges' own attitudes'.

Likert scales

Originally designed as a tool to measure the attitudes of general practitioners towards treatment of emotionally disturbed patients, this method has subsequently been used for many other purposes. The use of judges is avoided. Statements (items) are selected and respondents are asked to state how much they agree or disagree with each. Typically the scale of agreement involves five categories (strongly agree, agree, uncertain, disagree, strongly disagree); on occasion three or seven categories have been used, and approval–disapproval may be used as scale dimension as well as agree–disagree. Thus each item provides a number of possible scores (five in the case of a five-point scale), making possible the application of a number of statistical techniques for the evaluation of each item as well as of overall characteristics of the whole scale comprised by all items. This form of scale has often subsequently been referred to as a 'Likert' or 'Likert-type' scale.

Initial selection of items is based on criteria mentioned earlier: they should cover the full range of attitudes likely to be held in the population of respondents (but the items should not be so extreme that all respondents are likely to give the same response), and they should include favourable and unfavourable items – neutral items apparently do not discriminate well between respondents. Each scale for each item generates a score between one and five. Using the scores obtained from the responses of the pilot respondents, item analysis can be used to refine the overall 'scale' (questionnaire) by discarding items that correlate poorly with the majority of other items. By continual refinement, a high reliability (internal consistency) can be obtained. The refined scale can be used with subsequent groups of respondents. Although this type of scale is ordinal, giving an overall indication of the relative intensity of different respondents' attitudes, scores on single items can provide indications of respondents' views about a particular facet of the attitude (although scales for single items have low reliability). The scores also permit factor analysis to be applied to the resulting data, so that components of attitudes may be identified, and any subscales delineated.

It should be noted that this description of Likert scales resembles the account of personality measures – indeed Likert-type response categories are often used for responses to items on personality questionnaires and, as mentioned before, there is overlap between conceptions of personality and attitude.

A number of more sophisticated techniques for the measurement of attitude have been developed. Those of Guttman (1950) and Fishbein and Ajzen (1975) are just two examples.

There are many other techniques for gaining access to people's experience of the world, two of which deserve brief description. Both emanate from specific theoretical backgrounds, yet are often used without reference to their 'underpinnings'. These are repertory grids and Q-sort techniques.

Repertory grids

In its original conception, the role repertory grid technique for gaining access to a person's view of (a part of) his world was closely linked to George Kelly's (1955) theory of personal constructs, the fundamental postulate of which was 'a person's processes are psychologically channellized by the ways in which he anticipates events'. Kelly argued that we impose order on our experience and we use this 'order' to predict future events by means of developing systems of 'constructs' or categories. He denied that his theory simply argued the importance of cognitive structure/systems for passively making sense of the world.

According to Bannister and Fransella (1971) the use of a system of constructs was an active process; constructs and their relations to each other might change over time as a result of experience. Kelly's analogy was between 'man' and the 'scientist' – constructs were hypotheses; they were more-or-less integrated into hierarchical systems. Of particular interest is Kelly's stress on the uniqueness of each person's construct system, this position reflected in his 'sociality corollary', that only to the extent that a person understands ('construes') the construction processes of another person can he or she engage in social relationships with that person. Kelly was concerned to develop a method for gaining access to his clinical clients' (and his research students') construction processes. To this end he designed the role repertory test, formalized as the repertory grid. A fictitious example is shown in Figure 13.2.

| Constructs | ELEMENTS | | | | | | | | | |
✓	A	B	C	D	E	F	G	H	I	J
'Lazy–Busy'	✓O	✓O	xO	x	✓	✓	X	X	X	X
'Grey–White'	x	✓O	✓O	XO		✓	X	X	✓	✓
'Rich–Poor'	X		✓O	XO	✓O	X	X	X	✓	X
'.................'	X	X	✓	✓	✓	X	✓	X	✓	X

Figure 13.2: Fictitious example of repertory grid.

Elements are the concepts to be construed – people, buildings, abstractions, whatever. Kelly used role titles such as 'boss', 'close friend', 'someone disliked' and 'self', and asked respondents to insert the name of a particular person, who, for them, 'performed' this role. Having identified around 10 elements, the technique then requires the respondent to compare a triad of elements (for example, marked 'O' in Figure 13.2) and suggest a way in which two of them are alike and thereby different from the third. This 'way' is a 'construct' (typically a bipolar contrast). The researcher (or respondent) then assigns a symbol (such as – or x) to the relevant three cells in the grid to indicate which pole of the construct applies to each of the three 'elements'. The respondent may then apply the construct to other elements (signified further by use of – or x), before the next triad of elements is used to elicit the next construct, and so on. Although a grid such as that illustrated in Figure 13.2 allows a large number of triadic comparisons of elements, it is difficult to elicit a large number of constructs. In its least-structured form, the grid technique is valuable for exploring a person's construct systems. Not all cells need be filled (if an element falls outside a particular construct's 'range of convenience'), the number of – or x in a row need not be equal, and non-verbalizable constructs can be accepted. The resulting grid can be inspected for overlap and the degree of match between constructs and between elements, as well as providing some overall understanding of how a person construes his (in this example) interpersonal environment. The nature of the constructs themselves may be illuminating, especially if it is remembered that these arose from comparison of elements whose juxtaposition may never have been contemplated by the respondent before.

If statistical analysis (such as factor analysis) is to be applied to grids, either in order to pursue the structure of a single grid at a more sophisticated level, or to permit comparison between different respondents' construing, then constraints on grid completion need to be applied. These constraints include specifying the elements, requiring even distribution of different poles of a construct (equal numbers of – and x) requiring all cells to be completed, and ultimately, providing the constructs themselves. Researchers have increasingly required respondents to say not just which pole of a particular construct applies to an element, but how much (by assigning numbers signifying ranks) or by applying rating scales based on the construct to each element. These kinds of procedures generate quantitative grids for which programs for analysis have been developed. However, where both elements and constructs are specified, and grid completion is fully constrained, the differences between Kelly's original method and more conventional scaling techniques become evident.

Returning briefly to Kelly's conceptions of construct systems, later researchers have studied the unique hierarchical relationships of the repertoire of constructs in a person's system as discussed by Banister et al. (1994). Their techniques, like the repertory grid itself, may be particularly valuable in clinical settings.

Q-sorts

Q-sorting is the empirical technique forming part of Q-methodology, a theoretical position advanced by Stephenson (for example Stephenson, 1953). Somewhat like Kelly (see 'Repertory Grids') Stephenson acknowledged the diversity of people's subjective experience of phenomena (people, events, objects, abstracts, concepts and so forth). He was interested not only in the variety of individual experience but also in its social origins and expressions – people's interpretations may show considerable overlap. Further, he viewed interpretations as not simply being applied to, but as arising from phenomena (typically represented by textual material in Q-methodology), such as statements, 'positions'. Indeed the representations of the phenomena are the focus of the approach. The empirical technique is based on a ranking approach, rather than a rating approach; people are asked to order statements according to some specified criteria (for example, agree–disagree). As Stainton Rogers (1995) notes: 'Unlike the item checking required of a questionnaire, which is a sequential activity, ranking is a holistic or gestalt procedure in which all elements are interdependently involved'. The procedure initially involves selecting between 10 and 100 statements (the 'Q-set'), writing each on a card, providing a full set of cards to each of a number of participants, and asking them individually, to carry out a preliminary sort into roughly equal 'negative' and 'positive' groups. Participants are then asked to place the cards in a grid pattern approximating a normal distribution. For example, for 64 statements, marker cards (for example, +6 to –6, with centre 0) would be placed in a row and participants asked to place items above this, one at each extreme (+6 or –6) position, with 8 in the central neutral position, moving the cards around until they are satisfied that the 'sort' best represents their view of the statements presented on the cards.

Participants are chosen to represent groups believed to have access to particular attitudinal positions towards the topic addressed by statements as well as to represent the 'general population'. Each Q-sort is then correlated with each other Q-sort and the resulting intercorrelational matrix is factor analysed and rotated to simple structure. The main factors emerging are defined by virtue of the sorts loading heavily on them – that is, according to the participant producing the exemplary sorts (not according to the statements sorted). Factors are interpreted on the basis of theory and other related information, such as additional comments made by participants, background information about them, and so on. Thus the approach is, to some extent, idiographic but grounded in assumptions that Q-sorts derive from and are expressive of socially shared representations of phenomena. The initial part of the technique shares some superficial resemblance to that for constructing Thurstone scales. However, criteria for selection of 'items' differs; items ('propositions') to be Q-sorted may not only exhibit range but may vary in style, length and clarity. Instructions to participants involve ordering by ranking so as to approximate a normal distribution, rather than ordering according to a subjective assessment of 'equal interval' spacing. The integrity of individual Q-sorts is preserved – the entire sort being used in analysis, whereas the Thurstone method at this stage requires pooling of the individual judges' 'sortings', and discarding the non-consensual features of each individual judge's contributions to the overall group ordering of items.

Q-sort technique has been used to collect data about individuals – for example the relationship between Q-sorts of items reflecting 'self' and sorts reflecting 'ideal self' has been studied. Such research, however, may exploit the technique without acknowledging the Q-methodology context that justifies the approach as a unique means of exploring patterns of relationships within and between people's subjectivities.

Studying human development

Most of this chapter has focused on the measurement of those psychological variables involving inferences about subjective states and dispositions (be they characterized as personality or attitudinal), and some techniques for the objective assessment of behaviour about which inferences may subsequently be made. As noted at the beginning of the chapter, most research study designs fall within the categories: descriptive, correlational or experimental. It is usually argued that only in experimental studies where effects on dependent variable(s) following manipulation of independent variable(s) are assessed, can causal relationships be demonstrated. In correlational designs (typically involving measurement of variables whose intercorrelations are assessed or comparison of groups of people, each group representing a different level of a variable) it is not usually possible to infer causal relationships between variables unless one variable is logically or temporally prior to others. Such cases do arise in studies of development and change over time. A number of methodological approaches have been adopted: longitudinal, cross-sectional, cohort and individual studies will be discussed here.

Longitudinal approaches involve the study of people over time, usually by measuring the variables of interest at certain time intervals (for example, annually). Although they are useful for assessing the temporal stability of behaviour (for example, sociability) or the effects of early events (such as diet or trauma) on later behaviour or health, longitudinal studies do suffer problems arising from, for example, repeated testing and loss of members of the sample.

Cross-sectional research on development involves the comparison of the behaviour of groups of people, often children of different ages, such that 'age' is the independent variable. For example, a study to discover whether the ability to spell words increases with age might involve comparing the average ability of a group of six year olds with that of a group of nine year olds. Such a method would be relatively inexpensive and would take far less time than would a simple longitudinal study involving testing the spelling ability of one group of children at six years of age, the same group at seven years, at eight years and ultimately at nine years (three years after the initial testing). A cross-sectional approach would also avoid problems with *subject attrition* – subjects dropping out or being lost to the study through moving house, illness, loss of interest of parents and so on. The effects of repeated testing, and the fact that the measurement techniques used and research questions asked at the outset may be superseded by more sophisticated or better-informed ones by the time the study has been completed are further problems of longitudinal methods which do not arise when a cross-sectional approach is employed.

However, cross-sectional methods have the major problem that the groups compared may differ in important ways that are uncontrolled and unmeasured. An example is the *cohort effect*. A cohort is a group of people all sharing some common characteristic such as age. A cohort effect arises when some behaviour (such as the ability to spell) may be influenced by the particular conditions experienced by a particular generation (such as teaching methods). Groups of six year olds and nine year olds might thus have experienced different teaching styles and any performance difference in spelling between the two groups might be an effect of their education rather than their age per se.

The effects of individual differences between children within the two cohorts might also interfere with the clarity of results of cross-sectional studies; random sampling of children to become members of study groups is rarely feasible.

A partial resolution of these difficulties is to combine longitudinal and cross-sectional approaches into *cross-sequential* designs.

Cross-sequential designs (or 'cohort sequential studies') involve a cross-sectional approach in which two (or more) cohorts (for example children of different ages) are studied at the same time; a longitudinal approach is also taken, so that these cohorts are studied again on one or more later occasions. This design allows the presence of the major problem associated with cross-sectional designs (cohort effects) to be identified and assessed.

An example of a study using this approach is that of Svanborg (1996), cited by Bowling (1997). The effects of environment on health of people aged 70 years (born in 1901 and 1902) were studied over a period of 20 years; two more cohorts were later included (born in 1905 and 1906, and in 1911 and 1912 respectively). A sociomedical intervention was carried out for the third age cohort; the effects of this manipulation could therefore be studied.

These approaches study individuals as members of groups; other methods for studying development focus on changes in the individual over time.

Descriptive studies detailing changes in behaviour of individuals over time typically involve observation, and are necessarily limited to recording certain kinds of behaviour (such as problem-solving) and/or in specific contexts (such as emotional reactions to stressful situations).

Microgenetic studies are used to study a number of individual children intensively for a brief period of time. According to Vasta et al. (1995), they are designed to investigate important developmental changes, particularly discontinuous aspects of development, while they are taking place. For example children's approaches to solving certain types of problems may change sharply at the point when a child adopts a new strategy; problem-solving behaviour is studied at the point just before a strategy change is likely, and subsequently. While understanding of the change process may thus be increased, problems of the children's reactivity to the necessary intensive observation and repeated testing have to be acknowledged. Another approach to the individuals' long term development and change over time is the *life-course study*. Data obtained from archival sources (including, possibly, information from earlier longitudinal studies) and retrospective reports from the individuals themselves can permit research questions to be asked that had not been considered when the archives and/or earlier studies had been designed. Thus important questions about, for example, the effects of a particular event on later health, or about the stability of personality characteristics over time, may be tackled by examining existing data about individuals.

Case studies often focus on the individual case (but may examine the interrelationships or common experiences of a number of people in a particular setting or with shared characteristics). Case studies employ a variety of qualitative methodological techniques including unstructured interviewing, observation and exploitation of archival material.

The interest is often on the individual case itself, although case studies may be valuable sources of hypotheses that can be tested systematically with a larger sample of people in order to attempt generalizations.

In studying development over the life-course for example, a case-study approach to a small number of individuals can permit predictions about relationships between early experience and/or therapeutic intervention and later health states.

Identification and evaluation of influences

Interpretation of the results of both cross-sectional and longitudinal studies, is, as noted above, often difficult to achieve with confidence. Unless some intervention (manipulation) takes place, causal inferences are always cautiously made. Even when a manipulation apparently causes change (for example a new educational technique seems to improve the spelling performance of an experimental group in contrast to the spelling performance of the control group receiving the traditional educational input) this change may be due to factors associated with the manipulation (such as greater enthusiasm of teachers) rather than the educational technique itself.

Causal inferences are sometimes drawn in interpreting the results of longitudinal studies by virtue of the passage of time. That is, if change occurs it may be argued that it must be because of development over time. Such inferences are typically made on the basis of change scores. The evaluation of change is not simple. Firstly, if group measures rather than individual measures of the variables of interest are being used, variations in extent and direction of change between individuals would be ignored. Thus, total group scores showing an improvement in spelling performance over a period of time would not reflect the fact that some children had improved, some had not changed and a few had shown a decline in performance.

Thus a change score must be assessed for each group member and a summary of 'turnovers' made (the percentage changes in all directions). Obviously, the extent of change ('effect size') should be assessed by comparing measurements with those at baseline; a score of 60 on a spelling test is not a significant improvement on a baseline score of 59; a score of 30 is a significant improvement on a score of five.

The additional problem of 'regression to the mean' requires that great care be taken in the design of the study and the measurement of variables. A child's spelling performance may be poor on one occasion because he or she is tired and unwell, whereas on the second, later, occasion of testing, the child may be alert and well and perform much better. The reverse situation might even result in a decline in performance from the first to the later testing session. Multiple occasions and methods of assessment at both stages would reduce the possibility of this source of bias in the results. The difficulties arising from sample 'attrition', or 'drop out', in longitudinal studies also needs to be taken into account when evaluating their results. If attrition is due to random factors, the main problem is the reduction in sample size to levels that might prevent generalization of results, for example. More serious is the likelihood that attrition is systematically related to one or more variables (such as health, socioeconomic status, cognitive ability, motivation, gender). At each stage of a longitudinal study, the characteristics of non-respondents, and respondents ('dropouts' and 'survivors') should be assessed, to discover whether they differ in important (variables of interest-related) ways. This strategy might require encouraging/tracing a large enough sample of dropouts to participate in at least one further stage of the study, so that measures can be taken to permit comparisons between survivors and dropouts.

Final comments

It has not been the role of this chapter to review any areas of method and measurement in psychology exhaustively. Hopefully, the topics mentioned have been demystified to some extent and the essential similarities between many diversely labelled techniques have been successfully illustrated. Decisions about which methodological approach and which measurement techniques are appropriate for attempts to answer a particular research question or to undertake particular assessments of individuals will rest on matters concerning availability of human and material resources, time constraints and ethical issues. On the latter point, and particularly when using 'off the shelf' tests and assessment tools, it is crucial that the perspective of the naive test taker, study participant, assessee, is understood and confronted.

References

Adorno TW, Frenkel-Brunswick E, Levinson DJ, Sandford RM (1950) The Authoritarian Personality. New York: Harper.

Anastasi A (1998) Psychological Testing (6 edn). New Jersey: Prentice-Hall.

Banister P, Burman, E, Parker, I, Taylor M, Tindall C (eds) (1994) Qualitative Methods in Psychology. Buckingham: Open University Press.

Bannister D, Fransella F (1971) Inquiring Man: The Theory of Personal Constructs. Harmondsworth: Penguin Books.

Beigel A, Murphy DL, Bunney WE (1971) The Manic-state Rating Scale: scale construction, reliability and validity. Archives of General Psychiatry 25: 256–62.

Bowling Ann (1997) Research Methods in Health. Buckingham: Open University Press.

Cattell RB, Eber HW, Tatsuoka MM (1970) Handbook for the Sixteen Personality Factor Questionnaire. Champaign IL: Institute for Personality and Ability Testing.

Coopersmith S (1981) The Antecedents of Self-Esteem. Palo Alto CA: Consulting Psychologists Press.

Fishbein M, Ajzen I (1975) Beliefs, Attitude, Intention and Behaviour: An Introduction to Theory and Research. Reading MA: Addison-Wesley.

Fitzpatrick R (1997) The assessment of patient satisfaction. In C Jenkinson (ed.) Assessment and Evaluation of Health and Medical Care. Buckingham: Open University Press, pp. 85–101.

Guttman L (1950) The basis for scalogram analysis. In SA Stouffer (ed.) Measurement and Prediction. Princeton NJ: Princeton University Press.

Hamilton M (1967) Development of a rating scale for primary depressive illness. British Journal of Social and Clinical Psychology 6: 278–96.

Hathaway SR, McKinley JC (1943) The Minnesota Multiphasic Personality Inventory (revised edition). Minneapolis: University of Minnesota Press.

Kelly GA (1955) A Theory of Personality: The Psychology of Personal Constructs. New York: Norton.

Jenkinson C (ed.) (1997) Assessment and Evaluation of Health and Medical Care. Buckingham: Open University Press.

Moser CA, Kalton G (1971) Survey Methods in Social Investigation (2 edn). London: Heinemann.

Murphy KR, Davidshofer CO (1988) Psychological Testing: Principles and Applications. Englewood Cliffs NJ: Prentice-Hall.

Osgood CE, Suci GJ, Tannenbaum PH (1957) The Measurement of Meaning. Urbana: University of Illinois Press.

Peck DF (1993) Measurement in Psychiatry. In RE Kendall and AK Zeally (eds) Companion to Psychiatric Studies (5 edn). Edinburgh: Churchill Livingstone.

Rokeach M (ed) (1960) The Open and Closed Mind. New York: Basic Books.

Stainton Rogers R (1995) Q-Methodology. In JA Smith, R Harre and L Van Langenhove (eds) Rethinking Methods in Psychology. London: Sage.

Stephenson W (1953) The Study of Behaviour: Q-Technique and its Methodology. Chicago: University of Chicago Press.

Svanborg A (1996) Conduct of long term cohort sequential studies. In S Ebrahim, A Kalache (eds) Epidemiology in Old Age. London: British Medical Journal Publishing Group.

Thurstone LL (1931) The measurement of attitudes. Journal of Abnormal and Social Psychology 26: 249–69.

Vasta R, Haith MM, Miller SA (1995) Child Psychology: The Modern Science (2 edn) New York: Wiley.

Further reading

Bowling A (1997) Research Methods in Health. Buckingham: Open University Press.

British Psychological Society (1995) Psychological Testing: A User's Guide. Leicester: BPS.

Loewenthal KM (1996) An Introduction to Psychological Tests and Scales. London: UCL Press.

Part Two:
Human Development

Chapter 14
Human development

HELEN GRAHAM

Key concepts	Key names
Nature versus nuture	
Interactionism	
Attachment and bonding	Bowlby
Maternal deprivation	Harlow
	Bowlby
	Rutter
Post natal depression	
Temperament	
easy	Thomas and Chess
difficult	
...slow to warm	
Strange situation	Ainsworth
Parenting style	
Transitional object	
Development stages	Freud
	Erikson
	Piaget

In 1992 Jeffrey Dahmer was given 16 life sentences in a US court for the murder of 16 young men. He had lured each of them to his apartment and had then drugged and strangled them, exposed their internal organs, and engaged in various fetishistic behaviours before dismembering their bodies, and in some cases eating certain organs.

Afterwards he disposed of the remains, but kept some body parts as mementoes. There were several spray-painted skulls on a coffee table when police searched his apartment, three torsos in various stages of dismemberment, several containers of body parts, and human organs in the refrigerator.

Theories of human development: nature versus nurture

Inevitably, Dahmer's crimes prompt the question of how he became the kind of person for whom unspeakable acts were 'normal'. As his biographer observed, 'There would have to be some germ of his pathology, some seed out of which this poison tree grew' (Masters, 1993: 22). Such a view suggests that it was 'in his nature' (the seed) to become a serial killer – it was biologically determined and genetically based. Such a proposition is for many people unthinkable: 'his behaviour . . . was so unusual it would need to be the product of some trauma' (Masters, 1993: 22). Accordingly, Dahmer's pathology was nurtured – produced by the conditions in which he grew. These perspectives represent opposing strands of thought about development within psychology.

Traditionally, psychological theories differ in the importance they assign to nature and nurture, to biological and environmental factors. Biological theorists insist that development is governed by nature, and that all human traits are genetically based. Environmental theorists argue that upbringing – the way an individual is nurtured – influences development more strongly than genes. Although the former see development as determined by factors within the self, the latter view it as dependent on factors outside the self in the social environment.

In an attempt to shed light on the factors that influenced his behaviour, Dahmer spent hours in conversation with psychologists and psychiatrists. On the basis of the details that emerged, his biographer suggests that the key to Dahmer's strange personality lies in his early childhood experiences, notably his cool and distant relationship with a mother who was mentally ill, and traumatic invasive abdominal surgery when aged four. He argues that this led to an emotionally impoverished childhood which formed the basis of serious social inadequacies resulting in profound loneliness and isolation; and an obsessive fascination with the internal organs of the body. This combination of factors meant Dahmer could only find solace and sexual satisfaction in the company of the dead, or more precisely, their inner organs.

However, the same factors, particularly recognition of his mother's probable mental illness, could be used to argue for a genetic basis for Dahmer's pathology. Incredible as they were, his crimes are not unique. Ed Gein carried out similar atrocities in the US during the 1950s, as did Dennis Nilsen in Britain during the 1970s, suggesting the possibility of a genetic propensity, in some persons at least, to develop this kind of pathology. However, Dahmer has a 'normal' younger brother reared in the same home by the same biological parents. If Dahmer's pathology had a genetic basis or was the product of upbringing, his brother might be expected to show some signs of disturbance. On this basis, therefore, it does not seem possible to resolve the issue one way or another. Indeed, Dahmer's biographical details could be used to argue for an interactionist perspective – the idea that nature and nurture combined to influence the course of his development.

Theories of human development: interactionism

Most developmental psychologists today don't ask either/or questions, because research has confirmed that both biology and the environment work together to influence development. This interplay of biology and environment is constant. Furthermore, development is a dynamic process. Far from being passive recipients of environmental influences, children actively shape their world and help to create the very conditions that affect their own development. However, 'although the field has moved beyond the tired debate over whether nature or nurture is more important to a far more sensible appreciation of the need to look at how nature and nurture interact, most textbooks inadequately address the considerable evidence supporting biological and environmental interaction' (Sternberger and Mayer, 1995: xvii).

Developmentalists distinguish between an individual's *genotype* (the set of genes he or she inherits) and his or her *phenotype* (those observable physical and behavioural traits that emerge during development). There is no one-to-one correspondence between genotype and phenotype; rather, the phenotype is the expression of genetic endowment in a particular environmental context.

Some traits are so tightly controlled by genetic factors that the environment has little or no influence on their expression. Such *canalized* traits (McCall, 1981) are difficult to modify. So, for example, the timing of major motor developments of the first year of life, such as sitting up and crawling, is very similar in all normal babies. These behaviours occur as and when nature determines, irrespective of upbringing.

Most aspects of development are less well controlled by genetic factors, so phenotypic variation is considerable. A child's potential is determined by its genotype, but his or her attainment depends upon the interaction of that potential with the environment. A child may have the genetic potential, acquired from its parents, to grow tall. He or she may well do so if healthy and well fed, but may not grow to be tall – this potential may not be realized – if he or she suffers injury during childhood, is sickly or poorly nourished.

Intelligence, like height, also runs in families, and its expression is also determined by the environment. A child may not realize its high potential if deprived of appropriate environmental stimulation. He or she may be overtaken in terms of attainment by a child whose lower intellectual potential has been maximized in an enriching environment.

The active versus passive role of the individual in human development

It is now recognized that because of their genetic predispositions, children tend to evoke certain types of reactions from their environment. A child with the genetic potential for high intelligence is likely to act in ways that evoke intellectual stimulation from other people. He or she may ask questions, demand explanations and be keen to learn to read, whereas a child of lower intellectual development may not do so to the same extent. Furthermore, a child who inherits high intellectual potential is more likely to actively seek environments that encourage and reward intelligent behaviour. He or she is more likely than someone of lower intellectual potential to choose toys and books that are cognitively challenging, and friends who are as advanced, or more so, than himself or herself. In this way the child actively seeks and shapes an environment that fits his or her genetic predisposition, rather than passively responding to events in the environment, resulting in learned changes in behaviour, which is the way behavioural learning theorists have traditionally viewed development. Hence development of intelligence is not only a dynamic two-way interactive process between genetic and environmental factors, but these factors also tend to be correlated and work in the same direction.

Life before birth

It is now acknowledged that this complex interaction between biology and the environment occurs from the outset. However, what constitutes 'the beginning' of development has undergone revision in recent years. Previously it was assumed that traits present at birth were inherited or genetically determined. Little or no attention was given to the ways in which they might have been influenced by environmental factors. Until the mid-1980s developmental psychology was generally taught as though its starting point was birth. Life before birth had much the same status within psychology as life after death; it was dismissed from serious consideration. Technological advances have resulted in a more sophisticated appreciation of pre-natal life, and it is recognized that birth merely marks the transition from one environment to another, that is from the inner world of the uterus or womb to the outside world.

Normally the foetus exists within the womb for some 280 days or nine calendar months and it is now known that its experiences within the womb during that period may have important implications for subsequent psychological development. The uterine environment, like any other, influences and shapes the individual and has long-term implications for the development of personality, intelligence and behaviour.

Although it is still not possible to establish at what point the foetus may be said to commence life, it is clear that by the eighth week of life in the uterus it is capable of responding to many stimuli, and all sense receptors are capable of functioning. By the fourth month of life in the uterus all the responses of the newly born child can be elicited and a number of these pre-natal responses appear as precursors to later behaviour. Crying, sucking, eye reflexes, balancing, righting, and breathing movements and a trotting reflex are discernible. There is no sudden emergence of new behaviour after birth but rather a rapid and continuous development of behaviour. What seems to be the sudden appearance of behaviour after birth represents a reappearance of behaviour that has undergone gradual development and exercise prior to birth. This process of growth occurring in ordered sequences is referred to as *maturation* and considered to be unlearned (genetically determined or 'natural').

Learning *in utero*

However, although maturation obviously plays a major part in early development, it is becoming increasingly clear that the foetus learns from experiences in the womb. For example, if during pregnancy a woman regularly sits down to watch her favourite television 'soap opera' and relaxes, it appears that, after birth, the child recognizes the programme's theme tune. Studies have found that foetuses exhibit change in movement when they hear a tune they have heard previously during pregnancy. Moreover changes in heart rate, the number of movements and behaviour in response to the tunes are measurable 2–4 days after birth, although they are no longer evident by day 21. These effects cannot be attributed to postnatal exposure or genetic predisposition and are specific to the tune to which they were exposed, suggesting that the babies recognize the tunes and that foetal learning occurred before birth (Hepper, 1991).

Until recently foetal learning was thought to begin at 24 weeks. However, evidence now suggests that an unborn child can hear and remembers sounds in the womb as early as 20 weeks after conception. In one study (Evans, 1998) pieces of obscure folk music were played to pregnant women. One piece was played when they were 12 weeks pregnant, a second at 20 weeks, and a third at 36 weeks. Three weeks after the babies were born, the babies were played the tunes and their reactions, using kick rates, were recorded. The babies showed a significant reduction in kick rate when they heard the pieces that had been played to them at 20 and 36 weeks, suggesting that they recognized them.

Stress during pregnancy

The womb, like other parts of the mother's body is affected by hormones produced in response to stress, notably adrenaline, which enters the unborn baby's body via the placenta. High levels of stress hormones in the mother can reduce blood flow to the uterus and/or raise maternal blood pressure, and in extreme cases can cause severe risk to the foetus (Abell, 1992). Many women find pregnancy stressful. Worry, doubt and even dread are not unusual. The majority of women worry about the health of the unborn child; many are scared of childbirth; and over half of pregnant women fear losing their physical attractiveness (Light and Fenster, 1974). Anxious women are more likely to have difficult pregnancies. Their babies are also likely to be born prematurely, to suffer from respiratory and stomach problems and to be fidgety, irritable and difficult to soothe (Carlson and Labarba, 1979; Norbeck and Tilden, 1983; Omer and Everly, 1988). Women who experience severe and prolonged stress before or during pregnancy are more likely to have medical complications and to give birth to infants with abnormalities than women who do not. Stress has been associated with greater incidence of spontaneous abortion, difficult labour, premature birth and low birth weight, respiratory difficulties and physical deformities (Norbeck and Tilden, 1983; Omer and Everly, 1988).

Another source of stress during pregnancy is domestic violence. Studies of prenatal clinic patients report that between 7% and 8% of pregnant women are beaten by their partners and that these women have twice as many miscarriages as women who are not abused. Abuse during pregnancy is correlated with other stress factors such as unemployment, poverty, substance abuse and family dysfunction (Moran 1993).

Foetal insults

Stress during pregnancy may have other effects on the unborn child. Certain conditions can interfere with even the most highly canalized factors of foetal development. These *foetal insults* include not only stress but exposure to disease and other environmental hazards, many of which are stress-related. Unborn babies are extremely vulnerable, especially during the first few weeks of intrauterine life, to disruption if exposed to *teratogens*, harmful substances or other environmental influences that can interfere with or permanently damage their growth. They are most vulnerable at certain times known as *critical periods* when physical structures and organs are being formed. If development is disturbed or inhibited during these critical periods the changes scheduled to occur genetically may be disrupted or prevented from occurring. Teratogens include environmental hazards such as radiation, chemical pollutants, maternal diseases such as syphillis, gonorrhoea, chlamydia, and genital herpes, viruses such as rubella and AIDS, and drugs.

A pregnant woman may unwittingly ingest teratogens if, for example, she or the food she eats has been exposed to high levels of radiation, lead emissions from car exhausts, organophosphate crop sprays or industrial pollutants. Infants with higher-than-normal levels of lead in their umbilical cord blood have been found to show some slowing of mental development in infancy (Bellinger et al., 1987). Water is often a source of teratogens. Infants whose mothers had consumed fish contaminated by common industrial pollutants, such as polychlorinated biphenyls, only once or twice a month during pregnancy, showed poor muscle control and depression, and scored below their age level on tests of visual recognition at several months of age, and at the age of four had several cognitive difficulties that could affect their reading ability (Jacobsen et al., 1984, 1992). Like children exposed to other teratogens, they were more hyperactive and had less focused attention. Drinking water may also be contaminated with chemical substances such as nitrates, phenol and copper. A concentration of 100 mg of nitrates per litre can reduce oxygen levels in the mother's blood and produce blue baby syndrome, a cause of brain damage in newly born babies. Various fungi, spores, bacteria, organic solvents and chemicals can also present environmental hazards to the unborn child (Bernhardt, 1990), as can prescribed drugs.

During the 1950s, 8000 babies were born in several countries with severe physical deformities to mothers who had been prescribed the drug thalidomide for sleeplessness and nausea in the early stages of pregnancy, notably between the 38th and 46th days of pregnancy, the critical period for limb development *in utero*.

Commonly prescribed drugs such as antibiotics can produce deformities, and aspirin, a commonly available over-the-counter drug, is also potentially harmful to the foetus. Frequent use during pregnancy can lower birth weight and increase the risk of foetal or infant death before and shortly after birth (Corby, 1978). It is also associated with lower IQs and large muscle coordination in pre-school children (Barr et al., 1990).

However, many of the more common teratogens are those that a pregnant women knowingly ingests. What a pregnant woman ingests is likely to be determined, to a great extent, by how she feels, that is by her mood, and by her socioeconomic situation. If she is subject to stress as a result of poverty, poor living conditions, or insecure relationships, she may console herself with so-called 'junk foods', alcohol, cigarettes, prescription or illicit drugs – all of which have potentially damaging effects on the unborn child.

Deficiencies of vitamins and minerals have long been known to have physical effects on the child, which may in turn have psychological consequences. Essential vitamins and minerals are present in a balanced diet but fewer and fewer people in the developed world eat such a diet. Processed convenience foods may be lacking in some nutrients while having excessive amounts of some additives, notably sodium yellow and tartrazine, which are derived from coal tar. These have been implicated in excitation of the nervous system, resulting in hyperactivity and irritability in children, learning difficulties and behavioural disorders. It is possible that the babies of mothers who subsist on a largely junk-food diet produce more irritable and hyperactive babies, resulting in behavioural problems and subsequent psychological, emotional and cognitive difficulties.

Nutritionally deprived babies are less responsive to environmental stimulation and tend to be irritable when aroused.

Pregnant women may unknowingly ingest other substances that are teratogens without necessarily being aware of their adverse effects on the unborn child. Alcohol consumed by the mother passes into the unborn baby's bloodstream via the placenta and depresses central nervous system activity (Landesman-Dwyer, 1981); hence prenatal exposure to alcohol can affect subsequent physical, cognitive and social development. Women who drink heavily during pregnancy put their children at risk of developing foetal alcohol syndrome (FAS). Estimates of the proportion of babies born with FAS in the developed world vary from 1 in 600 to 1 in 1000 births. Affected babies show a group of physical and behavioural symptoms that include distinctive facial features, retarded growth both before birth and throughout childhood, mental retardation, poor motor development, hyperactivity and limited attention span (Streissguth et al., 1980).

The effects of prenatal exposure to alcohol show throughout childhood in every aspect of development. Babies affected by foetal alcohol syndrome are smaller than normal babies and remain in the tenth percentile of growth development. They do not 'catch up' with age. However it is not necessary for a mother to abuse or be addicted to alcohol for her child to develop FAS. No completely proven safe dosage of alcohol for a pregnant woman has yet been determined (Feinbloom and Forman, 1987). Even moderate drinking has effects that are evident in the first day of life. These include increased body tremors, decreased alertness and less vigorous body movements. Long-term effects are also discernible. The children of women who drink moderately to heavily during pregnancy have much in common with babies whose mothers are addicted to cocaine, which typically show signs of neurological damage, and may be overexcitable, jittery, irritable, may cry excessively with a distinctive high-pitched sound, show sleep and eating disturbances; or be depressed and withdrawn; and as they develop they may show retarded language development and less focused attention. At one year of age they tend to be more difficult to care for and less likely to receive the care they need (O'Connor, Sigman and Brill, 1987).

Babies whose mothers take heroin or methadone during pregnancy are born addicted and are at serious risk of death in the first few days of life. Those who survive suffer withdrawal symptoms such as sleeplessness, irritability and tremors (Fricker and Segal, 1978) and are difficult to care for.

The effects of marijuana or cannabis use during pregnancy are less clear, although frequent use during pregnancy can lead to retarded foetal growth, low birth weight and prematurity; and there is evidence that longer term effects on the children may include sleep difficulties and poor performance on preschool verbal and memory tests.

It is difficult to isolate the effects of cannabis from nicotine as usually the two substances are smoked together. The evidence that nicotine is harmful to the foetus is overwhelming. Smoking during pregnancy increases the risk of spontaneous abortion and stillbirth by 30% to 50%, and full-term babies of smokers are typically smaller and have lower birth weights, indications of retarded intrauterine growth (Handler et al., 1991). Babies of smokers may also be at higher risk from sudden infant death syndrome, which occurs in early infancy for no apparent reason (Taylor and Emery, 1988).

Caffeine, found in tea, coffee, cola-type drinks, and many medications, also increases the risk of retarded growth and low birth weight (Fenster et al., 1991). There is no evidence that caffeine causes birth defects in humans, although they have been found in rats fed high amounts of caffeine (Fried, 1983). However it has been found to relate to clumsiness in children (Barr et al., 1990).

Pregnant teenagers are much less likely to maintain nutritious diets than pregnant adults, and more likely to be stressed and to resort to use of prescribed and illicit drugs (Lawson and Rhode, 1993). They are more likely to suffer complications, and babies born to teenagers are often premature and suffer low birth weight and associated problems.

To help them cope with stress during pregnancy, many women are prescribed tranquillizers that can produce birth defects such as cleft palate. However, these anxiolytic drugs have more subtle but equally damaging effects. The tranquillizer builds up in the blood stream of the baby and can lead to the so-called 'floppy child syndrome', where the newly born baby lacks muscle tone and is dozy, unable to feed or interact with the mother.

It is not necessary to take tranquillizers throughout pregnancy for the baby to be adversely affected by them. Women who do not ordinarily take these drugs are often given them in the final stages of labour to help them to cope with anxiety and as a muscle relaxant. When tranquillizers are given 15 hours before birth, babies are found to have lower scores on tests of mental and physical ability conducted immediately after birth. They often need tube feeding because they lack muscle tone and strength, and cannot suck. This can create difficulties in the bonding or attachment process between mother and child and may have serious long-term implications.

The development of attachment

Attachment is an affectionate tie between individuals that keeps them together over time. The process by which attachment develops between infants and parents or other caregivers is termed bonding. In the 1950s,

John Bowlby claimed that the child is monotrophic, that is, it becomes attached to one caregiver, normally the mother, and should have a continuous unbroken relationship with her. He insisted that any separation from the mother in early life constitutes a bereavement for the child, which gives rise to grief and distress in the short term and consequent psychiatric and behavioural disorders. This *maternal deprivation hypothesis* was presented in a report to the World Health Organization Expert Committee on Mental Health in 1951 and subsequently proved to be highly influential. Subsequent research on animals appeared to lend support to Bowlby's claims (Harlow, 1961). However, a review of the research evidence relating to children (Rutter, 1981) concluded that although the syndrome of distress following separation is fairly well established, it is also clear that children form and benefit from multiple attachments, and differ greatly in their response to separation. Moreover, distress is less severe in all infants that remain in a familiar environment following separation. As regards the long-term effects of separation, there was found to be insufficient evidence to justify any firm conclusions. In the light of research that largely discredited his theory, Bowlby reviewed his position (1969) and accepted that separation from the mother did not inevitably give rise to serious psychopathology. It is now generally accepted that the quality and stability of care a child receives is more important than its source or 'quantity'.

The development of social relationships

Research during the 1970s and subsequently was greatly stimulated and facilitated by developments in audio-visual recording techniques that enabled precise analysis of the behaviours of mothers and infants. A number of studies suggested that the behaviours of newly born infants are not random but are perfectly articulated to serve their survival needs. They emit clear signals of need, which are recognized, albeit intuitively for the most part, by the mother as attempts at communication, and to which she responds accordingly. Mother and infant are thus engaged in a two-way communication process or dialogue. It has been suggested (Sluckin et al., 1983) that the mother's attempt to engage in this dialogue and respond to the infant's needs constitutes the first signs of maternal–child attachment or bonding, and that being able to respond to the infant's basic needs is an indication that the bonding process is under way. An important implication of these findings is that mothering emerges as a skill – that of recognizing and responding to the infant's attempts to communicate its needs. From such a perspective, mothering is monitoring and a skill that can be learned by anyone, whether or not they have given birth to a child, or whether female or male. A further implication of this research is that if the needs the child is attempting to communicate are not attended to (as a result of inadequate monitoring) or if for any reason the infant's attempts at communicate are impaired, then the infant is less likely to thrive. Furthermore if no one is attending to the infant or attempting to interact with it, its needs to communicate will not be reinforced and will extinguish over time. Additionally, the infant is likely to suffer a reduction in stimulation – social, perceptual and physical – as a consequence of this lack of attention. It is probable that this constellation of factors accounts for the subsequent impoverishment of social and emotional development that concerned Bowlby, as well as much of the physical ill health and distress noted in studies of separation. Moreover, rather than being affected by different psychological mechanisms they would seem to be the result of a fundamental disturbance in the social interaction between the infant and its caregiver.

It has been suggested (Klaus et al., 1972) that separation of the mother and child during the first three days after birth has an adverse effect on the mother because she loses intimate contact with her child at a time when she is maximally sensitive to it. On the basis of observational studies, it is claimed that mothers separated from their infants in the first few hours after birth show a greater tendency towards post-natal depression and subsequent rejection of their offspring than mothers who have not experienced this separation. One of the most striking differences noted between mothers separated from their infants and those not is that the former tend to hold their infants at a greater distance, rarely look them in the face and generally touch them less. These differences are still apparent after 12 months (Kennell et al., 1974). Moreover, mothers separated from their infants immediately after birth are subsequently more likely to chastise them physically. This is particularly significant in the light of statistics that suggest that premature babies, those most usually separated from their mothers after birth, represent 30% to 40% of physically abused children although they constitute only 8% of the live birth total. Women who have taken tranquillizers throughout pregnancy also have a greater tendency to physically abuse their children, not only because these babies are more likely to have birth complications leading to initial separation from the mother, but also because the effects on the tranquillizer on the child make it unresponsive and uncommunicative in the first few days of life (Kempe and Kempe, 1978).

Bowlby viewed attachment as a canalized developmental process, an instinctive and immediate repertoire of behaviours directed towards survival. Others put more emphasis on processes of learning in the development of attachment, and on the communication that occurs in its context. From such a perspective, attachment develops as in any other personal relationship, slowly, but in most cases surely. However, the instinctive repertoire of the newborn and learning are both important in early social interactions, and both can be disrupted by the birth process and its immediate aftermath.

The effects of birth trauma

Separation of mothers and babies immediately after birth is invariably a consequence of traumatization of one or both of them during delivery, or technological intervention ostensibly for the purpose of preventing or reducing trauma. According to an editorial in the *Lancet* (1988) 25% of births in the USA and 20% in Canada are achieved by Caesarian section and the number is rising. Britain appears to be following this trend. Yet, at all levels of obstetric risk, giving birth at home is safer than doing so in hospital (Tew, 1995). This is largely because the medical technology surrounding hospital childbirth is not as safe as is generally supposed. There is ample evidence that most of the hi-tech forms of care offered during pregnancy and childbirth, including ultrasound scans and foetal monitoring, are unnecessary and potentially dangerous. Foetal monitors, for example, have been shown to increase the rate of surgical intervention without a corresponding decrease in morbidity, and may contribute to maternal and foetal distress (Chalmer, Enkin and Kirse, 1989). Moreover, despite modern surgical techniques and drugs, infection and fever still occur in one in five mothers who undergo Caesarian section, and psychological disturbance is common. Mothers given general or local anaesthesia before delivery often take several days to recover from the effects (Hamilton, 1984), and babies born by general anaesthesia tend to show decreased responsiveness and alertness following birth (Feinbloom and Forman, 1987). Analgesia administered to the mother may also cause drowsiness and decreased responsiveness for the first few hours following birth or longer. Therefore, following surgical, technological and chemical intervention the bonding between mother and child may be delayed while both are recovering from their effects.

Temperament

As a result of prenatal and/or birth stressors it is fair to say that some children are highly stressed by the time they are born, whereas others are less so, and these differences are evident in patterns of tension, reactivity and pain at birth. Some children are physically soft and compliant, but others are tense and rigid. The latter tend to have a lower pain threshold, to be irritable and to cry more than relaxed babies. These differences influence how susceptible babies are to physical and emotional stimulation, how quickly and intensely they respond, their general mood and changeability of mood. On the basis of these patterns of responsiveness and mood, three types of baby have been identified (Thomas and Chess, 1977, 1980): the difficult child who cries a lot, is easily distracted, highly active and inhibited socially and can be characterized as negative, irregular and unadaptable; the easy child who is calm, easygoing, predictable and highly sociable, and characteristically positive, regular and adaptable; and the slow-to-warm-up child whose reactions tend to be less intense and extreme. These differences are viewed as inborn temperamental characteristics and linked to heredity by some developmentalists (Thomas and Chess, 1977; Bornstein, Gaughran and Segui, 1991). However, it is too simplistic to view these temperamental qualities as inherent in the child, partly because they are based on caregiver ratings and the relationship is dyadic and reflects the mother's own psychological state and understanding of her child's behaviour (St James-Roberts and Wolke, 1984), and partly because the possible effects on the unborn child of the mother's mood and behaviour during pregnancy cannot be underestimated.

However whether inherent or not, this 'inborn temperament is the raw material out of which personality is shaped' (Sternberger and Meyer, 1995: 174), because it sets up patterns of interactions with caregivers. Temperament influences the responses babies evoke from others (Scarr and McCartney, 1983). Mothers spend less time with and are less responsive to difficult infants, find it harder to cope with such babies and feel less satisfied as mothers (Campbell, 1979; Maccoby, Snow and Jacklin, 1984; Van den Boom and Hoeksma, 1993). Difficult babies are more of a challenge for parents and are more at risk of developing later behaviour problems.

However, both the child's temperament and the environment it is born into affect development. The parents' behaviour cannot be separated from that of the child: it is the interaction between infant temperament and parental characteristics that influences development. The emotional and psychological experiences of the mother during pregnancy, her overall levels of stress, tension or relaxation, (which are probably embedded in her ongoing psychosocial situation) are likely to continue after the child's birth and contribute to her coping strategies. Studies of 'goodness of fit' between infants and their parents have found that difficult infants raised by easygoing and patient parents are seemingly 'normal' at age 10, whereas difficult infants raised by nervous and angry parents showed signs of psychological disorder at the same age (Thomas and Chess, 1977).

Security of attachment

However, 'with easy babies or difficult ones, with mothers who are relaxed or tense, warm or rejecting, no matter how good the fit, an attachment relationship develops. What differs is their quality. And for infants, the critical difference is in the strength of their security' (Sternberger and Meyer, 1995: 188). Security of attachment is the extent to which a child can rely on his or her mother's being there to meet its needs.

The 'strange situation' (Ainsworth et al., 1978) is a standardized method for assessing a child's attachment to its caregiver by observing how well the child uses the caregiver as a secure base for exploration, and is comforted by the caregiver after a mildly stressful experience (in which a stranger enters an unfamiliar room from which the mother exits, leaving the baby alone with the stranger). On the basis of such measures a number of attachment types have been identified. The primary ones are *type A* (anxious/avoidant), where distress appears due to being left alone rather than to the mother's absence and where after separation the mother is ignored; *type B* (secure), where the child may or may not show distress during separation, though any distress is clearly related to the mother's absence, and the child actively seeks and maintains proximity, contact or interaction with the mother, especially upon being reunited with her; *type C* (anxious/resistant), where the child seeks proximity and contact with the mother but resists contact and interaction upon reunion with the mother after separation; and *type D* (disorganized), where babies show a disoriented pattern of behaviour.

There is now considerable evidence that these attachment types are predictive of other aspects of development. Secure attachment at 12 months has been correlated with the quality and sensitivity of mother-infant interaction at 6 to 15 weeks; curiosity and problem solving at age two; social confidence at nursery school at age three; empathy and independence at age five (Oppenheim et al., 1988) and with lack of behaviour problems (in boys) at age six (Lewis et al., 1984). Anxious/resistant attachment has been related to the likelihood of infant abuse: 70% of maltreated infants are found to have insecure attachments to their caregivers compared with only 26% of infants with no history of maltreatment (Browne, 1989). The research evidence suggests that secure attachments are linked with many kinds of favourable outcomes in later years and that insecure attachments undermine competence and are associated with developmental problems. However, there is no direct, inevitable link between attachment and later development. 'In reality, that link is only as strong as the child's experience. In other words, securely attached infants who continue to have good experiences continue to develop well. But insecurely attached infants whose experience improves can also improve emotionally. How attachment develops depends on the quality of care the infant receives over time' (Sternberger and Meyer, 1995: 195).

Family type

An important determinant of the quality of care given to a child is the type of family they are reared in. Conflict between parents, whether or not it precedes divorce or separation, has adverse effects on children (Davies and Cummings, 1994). Maritally distressed couples have been found to have more stressed children who show more negative peer interactions and more illness (Gottman and Katz, 1989).

Security of attachments can be undermined by separation and divorce. The effects vary considerably with the child's age when divorce or separation occur (Hetherington, 1988), and some of the ill effects, which can include long-term depression (Wallerstein, 1987) and maladjustment (Luepnitz, 1986), especially in young boys, are probably attributable to conflict between partners preceding the separation or divorce. Indeed it has been concluded that at least as much attention needs to be given to the processes that occur in troubled, intact families as to the trauma children suffer after their parents separate (Cherlin et al., 1991). Mother–daughter relationships tend to remain much the same as in non-divorced families, and mother–son relationships tend to be tense for divorced mothers who do not remarry. Despite warmth in the relationship, sons are often non-compliant and beyond their mothers' control. Remarriage and the presence of a stepfather can improve mother–son relationships but lead to deterioration in those between mothers and daughters (Hetherington, Cox and Cox, 1982). Forming strong relationships in a reconstituted family is often a gradual and difficult process (Ferri, 1984).

Increasingly children are not being raised in traditional family units. Child abuse tends to be more common in lone parent families (Daly and Wilson, 1996). The effects of abuse can be wide-ranging and long lasting. The research evidence suggests links between childhood physical abuse and adolescent criminal behaviour, adult family violence, and non-familial violence (Malinosky-Rummell and Hansen, 1993). Parents who do not react negatively towards difficult babies often have the support of others, and this is more easily provided in extended families. Hence wider cultural factors influence child development. Childhood sexual abuse is a risk factor for long-term effects on mental health (Spaccerelli, 1994). To date, research on children reared by homosexual couples of either sex does not suggest that they develop differently in any significant way (Patterson, 1992).

Parenting style

Attachment cannot be considered independently of parenting style, although research on parenting styles has been largely independent of that on attachment. Three global styles of parenting have been identified (Baumrind, 1967, 1980): authoritarian – where parents have strict and non-negotiable ideas about discipline and behaviour; authoritative – where parents have ideas about behaviour and discipline they are willing to explain and discuss with children and at times adapt; and permissive, where parents' ideas about behaviour and discipline are liberal and relaxed. Studies using this schema have found that authoritative parents tend to have popular, prosocial children, whereas authoritarian parents tend to have sociometrically rejected children (Dekovic and Janssens, 1992), as do the children of permissive parents.

Parenting style has also been identified as a major influence on the development of self-esteem (Coopersmith, 1967). Where parents are liberal and establish no clear guidelines or boundaries, the child tends to feel that it is not worthy of their care and love and is highly likely to place a low value on itself and to have poor self-esteem. Authoritarian parenting, where the parents establish clear and usually rigid boundaries for the child and punish transgressions, often physically, and where the child is not expected to express itself in any way, also produces children with poor self-esteem; whereas authoritative parenting, which is intermediate between the other two styles, in which parents clear guidelines for the child and enforce these with praise rather than punishment so that the child feels secure, and also encourage self-expression, produces high self-esteem.

The temperament of parents and the quality of their relationship influences parenting style. Adequate mothers generally have warm and secure relationships with both their children and partner whereas abusing mothers appeared to view relationships in terms of power struggles, to be controlling and hostile with anxiously attached children, and to have angry and unstable adult relationships (Crittenden, 1988). Typically children with high self-esteem tend to have mothers with high self-esteem; women who are confident in themselves and whose self-worth is not threatened by their children. By comparison mothers with low self-esteem are likely to interpret their children's challenges to their authority and its transgressions as a reflection of their being poor mothers and will forcefully stop them (Coopersmith, 1967). Importantly, therefore, different styles of parenting tend not only to produce different kinds of behaviour but different kinds of person.

Nevertheless, the child is not a passive recipient of parenting. Temperament not only influences the responses that the child evokes from others but also the activities and experiences that infants choose for themselves (Scarr and McCartney, 1983). This insight is implicit in psychodynamic theories of child development.

Psychodynamic developmental theories

Psychodynamic theories, which view development as an active, dynamic process that is influenced by both a person's inborn, biological drives and his or her conscious and unconscious social and emotional experiences, originate in the thinking of Sigmund Freud (1856–1939). His theory views development as a series of discrete, discontinuous stages. In this respect it is similar to the theories of Erik Erikson (1963) and Jean Piaget (1959) who also assume that development occurs in stages; that all individuals follow the same sequence or order; each successive stage is qualitatively distinct from all other stages, is increasingly complex, and integrates the developmental changes and accomplishments of earlier stages.

These *stage theories* contrast with *learning theories*, which view development as a relatively smooth and continuous process consisting of many small, incremental changes.

Freud conceptualized early child development in terms of three major stages: *oral*, from birth to one year when the mouth is the focus of stimulation and interaction during feeding and weaning; *anal*, from one to three years, when the anus is the focus of stimulation and interaction during elimination and toilet training; and *phallic*, from three to six years, when during gender role and moral development the genitals are central. According to this theory the major orifices of the body, by which the child experiences erotic pleasure, are the interfaces between the child and its environment. It is by way of these that the child develops a basic sense of its own identity as distinct from its environment. Its experiences of pleasure or frustration at each of these focal areas act as a template for later learning, and for different kinds of personality. So, for example, a child who during toilet training receives encouragement and praise, learns that giving is a rewarding and pleasurable experience, and is likely to develop an open and generous personality, whereas a child whose elimination is punished develops a withholding pattern of behaviour that subsequently comes to characterize his or her personality. If a child is denied gratification at any of these stages, he can become fixated and continue striving for erotic satisfaction there. The psychoanalytic theorist Erik Erikson observed different societies and claimed that the principles of Freudian theory were evident in practice, and that different styles of child rearing do indeed produce different kinds of children, and ultimately, different kinds of society.

Applying developmental theories and research findings

The question remains as to whether the theories and findings relating to human development provide any insight into the puzzling case of Jeffrey Dahmer. There can be no conclusive answer. Nevertheless, Dahmer's mother suffered from post-natal depression after his birth, refused to breast feed him, became increasingly depressed, was reliant on sedatives, laxatives and sleeping pills, and was unstable and self absorbed. His father was distant and busy. Thus, while by all accounts Dahmer was an easy baby, his parents were both 'difficult', and there was little 'goodness of fit' between them. As Dahmer's mother's health deteriorated she became unable to do anything; the domestic atmosphere was bad, and she and his father fought and threatened each other in front of their son. Dahmer saw his father hit his mother on numerous occasions throughout his childhood. Following several relapses, his mother spent a month in a mental hospital and this was followed by lengthy psychotherapy, but her intake of sedatives was not reduced, nor her instability. The family moved area several times, so there was no security for Dahmer in or outside the home. As a young child he was extremely shy, utterly isolated, lonely and withdrawn. Aged four he underwent surgery for a double hernia, and

afterwards experienced so much pain that, 27 years later, he reported that
he thought his genitals had been cut off. He never forgot the experience.
As his biographer observes, 'For a very long time, this would be the most
intimate event of his life' (Masters, 1993: 30). He subsequently developed
an erotic fascination with the insides of the body.

By the time he was school age Dahmer's mother 'appeared to have
"switched off" . . . The threads which bound mother to son, never very
strong, had virtually worn away to nothing' (Masters, 1993: 43). Dahmer
became progressively more withdrawn, remote and private. 'Like his
mother, he was dangerously self-centred; like his father he was unnaturally
reticent. He became silent and broody as a result' (Masters, 1993: 33). He
never learned to be open with his feelings, especially his frustration, and
increasingly retreated into a fantasy world. Eventually, Dahmer's parents
divorced following a psychological evaluation of his mother that found
that she suffered from very severe emotional problems and was constantly
angry, frustrated and demanding in her interpersonal relationships. By
this time, Dahmer was described by his high school counsellor as solemn
and depressed. He had also developed a drink problem. Shortly afterwards, aged 18, he committed his first murder, and his fantasy became
real. A serial killer was 'born'.

References

Abell T (1992) Low birth weight, intrauterine growth-retarded, and pre-term infants.
    Human Nature 3: 335–78.
Ainsworth MDS, Blehar M, Waters E, Wall S (1978) Strange-Situation Behavior of One
    Year Olds. Its Relation to Mother–Infant Interaction in the First Year and its
    Qualitative Differences in the Infant–Mother Attachment Relationship. Hillsdale NJ:
    Erlbaum.
Barr H, Streissguth A, Darby B, Sampson P (1990) Prenatal exposure to alcohol, caf-
    feine, tobacco and aspirin: effects on fine and gross motor performance in four year
    old children. Developmental Psychology 26: 339–48.
Baumrind D (1967) Child care practices anteceding three patterns of preschool behav-
    ior. Genetic Psychology Monograph 75: 43–88.
Baumrind D (1980) New directions in socialization research. Psychological Bulletin 35:
    639–52.
Bellinger D, Leviton A, Waternaux C, Needleman H, Rabinowitz M (1987) Longitudinal
    analyses of prenatal and postnatal lead exposure and early cognitive development.
    New England Journal of Medicine 316: 1037–43.
Bernhardt JS, (1990) Potential workplace hazards to reproductive health. Journal of
    Obstetrical Nursing 19(536): 53–62.
Bornstein MH, Gaughran JM, Segui I (1991) Multimethod assessment of infant tem-
    perament: mother questionnaire and mother and observer reports evaluated and
    compared at five months using the Infant Temperament Measure. International
    Journal of Behavioral Development 14: 131–51.
Bowlby J (1969) Attachment and Loss, vol. 1. London: Hogarth.
Browne K (1989) The naturalistic context of family violence and child abuse. In J
    Archer, K Browne (eds) Human Agression: Naturalistic Approaches. London:
    Routledge.

Campbell S (1979) Mother–infant interactions as a function of maternal ratings of temperament. Child Psychiatry and Human Development 10: 67–76.

Carlson D, Labarba R (1979) Maternal emotionality during pregnancy and reproductive outcome: a review of literature. Int Journal of Behavioural Development 2: 343–76.

Chalmer I, Enkin M, Kirse M (eds) (1989) Effective Care in Pregnancy and Childbirth. Oxford: Oxford University Press.

Cherlin AJ, Furstenberg FF, Chase-Lonsdale PL, Kiernan KE, Robins PK, Morrison DR, Teitler JO (1991) Longitudinal studies of effects of divorce on children in Great Britain and the United States. Science 252: 1386–9.

Coopersmith S (1967) The Antecedents of Self-Esteem. San Francisco: Freeman.

Corby DG (1978) Aspirin in pregnancy: maternal and fetal effects. Pediatrics 62 (Supplement): 930–7.

Crittenden PM (1988) Relationships at Risk. In J Belsky, T Nezworski (eds) Clinical Implications of Attachment. Hillsdale NJ: Erlbaum, pp. 136–74.

Daly M, Wilson M (1996) Violence against step children: Current Directions in Psychological Science 5: 77–81.

Davies G, Cummings EM (1994) Marital conflict and child adjustment. Psychological Bulletin 116: 387–411.

Dekovic M, Janssens JMAM (1992) Parents'child rearing style and child's sociometric status. Developmental Psychology 28: 925–32.

Erikson E (1963) Childhood and Society (2 edn). New York: Horton.

Evans S (1998) The ontogenesis of auditory perception and memory at 20 weeks gestation. Paper presented at the conference of The British Psychological Society, 29 March, Brighton.

Feinbloom RI, Forman BY (1987) Pregnancy, Birth and the Early Months: A Complete Guide. Reading MA: Addison-Wesley.

Fenster L, Eskenazi B, Windham G, Swan S (1991) Caffeine consumption during pregnancy and fetal growth. American Journal of Public Health 81: 458–61.

Ferri G, (1984) Stepchildren: A National Study. Reading: NFER-Nelson.

Fricker H, Segal S (1978) Narcotic addiction, pregnancy and the newborn. American Journal of the Diseases of Children 132: 360–6.

Fried PA (1983) Pregnancy and life-style habits. New York: Beaufort Books.

Gottman, JM, Katz LF (1989) Effects of marital discord on young children's peer interactions and health. Developmental Psychology 25: 373–81.

Hamilton PM (1984) Basic Maternity Nursing (5 edn). St Louis: Mosby.

Handler A, Kistin N, Davis F, Ferre C (1991) Cocaine use during pregnancy: perinatal outcomes. American Journal of Epidemiology 133: 818–25.

Harlav HF (1961) The development of affectional patterns in infant monkeys. In Fors BM (ed.) Determinants of Infant Behaviour, vol. 2, London: Methuen.

Hepper PG (1991) An examination of fetal learning before and after birth. The Irish Journal of Psychology 12(2): 95–107.

Hetherington EM (1988) Parents, children and siblings six years after divorce. In R Hinde and J Steveson-Hinde (eds) Relationships Within Families. Cambridge MA: Cambridge University Press, pp. 311–31.

Hetherington EM, Cox M, Cox R (1985) Long-term effects of divorce and remarriage on the adjustment of children. Journal of the American Academy of Psychiatry 24: 518–30.

Hoffman LW (1983) Work, family and the socialization of the child. In R. Parke (ed.) Review of Child Development Research, vol. 7. The Family. Chicago: University of Chicago Press, pp. 223–82.

Jacobsen J, Jacobsen S, Fein GG, Schwartz PM (1984) Factors and clusters for the Brazelton Scale: an investigation ofthe dimensions of neonatal behaviour. Developmental Psychology 20: 339–53.

Jacobsen J, Jacobsen S, Padgett R, Brumitt G, Billings R (1992) Effects of prenatal PCB exposure on cognitive processing efficiency and sustained attention. Developmental Psychology 28: 297–306.

Kempe RS, Kempe H (1978) Child Abuse. London: Fontana.

Kennell JH, Jerauld R, Wolfe H, Chester D, Kreger NC, McAlpine W, Steffa N, Klaus MH (1974) Maternal behaviour one year after early and extended post-partum contact. Developmental Medicine and Child Neurology 16: 172–9.

Klaus M, Jerauld R, Kreger N, McAlpine W, Steffa M, Kennell J (1972) Maternal attachment: importance of the first post-partum days. New England Journal of Medicine 286: 460–3.

Landesman-Dwyer S (1981) Drinking during pregnancy: effects on human development (monograph). Alcohol and Health, vol. 4.

Lawson A, Rhode DL (1993) The Politics of Pregnancy: Adolescent Sexuality and Public Policy. New Haven CT: Yale University Press.

Lewis M, Feiring C, McGuffog C, Jaskir J (1984) Predicting psychopathology in six year olds from early social relations. Child Development 55: 123–36.

Light H, Fenster C (1974) Maternal concerns about pregnancy. American Journal of Obstetrics and Gynecology 118: 46–50.

Luepuitz DA (1986) A comparison of maternal, paternal and joint custody: understanding the varieties of post-divorce family life. Journal of Divorce 9: 1–12.

McCall R (1981) Nature–nurture and the two realms of development: a proposed integration with respect to mental development. Child Development 52: 1–12.

Maccoby E, Snow M, Jacklin C (1984) Children's dispositions and mother–child interaction at 12 and 18 months: a short-term longitudinal study. Developmental Psychology 20: 459–72.

Malinosky-Rummel R, Hansen, DI (1993) Long-term consequences of childhood physical abuse. Psychological Bulletin 114: 68–79.

Masters B (1993) The Shrine of Jeffrey Dahmer. London: Hodder and Stoughton.

Moran EG (1993) Domestic violence and pregnancy. In BK Rothman (ed.) The Encyclopedia of Childbearing. New York: Henry Holt.

Norbeck, JS and Tilden, VP (1983) Life stress, social support and emotional disequilibrium in complications of pregnancy: a prospective multivariate study. Journal of Health and Social Behaviour 24: 30–46.

O'Connor M, Sigman M, Brill N (1987) Disorganization of attachment in relation to maternal alcohol consumption. Journal of Consulting and Clinical Psychology 55: 831–6.

Omer H, Everly G (1988) Psychological factors in preterm labor. American Journal of Psychiatry 145: 1507–13.

Oppenheim D, Sagi A, Lamb ME (1988) Infant–adult attachments on the Kibbutz and their relation to the socioemotional development four years later. Developmental Psychology 24: 427–33.

Patterson CJ (1992) Children of lesbian and gay parents. Child Development 63: 1025–42.

Piaget J (1959) The Language and Thought of the Child (3 edn). London: Routledge & Kegan Paul.

Rutter M (1981) Maternal Deprivation Reassessed. Harmondsworth: Penguin.

Scarr S, McCartney K (1983) How people make their own environments: a theory of genotype–environment effects. Child Development 53: 424–35.

Sluckin W, Herbert M, Sluckin A (1983) Maternal Bonding. Oxford: Blackwell.

Spaccerelli S, 1994 Stress, appraisal, and coping in child sexual abuse. Psychological Bulletin 116: 340–62.

St James-Roberts I, Wolke D (1984) Comparison of mothers' with trained observers' reports on neonatal behavioral style. Infant Behavior and Development 7: 299–310.

Sternberger L, Meyer R (1995) Childhood. New York: McGraw-Hill.

Streissguth AP, Landesman-Dwyer S, Martin DC, Smith DW (1980) Teratogenic effects of alcohol in humans and laboratory animals. Science 209: 355–61.

Taylor E, Emery J (1988) Trends in unexpected infant deaths in Sheffield. The Lancet 13: 1121–2.

Tew M (1995) Safer Childbirth? London: Chapman & Hall.

Thomas A, Chess S (1977) Temperament and Development. New York: Brunner/Mazel.

Thomas A, Chess S (1980) The Dynamics of Development. New York: Brunner/Mazel.

Van den Boom D, Hoeskma J (1993) The interaction of mothers and their irritable and non-irritable infants. University of Leiden manuscript. Cited in Sternberger L, Meyer R (1995) Childhood. New York: McGraw-Hill.

Wallerstein JS (1987) Children of divorce: report of a ten-year follow-up of early latency-age children. American Journal of Orthopsychiatry 57: 199–211.

Further reading

Smith PK, Cowie II, Blades M (1998) Understanding Children's Development (3 edn). Oxford: Blackwell

Chapter 15
The development of sociability and fears

N.J. BANKS

Key concepts	Key names
Social competence	Izard
Friendships	Shaffer, Bronfenbrenner
Isolation and rejection	
Components of popularity	
Development of fears	
Behaviourism	Watson
Social learning theory	Bandura
Ethology	Hinde, Bowlby
Social cognition	Paiget and Inhelder, Selman
Empathy	Feshbach

Introduction

This chapter will consider the development of social competence, popularity and friendships/relationships, isolation, rejection, group formation and the development of fears in childhood and adolescence. Broad theoretical considerations are provided to aid the conceptualization of selected issues.

Social competence

The secure development of attachments with nurturing responsive caregivers, discussed in Chapter 14, is an important influencing factor in the development of social competence. With this in mind, the relevant section on attachment should be consulted in conjunction with this chapter. Early social competence is related to the infant's early ability to emit, recognize and respond to social signals. The later development of social competence is related to a child's environmental/social experience, personality and emotional security. Children's emotional responses to caregivers have a reciprocal effect in that there is a linked feedback response to cues and these signals effect the response of the sender and receiver. Responsiveness to emotional communication has been found to exist as early as three months of age (Malatesta and Haviland, 1982; Tronick and Cohn, 1989).

Theoretical considerations

There are different ways of conceptualizing the development of social competence. This will be discussed briefly so that the reader is aware of the variance of explanation. A full discussion of the different theoretical models is beyond the scope of this chapter.

Behaviourism

Behaviourism sees people as responding to their environment. Behaviourists believe that people can only produce the responses they have learned when the stimulus conditions are appropriate. Individuals are seen as products of their conditioning with the stimulus–response paradigm being the fundamental premise of learning. Watson, an early behaviourist, writing in 1913, suggested three innate emotions in infants: fear brought on by loud noises or loss of body support, rage brought on by a frustration or restriction of movement or goal, and love brought on by being cuddled or caressed. Watson believed that responses were learned through 'classical conditioning'. Later behaviourists found that responses in infants such as smiling, vocalizing and crying could be initiated or inhibited through the process of 'reinforcement'.

Social learning theory

Bandura (1986, 1989) is seen as the originator of social learning theory. *Social learning theory sees behaviour as being learned by observation, 'modelling' and 'cognitive appraisal'.* Modelling of another's emotions is seen as a means by which people learn to react to their environment. This process involves that of associating specific stimuli with the reactions of others – for example, an observed fearful response to a dog creates a fear of dogs. The cognitive appraisal aspect is reflected in the fact that, as children's cognitive capacities develop, they can recall early associations and engage in emotional self-arousal by considering their own or others' previous emotional responses to stimuli.

Ethology

The ethological perspective for which researchers such as Hinde (1989) and Bowlby (1969) are well known, argues that the infant is a motivated and responsive social being. The perspective argues that infants are what could be termed 'biologically pre-programmed' to give out social signals and respond to the social signals of others, particularly carers, as this promotes survival as responsiveness ensures care and attention. An example of this 'biological pre-programming' would be that of the reflex actions children are born with or develop soon after birth, such as smiling, that bring about proximity seeking and nurturing behaviour in carers.

Social cognition approaches

Emotional development in children is linked to self-expression and recognition of emotions in others. The ability to recognize emotions in others and respond appropriately is linked to the development of empathy. This recognition involves both a cognitive appraisal of another's situation and the emotional appraisal of one's own response. Feshbach (1978) saw empathy as 'shared emotional responses which the child experiences on perceiving others' emotional reactions'. Empathy is believed to begin during the preschool years and is seen as an important precursor of prosocial behaviour (Eisenburg and Strayer, 1987). Thompson (1990) in a review of the early development of empathy suggests that the psychoanalytic perspective sees the development of empathy 'in the context of the mother infant bond'. He suggests a more influential perspective is the work of cognitive development researchers. This work has been stimulated by Piaget and Inhelder's (1969) cognitive development theory. Here, the development of empathy is dependent on the existence of certain cognitive reasoning abilities such as person (object) permanence, an ability to see self as separate from others and the initial emergence of an ability to see the world from another's perspective. The development of this was tested by Feshbach (1978) who used slides accompanied by stories about a boy and his dog. In one slide children were shown a boy and his dog and told that the boy went everywhere with his dog but the dog sometimes tries to run away. In the next slide, the dog was seen running away. In the third slide, the boy was unable to find the dog and the children were told that the dog may be lost and gone forever. Feshbach then asked the children how they felt about what they had seen and heard. *An empathic response was seen to be one which included both a cognitive understanding of the boy's feelings and point of view and an emotional response to the boy's feelings.* Here the cognitive components were the ability to distinguish and label the feelings of the boy. The affective or emotional component was the capacity for emotional responsiveness.

Distinct from the psychoanalytic viewpoint, the social-cognitive theorists do not believe true empathy, as opposed to pseudo-empathy, occurs until the later preschool years (four to five years). The social-cognitive theorists essentially see a child as having to develop beyond its egocentric limitations before it can begin to be a 'true' social being (six to seven years). Investigators of social competence have tended to be strongly influenced by Piaget's (1969) cognitive development theory. The influence of this cognitive stage theory view is that many researchers maintain that children's conceptualizations or understanding of people progresses through qualitatively distinct stages in invariant order closely linked to Piaget and Inhelder's (1969) cognitive development model. The order of the stages is argued to be invariant although they may emerge earlier or later in different children. Mussen et al. (1984) have stated that:

> At the most general level, children's social thinking can be described as developing in several independent directions: (a) from 'surface to depth,' that is, from attention to appearances to consideration of more enduring qualities (e.g. from thinking about friends in terms of attractiveness to judgements about personal motives); (b) from simple to complex, that is, from narrow concentration on one aspect of an issue or problem to concentration to a broader perspective that takes account of many dimensions simultaneously; (c) from rigid to flexible thinking; (d) from predominant concern with oneself and the here and now to concern with the welfare of others and with the future; (e) from concrete to abstract thinking; and (f) from diffuse, sometimes inconsistent, ideas to systematic, organized, integrated thoughts. (p. 308)

The influence of Piaget's (1970) cognitive development theory has meant that much research takes 'as given' that *children in the preoperational stage are 'egocentric' which means they tend to be unable to understand that their own viewpoints may be different from others' points of view.* Egocentric thought is said to decline in its influence from the ages of six to seven years when the stage of concrete operational thought emerges and children are able to conceptualize the thought content of others as being potentially different from their own. The reader may like to consider the questioning of young concrete operational children about what they did at school on that particular day and receiving a reply of 'you know'. This may appear a 'brush off' or an attempt to avoid the questioning. However, if one takes a cognitive development view, it may be that children, wrapped in their own egocentric thought, actually believe the questioning adult has access to the same information they have even though the adult was not present on the school premises.

Social behaviour

Early social competence can be seen in mother–infant face-to-face play which begins at two to three months of age. This activity tends to be mainly social in origin without being involved in formal caregiving tasks. Thompson (1990) notes that the development of mother–infant face-to-face play is seen as an important activity for the infant's development of social skills and social expectations. Malatesta et al. (1986) has shown that caregivers and infants involve themselves in play exchanges that are called 'non-verbal conversation' or 'behavioural dialogue'. The aim of these exchanges is said to be emotional synchrony between caregiver and infant, which is seen as a mutual sharing of positive emotional arousal. Simply put, caregiver and baby are having reciprocal 'fun' and this sharing of intimate activity lays the foundation for caring and sharing, playful intimacy and sociability in later life. Izard's work (Izard, 1982; Izard et al., 1987), which involved videoing babies' responses to a variety of events, suggests that various emotions develop at different points over the first two years of age. Angry expressions appear at three to four months. Sadness is displayed at about the same age. Fear shows itself at about the age of five to seven months followed by shame and shyness. The socially complex emotions of guilt and contempt can be seen during the second year of life. By the age of 18 to 24 months there is little doubt that children are emotional beings and indeed some work has suggested that older toddlers can pretend emotions to manipulate another person (Bretherton et al., 1986). There appears to be a developmental consistency among young children in their emotional sensitivity and responsiveness to others. Children of 12 months to 18 months may respond to the distress of others by focusing on their needs and showing sympathetic distress and seeking their own caretaker. An older child at 24 months is more likely to show concern by some physical action to reduce the distress of the other child (Radke-Yarrow and Zahn-Waxler, 1984). These responses have been reported as being stable qualities among about two-thirds of individuals at least until seven years of age (Radke-Yarrow and Zahn-Waxler, 1984).

Selman (1976, 1980), in an early investigation of social competence and children's ability to understand and take another's perspective (social role-taking ability), gave children stories of social situations where there existed social or moral dilemmas. One example of such a dilemma presented to children age between 4 and 10 years was the story of 'Holly':

Holly is an 8 year old girl who likes to climb trees. She is the best tree climber in the neighbourhood. One day while climbing down from a tall tree, she falls off the bottom branch but does not hurt herself. Her father sees her fall. He is upset and asks her to promise not to climb trees anymore. Holly promises. Later that day, Holly and her friends meet Shawn. Shawn's kitten is caught up in a tree and can't get down. Something has to be done right away, or the kitten may fall. Holly is the only person who can climb trees well enough to reach the kitten and get it down, but she remembers her promise to her father. (Selman and Byrne, 1974: 805)

Questions examining the social perspective of the children included 'Does Holly know how Shawn feels about the kitten? Why?' 'How will Holly's father feel if he finds out she climbed the tree?' 'What does Holly think her father will think of her if he finds out?' The responses were analysed according to the children's ability to consider the position of the characters in the story. To be seen as non-egocentric children had to be able to verbalize about Holly's situation. Selman devised a framework that allows us to understand the discrete levels or stages in a child's development of social perspective taking:

- Stage 0 – egocentric thinking (3 to 6 years). Here children are not able to distinguish between their own view and the view of others (the child is 'stuck' in a view of 'they know what I know'). Asked 'how will Holly's father feel when he finds out (that she climbed the tree)?' a child at this stage may say 'happy, he likes kittens'.
- Stage 1 – social informational role taking (ages 6 to 8 years). Children have an understanding that others have a different perspective (they may not know what I know). A child at this stage may say Holly's father will be angry because he told her not to climb trees.
- Stage 2 – self-reflection (ages 8 to 10 years). At this stage children are able to understand both that each person may have a different view point and that each person may be aware of this (they may not know what I know and they may be as aware of this as I am). If asked if Holly's father will punish her, children at this level may respond that this depends whether her father understands why she climbed the tree. If he has this information, he will understand and be unlikely to punish her.
- Stage 3 – mutual role taking (ages 10 to 12). Children at this age can understand people from a third person perspective such as a neutral bystander or family friend. A child is able to conceptualize that 'Holly and her father trust each other, so they can talk about why she climbed the tree'. (We have a shared perspective that has developed into a mutual understanding.)
- Stage 4 – social and conventional system role taking (ages 12 to 15+). At this stage children are capable of understanding that beliefs may be determined and operate within a system of shared perspectives. They may interpret things from a cultural or religious view – for example, the Muslim perspective on alcohol or the Jehovah's Witness perspective on blood transfusions. Selman (1976) argued that the subject realises that each considers the shared point of view of the social system in order to facilitate accurate communication with and understanding of others.

This framework reflects children's ability to consider hypothetical social situations and to be able to verbalize their reasoning. The methodological difficulties with this method are that it may be more difficult for children to understand the position of another in a test situation than when seeing the situation in real life and/or with a person the child knows. Children often understand more than they can accurately verbally express (to a researcher formally investigating in a one-off situation). Mussen et al. (1984) note that when investigators use methods that do not rely excessively on language, or when children's responses are considered in real life situations, they often find signs of perspective taking at an earlier age. Despite these observations, Selman's work is still seen as valid and a useful contribution to our understanding of children's development of social competence. An anecdotal example of children's ability to accurately assess and respond to the needs of others was provided by Hoffman (1981) in a story about a 15-month-old boy fighting with his friend over a toy, making the friend cry. The 15-month-old boy lets go but the friend continues to cry. The 15-month-old boy then brings his toy to his friend but this does not stop the crying. The 15-month-old boy then gets his friend's comfort blanket. Hoffman has argued that this anecdote illustrates that the abilities of children can be underestimated by a sole reliance on language or verbal methods to assess their understanding. Mussen et al. (1984) note that empathy is not an all-or-nothing quality. It may be a specific situational quality related to a child's experience and the people to whom the child is responding. It seems that children may show a greater empathic response to people who are more similar to themselves, such as members of their own gender or ethnic group. They are more able to empathize with people who are in a situation they have experienced themselves than one that they have not experienced. The extent of a child's empathy development may be a key factor in their overall social-emotional development. Feshbach (1982) has suggested that there is a range of effects, mediated by empathy, which include 'social understanding, greater emotional competence, heightened compassion, caring and related behaviours; regulation of aggression and other antisocial behaviours; increased self-awareness; enhanced communication skills; and greater cohesion between the cognitive, affective and interpersonal aspects of the child's behaviour' (p. 320).

There is some evidence of gender differences in empathy display and development. One study of four-to-six year olds found that when a mother was rated as having a higher measure in empathy than the father, the display of empathy was seen as more appropriate for girls, and when this occurs with mothers the development and display may be heightened in girls as it is seen as sex-stereotypical behaviour. Boys' scores on the empathy measures did not correlate with either parent's scores (Barnett et al., 1980). In another study (Strayer, 1983), the scores of mothers, but not fathers, on an empathy measure were found to be statistically correlated to children's scores of empathy. These results suggest that mothers in particular may play an important role in the socialization and display of empathy in children. However, one must take a cautious view as fathers are not always comprehensively included, if at all, in the investigations.

Social perspective ability increases with age. This is most probably a result of cognitive development and social experience. Difficulties in taking the perspective of another are one aspect of children who have social interaction difficulties. This can be helped by training in social skills (Chandler, 1973; Shure and Spivack, 1980). A study of preschool children (Friedrich and Stein, 1973) revealed a paradox in children's social behaviour. This was that children who are often seen as being the most helpful in their ability to share and care for others may also be the most aggressive in the classroom. The study was in the USA and involved children of different social classes, localities and ethnic groups. The findings were that children who were the most co-operative, generous and helpful were also more assertive, aggressive and generally sociable. It was suggested that one explanation for this was that some children might simply show more of all types of social behaviour. Radke-Yarrow et al. (1983) suggested that it might be moderately aggressive children who are more helpful and kind with the very aggressive children being less prosocial. Aggressive behaviour was seen more in preschool children who may assert themselves more aggressively. As children develop it is likely that they distinguish between what is socially acceptable and what is not socially acceptable and use less inappropriate 'communicative' behaviour such as hitting. Those children of age five to eight years who were seen as more empathic used both assertiveness and socially acceptable behaviour (sharing and negotiating) in peer interactions and were more popular with their peers. Children who continued to use physical aggression tended to be unpopular and rejected by others (Parke and Slaby, 1983). This leads us to consider popularity.

The components of popularity

As well as personality traits, body-build characteristics have been found to affect popularity with peers. Staffieri (1967) showed six-to-ten year olds full-length ectomorphic (thin), endomorphic (plump) and mesomorphic (athletic build) silhouettes. After choosing the one they preferred they were given a list of adjectives and asked to attach those that applied to each body type. The children were then asked to give the names of five class peers who could be considered as good friends and three classmates whom the child did not like. It was found that most children preferred the mesomorphic silhouette and attached the positive adjectives such as 'helpful', 'brave', and 'strong' to this physique. Less positive adjectives were attributed to the ectomorphic figure with even less benign adjectives assigned to the endomorphic figure type. The researchers also found that friendships between the actual children in the classroom showed a definite correlation between body physique type and popularity. As would be expected, the findings were like those found with the silhouette figures: the mesomorphic children were the most popular and the endomorphic children were the least popular.

Later research with adults and adolescents has shown similar findings (e.g. Clausen, 1975). Early research in the USA (Jones and Bayley, 1950) followed 16 early-maturing and 16 late-maturing male adolescents over six years and found how early-maturing males tended to be more confident and more popular with their peers. This may relate, in part, to competence in sports and being personally associated with physical prowess and masculinity. Follow up studies (Jones, 1965) of the same group of adolescents found that some of the social differences disappeared although the late maturers were still less confident and less popular with their peers than the early maturers. This continuing lack of confidence in late maturers may relate to having a late start compared with their peers and less time for social competence practice and resultant building of self-esteem. With girls it appears that early maturation is less advantageous. Many studies have found that early-maturing females are less popular and less self-confident than late maturers (Aro and Tipale, 1987; Duncan et al., 1985). However, Brooks-Gunn and Warren (1988) found with girls 9 to 11 years of age, breast development correlated with a more positive view of self and greater feelings of peer acceptance and superior psychological adjustment.

Perceived facial attractiveness is related to body characteristics as a facet of popularity. Although 'attractiveness' can be subjective and culturally defined, it appears that even infants can show different responses to faces that are seen as attractive and less attractive (Langlois et al., 1987). It also seems that children who are seen as attractive are described in more favourable terms than less attractive children by both their peers and teachers (Langlois, 1986). This may be related to a self-fulfilling prophecy as subtle cues may be passed on in interaction of how favourable the child is perceived to be by others.

Parenting styles also appear to have an influence on popularity. This would seem related to the process of socialization and the effect of parenting style on children's behaviour. Sensitive authoritative caregivers tend to socialize children who are securely attached and can establish positive relationships with adults and their age peers. Unresponsive caregivers who are too permissive, providing poor boundaries and low social expectations, have been found to raise children who are hostile and aggressive. Children raised by authoritarian caregivers tend to be anxious, reserved and temperamental (Putallaz, 1987). There has been early evidence that overprotective parents may create children who are unsure of their role with children although they appear socially able when mixing with adults. Overprotected children may avoid the company of other children and seek out the company of adults whom they perceive as more accepting of them and less rejecting than their peers (Martin, 1975).

The child's birth position appears to have an effect on sociability. Being a younger child may bring about a situation where one must learn to communicate, co-operate and negotiate with older and more dominant siblings. If this is so, then one would expect many younger children, because these skills are nurtured, to become more popular than first-born children. This would be rather a broad generalization and may not be applied to all.

Friendships

Hartup (1983) has argued that friendships are reciprocal relationships that tend to resemble the attachments between children and their mothers. In order to discover what children think about friendship Bigelow and LaGaipa (1975) asked children in Canada and Scotland aged between 6 to 14 to tell them which characteristics friends should have and what they believed they should expect from a friend. Three stages were discovered:

*   Reward–Cost stage (age 7 to 8 years). This is characterized by geographical proximity, the availability of interesting toys, and co-operative playing in mutually liked games and activities.
*   Normative stage (ages 10 to 11 years). At this stage, common values and beliefs become important. Loyalty is seen as important and sharing, support and co-operation are required.
*   Empathic stage (age 10 to 12). At this stage children see friends as those who share common interests, make active attempts to understand one another, share personal information about each other and respond with sensitivity to one another's disclosures. It seems that adolescents' views on the expectations of friendship are closely linked to the development of the empathic stage with a clear emphasis on reciprocal emotional relations. From age 10 to 11 the emphasis is on mutual help and support, whereas at age 16 to 17 this view has developed into emotional availability and intimate exchange (Smollar and Youniss, 1982; Tesch, 1983). Hartup (1983) sees close friendship in adolescence as reflecting a 'shared identity' in which 'you' and 'me' have become 'we'.

Group formation and peer relationships

Most children of preschool age enjoy interaction with their peers. During the preschool years social mixing becomes closer, more regular and more sustained than in younger years. From about the age of three onwards, children seek out and associate more frequently with peers of the same sex. Children of this age appear to be more able to co-operate and collaborate than previously, although *solitary play* (where children play alone) and *parallel play* (where children play side by side) are still the norm.

Between three to four years of age, attachments to playmates increase and given the opportunity the number of friendships increases. Make-believe play is more complex and includes role-taking mimicking the roles of significant adults (Almy et al., 1983). With school-age children their behaviour becomes task orientated, and goal related with greater structure and social organization. During the ages of six to eight years, group formation is more evident and at the ages of 10 to 14 years children's groups are more formal and can be highly complex. Shaffer (1989) states that peer groups are generally seen to have the following characteristics. They

- interact on a regular basis;
- have a sense of belonging;
- share implicit or explicit norms that determine how its members are supposed to behave; and
- have or develop a structure or social organization that enables the group to work together towards shared goals.

It would seem that children between the ages of 6 to 10 begin to assume membership in true peer groups as they begin to identify with groups such as cub scouts or a football club. Children do not necessarily conform to the expectations of a group if these go against their beliefs. With anti-social behaviour it seems that children are more likely to go against parentally instilled values between the ages of 6 to 15 but are less likely to go against their socialized moral code after this age band (Brown et al., 1986; Steinberg and Silverberg, 1986).

Bronfenbrenner (1967) in a cross-cultural study of North American, Russian, English and German children aged between 11 and 12 found that, overall, the English children were more likely to take part in peer-influenced misconduct (involving the non-disclosure of the discovery of a teacher's test answer sheet) and that, in all the cultures, boys were more likely to be subject to deviant peer influence than girls. Russian children raised in a strong group-conformity culture showed the least influence to deviant peer pressure.

Isolation and rejection

Generally, when children are asked about reactions to their classmates, factors such as immaturity tend to be related to rejection and positive traits such as physical attractiveness, intelligence and peer sensitivity are associated with popularity. Some research has suggested that poor relationships with peers during childhood are a significant predictor of later maladjustment and offending behaviour (Achenbach and Edelbrook, 1981). Sociometric assessments where children are asked to self-report their peers' popularity show that such assessments tend to remain stable over childhood and adolescence (Howes, 1988; Ladd and Price, 1987) with the rejected category remaining the most stable over time (Coie and Dodge, 1983). Rejected children tend to be miserable, alienated, low achieving and have low self-esteem. Much of the evidence for rejected children's difficulties is correlational and peer relationships may not necessarily be a causal factor in major life difficulties. It may be that peer rejection is related to personality characteristics and the influence of child-rearing practices affecting sociability. Rejection tends to be associated with a wide range of negative social behaviours in children such as aggression, disrupting playmates' activities, conflict and immaturity (Ladd and Price, 1987; Shantz, 1986).

Development of fears in childhood and adolescence

The ICD-10 Classification of Mental and Behavioural Disorders (1992) lists three categories related to fears in children:

- 'separation anxiety';
- 'social anxiety disorder'; and
- 'phobic anxiety disorder'.

The common factor of these categories is anxiety as the related symptom. The difference between the categories is that the anxiety has a different cause in each. Readers should be aware that in order to attract the label of 'disorder' the displays of behaviour should be intense and persistent reactions that interfere with daily living or that have lasted for more than five months (Graziano et al., 1979). Barrios and O'Dell (1989) note that various texts use different terms, such as anxiety, fear, phobia, phobic reaction and anxiety state. They take the view that this distinction may help predict which treatment is most effective although, in practice, the distinction may be of little real value. Barrios and O'Dell use a working definition of children's fears and anxieties as 'a complex pattern of motor, subjective and physiological reactions to a real or imagined threat' (p. 169). It would appear that a fear of a real situation that poses some objective threat to a child would give rise to a different response than a fear that posed no objective threat to a child (other than the fear itself). Barrios and O'Dell note that fears show a behavioural pattern of anxiousness, fearfulness, tension, shyness, timidity, bashfulness, withdrawal, seclusiveness, social isolation, depression, aloofness, and secretiveness. It may be that not all children show the same symptoms as a 'total cluster' and some children may show some symptoms more intensely than others.

The most common fear in early childhood develops when the child is about 7 to 11 months and is referred to as *fear of strangers* or *stranger anxiety*. This development appears to occur as a result of two cognitive abilities:

- the child obtaining *(social) object permanence* (Piaget, 1969). Here the child is able to conceive that social and inanimate objects have permanence when they disappear from view and that the attached caregiver is different from the stranger; and
- the child's ability to compare the pattern of a known person's face with an unknown person's face.

If the face does not resemble the known pattern or schema the difference causes uncertainty, resulting in distress. The proximity of a stranger at this time may not always be distressing to a child if they approach slowly and offer soothing communication to the child. This fear is a normal and expected part of a child's development and would not normally warrant psychiatric intervention unless it continues beyond the expected age and shows itself as being persistent and limiting of a child's social experience. In the context of being an older age-related 'disorder', the psychiatric label is one of 'social anxiety disorder' or 'avoidant disorder' where the anxiety-provoking stimulus is contact with strangers. There is excessive and persistent avoidance of contact with strangers and new social situations, resulting in a child's social experiences and contact with peers being so inhibited and reduced that the child's social development is impaired. To be seen as a 'disorder', the resistance to new social situations (and people) should be persistent, generalized, and not specific to one particular social situation (or person), arising before the age of six years towards adults, peers or both. There is normally selective attachment to parents and familiar people. The common symptoms are:

- unrealistic, excessive and persistent fear about what the future holds;
- unrealistic, excessive and persistent concern about the child's past behaviour;
- unrealistic, excessive and persistent concerns about the one's social, educational and practical skills; and abilities with much undermining self-doubt leading to a self-fulfilling prophecy resulting in a;
- loss of self-confidence and gross self-consciousness;
- somatization;
- emotional and physical tension;
- persistent demands for reassurance.

Four or more of the symptoms are normally present to attract the label of 'social anxiety disorder'. Hoghughi (1992) suggests that social phobias become more evident in mid-adolescence and grow beyond late adolescence into early adulthood. This may be related to cognitive development and the ability to reflect on others' views of one's self and concerns with an imaginary audience.

Another common fear with infants is *separation fear* or *separation anxiety*. This appears most often when the child is left with a stranger in an unfamiliar environment – for example, being left in day care for the first time with no prior preparation. As with stranger anxiety, this fear usually appears around 7 to 11 months. It peaks at about 15 to 18 months. The explanation given for its occurrence is similar to that of stranger anxiety. This fear appears to reduce after the age of two years in a securely attached child as the child is able to comprehend the event and predict the return of the caregiver. The fear of separation from a caregiver to whom the child is attached shows itself as a disorder after the age of two to three years under the following conditions:

- unrealistic, excessive and persistent fear about harm to the caregiver(s);
- unrealistic, excessive, preoccupying and persistent fear about harm to the child – for example that the child might be lost, kidnapped, or suffer a road traffic accident or go in to hospital;
- unrealistic, excessive and persistent fear about loss of or abandonment by the caregiver(s);
- opposition towards school attendance due to fear of separation but not other school-linked events;
- unrealistic, excessive, and persistent fear about sleeping alone or away from home;
- unrealistic, excessive and persistent fear about being alone;
- persistent and regular nightmares or difficulty in going to sleep due to fear of separation from or loss of the caregiver(s);
- somatic or physical complaints related to separation, for example, headache, vomiting;
- unrealistic, excessive and persistent distress in relation to actual or anticipated separation. This distress may show itself as crying, apathy, misery, tantrums or social withdrawal.

At least three or more of the above conditions are usually present to attract the label of 'disorder'. In addition there should be no general disturbance of personality development or personality functioning and the fear should not be part of generalized anxiety about multiple issues. The disorder usually arises in early childhood after four years of age. Development in adolescence requires additional considerations and may not be appropriate to attract the diagnostic label.

The other phobias or fears in children are: *agoraphobia (without history of panic disorder)*, *social phobia*, and *simple phobia*. With these the fear is the result of a specific stimulus although the particular stimulus may be different with each. With agoraphobia (without history of panic disorder) the fear is one of being alone in a public place or outside of the home without social support. With social phobia the issue is one of being excessively self-conscious and fear of being observed by others. This may show itself in a refusal to speak (although this may be a symptom of 'elective mutism') or to eat in the presence of strangers. With a simple phobia the trigger may be a specific fear such as fear of particular animals – dogs, spiders, darkness, water (swimming or washing), or particular noises when this is irrational, persistent and leads to a block in the social development of the child. The ICD-10 states that the onset should be during a developmentally appropriate age period, the degree of anxiety should be clinically abnormal and the anxiety should not be part of a more generalized disorder.

Other generalized disorders such as *panic disorders* or *panic attacks* show symptoms of dizziness, profuse sweating, intense feelings of loss of control, mental confusion, and muscle tension, sometimes with chest pain. These attacks may happen spontaneously and may not be the result of an identifiable trigger.

With post-traumatic stress disorder anxiety is the result of a specific and particular direct or observed experience such as a road traffic accident, physical attack, or sexual attack on either self or another. The memory of the traumatizing event is continually 'experienced' and 'relived' in the child's memory as evidenced by 'flashbacks', nightmares, and 'stuck (excessively repetitive/stereotyped/developmentally regressed) play'. Children's social development is inhibited by the constant anxiety, which may make them appear irritable and tense and may cause them to lose interest in social activities, including play with peers. There may be some emotional and educational regression.

It would seem that it is a fairly common occurrence for children to have a number of fears. For example, in a study of 213 children aged eight to 11, Ollendick (1983) found a mean of between 9 and 13 fears existing. Ninety-nine 10-year-old children in a study by Croake and Knox (1973) were found to have an average of 43 to 54 fears. It is unclear whether children's fears decline or increase with age. Some research that has been undertaken in this area has not found evidence of specific age trends – for example Barrios et al. (1983). Kirkpatrick (1984) found that with young infants, heights, loss of physical support, and sudden loud noises were the most commonly feared stimuli. For children aged between one and three years the common fears appear related to strangers, separation from caretakers and loud noises. With older children, between the ages of five and seven, the more common fears are related to animals, darkness, fear of separation, 'monsters' and thunder. The present writer had a case involving a seven year old who would not attend birthday parties as she feared bursting balloons. With adolescents, fears appear related to examinations and tests, personal abilities, health and sexual matters. Hoghughi (1992) has noted that phobic reactions show themselves in about 7% of adolescents but that treatment is likely to be indicated in only 2%. There appear to be gender differences. Girls tend to fear animals and physical illness or injury more than boys and fears of economic and academic failure are more common with boys (Kirkpatrick, 1984; Ollendick, 1983). The existence of these gender-specific fears may require further investigation.

Some studies have noted a link between the fears of caregivers – specifically the mother – the fears of children (Peterson and Brownlee-Duffeck, 1984; Winer, 1982) and the fears of siblings (Winer, 1982). Hoghughi (1992) suggests that this may indicated a genetic disposition rather than socialization or learning.

As can be seen, the social development of children involves biological predisposition, and social and environmental factors in interaction and rarely in mutual exclusivity. One must remember that biological predisposition can be environmentally and socially influenced by an accurate formulation and appropriate choice of intervention.

References

Achenbach TM, Edelbrook CS (1981) Behavioural Problems and Competencies Reported by Parents of Normal and Disturbed Children Aged 4–16. Monographs of the Society for Research in Child Development, 46 (Serial No. 188).

Almy M, Monighan P, Scales B, Van Hoorn J (1983) Recent research on playing: a perspective of the teacher. In L Catz (ed.) Current Topics in Early Childhood Education, vol. 5. Norwood: NJ Ablex.

Aro Hand Taipale V (1987) The impact of timing of puberty on psychosomatic symptoms among 14–16 year old Finnish girls. Child Development 58: 261–68.

Bandura A (1986) Social Foundations of Thought and Action: A Search for Cognitive Theory. Englewood Cliffs NJ: Prentice Hall.

Bandura A (1989) Social Cognitive Theory. In R Vasta (ed.) Annals of Child Development, vol. 6. Greenwich CT: JAI Press, pp. 1–60.

Barnett MA, King LM, Howard JA, Dino GA (1980) Empathy in young children: relation to parents' empathy, affection, and emphasis on the feelings of others. Developmental Psychology 16: 243–4.

Barrios BA, O'Dell ST (1989) Fears and anxieties. In EJ March, RA Barkley (eds) Treatment of Childhood Disorders. New York: Guilford Press, pp. 167–222.

Barrios BA, Replogle W, Anderson-Tisdelle D (1983) Multi-System Unit-Method Analysis of Children's Fears. Paper presented at the meeting of the Association for Advancement of Behaviour Therapy, Washington DC.

Bigelow B, LaGaipa J (1975) Children's written descriptions of friendship: a multidimensional analysis. Developmental Psychology 11: 858.

Bowlby J (1969) Attachment and Loss. New York: Basic Books.

Bretherton I, Fritz J, Zahn-Waxler C, Ridgeway D (1986) Learning to talk about emotions: a functionalist perspective. Child Development 57: 529–48.

Bronfenbrenner U (1967) Response to pressures from peers versus adults in Soviet and American Schoolchildren. International Journal of Psychology 2: 199–207.

Brooks-Gunn J, Warren MP (1988) The psychological significance of secondary sexual characteristics in 9–11 year old girls. Child Development 59: 1061–1069.

Brown BD, Clasen DR, Eicher SA (1986) Perceptions of peer pressure, peer conformity, dispositions and self-reported behaviour among adolescents. Developmental Psychology 22: 521–30.

Chandler MJ (1973) Egocentrism and anti-social behaviour: the assessment and training of social perspective taking skills. Developmental Psychology 9: 326–32.

Clausen (1975) The social meaning of differential physical and sexual maturation. In SE Dragastin, GH Elder (eds) Adolescence in the Life Cycle: Psychological Change and the Social Context. New York: Halstead.

Coie JD, Dodge KA (1983) Continuities and changes in children's social status: a five year longitudinal study. Merrillpalmer Quarterly 29: 261–82.

Croake JW, Knox FH (1973) The changing nature of children's fears. Child Study Journal 3: 91–105.

Eisenberg N, Strayer J (1987) Empathy and its Development. Cambridge: Cambridge University Press.

Feshbach ND (1978) Studies of empathic behaviour. In Bamher W (ed.) Progress and Experimental Personality Research, vol. 8. New York: Academic Press.

Feshbach ND (1982) Sex differences in empathy and social behaviour in children. In N Eisenberg (ed.) The Development of Pro-Social Behaviour. New York: Academic Press.

Friedrich LK, Stein AH (1973) Aggressive and Pro-Social Television Programmes and the Natural Behaviour of Pre-School Children. Monographs of the Society for Research in Child Development, 38 (4 Serial No. 151).

Graziano AM, Degiovanni IS, Garcia KA (1979) Behavioural treatment of children's fears: a review. Psychological Bulletin 86: 804–30.

Hartup WW (1983) The peer system. In P Mussen (ed.) Handbook of Child Psychology, vol 4. Socialism, Personality and Social Development. New York: Wiley.

Hinde RA (1989) Ethnological and relationships approaches. In R Vasta (ed.) Annals of Child Development, vol. 6. Greenwich CT: JAI Press, pp. 251–85.

Hoffman ML (1981) Development of the motive to help others. In JP Rushton, RN Sorrentino (eds) Altruism and Helping. Hillsdale NJ: Erlbaum.

Hoghughi M (1992) Assessing Child and Adolescent Disorders: A Practice Manual. London: Sage.

Howes C (1988) Relations between early child care and schooling. Developmental Psychology 24: 53–7.

Izard CE (1982) Measuring Emotions in Infants and Children. New York: Cambridge University Press.

Izard CE, Henbree EA, Huebner RR (1987) Infants emotion expressions to acute pain: developmental change and stability of individual differences. Developmental Psychology 23: 105–13.

Jones MC (1965) Psychological correlates of somatic development. Child Development 36: 899–911.

Jones MC, Bayley N (1950) Physical maturing as related to behaviour. Journal of Educational Psychology 41: 129–148.

Kirkpatrick DR (1984) Age, gender and patterns of common intense fears among adults. Behaviour Research and Therapy 22: 141–50.

Ladd GW, Price JM (1987) Predicting children's social and school adjustment following the transition from pre-school to kindergarten. Child Development 58: 1168–89.

Langlois JH (1986) From the eye of the beholder to behavioural reality. Development of social behaviours and social relations as a function of physical attractiveness. In CP Firman, MP Zanna, ET Higgins (eds) Physical Appearance, Stigma and Social Behaviour: Ontario Symposium, vol. 3. Hillsdale NJ: Erlbaum.

Langlois JH, Roggman LA, Casey RJ, Ritter JM, Rieser-Danner LA, Jenkins VY (1987) Infant preferences for attractive faces: rudiments of a stereotype. Developmental Psychology 23: 363–9.

Malatesta CZ, Grigoryev P, Lamb C, Albin M, Culver C (1986) Emotion, socialisation and expressive development in pre-term and full-term infants. Child Development 57: 316–330.

Martin B (1975) Parent and child relations. In FD Horowitz (ed.) Review of Child Development Research, vol 4. Chicago: University of Chicago Press.

Mussen PH, Conger JJ, Kagan J, Huston AC (1984) Child Development and Personality (6 ed.). New York: Harper & Row.

Ollendick TH (1983) Reliability and validity of the Revised Fear Survey Schedule for Children (FSSCR). Behaviour Research and Therapy 21: 685–92.

Parke RD, Slaby RG (1983) The development of aggression. In PH Mussen (ed.) Handbook of Child Psychology, vol. 4. Socialisation, Personality and Social Development. New York: Wiley.

Peterson L, Brownlee-Duffeck M (1984) Prevention of anxiety and pain due to medical and dental procedures. In MC Roberts, L Peterson (eds) Prevention of Problems in Childhood. Psychological Research and Application. New York: Wiley, pp. 267–308.

Piaget J (1970) Piaget's theory. In P Mussen (ed.) Carmichael's Manual of Child Psychology, vol I. New York: Wiley.

Piaget J, Inhelder B (1969) The Psychology of the Child. London: Routledge & Kegan Paul.

Putallaz M (1987) Natal behaviour and children's sociometric status. Child Development 58: 324–40.

Radke-Yarrow M, Zahn-Waxler C (1984) Routes, motives and patterns in children's pro-social behaviour. In E Staub, D Bartal, J Karylowski, J Reykowski (eds) The Development and Maintenance of Pro-Social Behaviour. New York: Plenum.

Radke-Yarrow M, Zahn-Waxler C, Chapman M (1983) Children's pro-social dispositions and behaviour. In PH Mussen, EM Heatherington (eds) Handbook of Child Psychology, vol. 4. Socialization, Personality and Social Development (4 edn). New York: Wiley.

Selman RL (1976) Social/cognitive understanding: a guide to educational and clinical practice. In T Likona (ed.) Moral Development and Behaviour: Research and Social Issues. New York, Holt Rinehart and Winston, pp. 299 316.

Selman RL (1980) The Growth of Interpersonal Understanding. New York: Academic Press.

Selman RL, Byrne DF (1974) A structural/developmental analysis of levels of role taking in middle childhood. Child Development 45: 803–6.

Shaffer D (1989) Developmental Psychology: Childhood and Adolescence. California: Brooks/Cole Publishing.

Shantz DW (1986) Conflict, progression and peer status: an observational study. Child Development 57: 1322.

Shure MB, Spivack G (1980) Interpersonal problem-solving as a mediator of behavioural adjustment in pre-school and kindergarten children. Journal of Applied Developmental Psychology 1: 29–44.

Smollar J, Youniss J (1982) Social development through friendship. In KH Rubin, HS Ross (eds) Peer Relations and Social Skills in Childhood. New York: Springer-Verlag.

Staffieri JR (1967) A study of social stereotype of body image in children. Journal of Personality and Social Psychology 7: 101–4.

Steinberg CS, Silverberg SB (1986) The vicissitudes of autonomy in early adolescence. Child Development 57: 841–51.

Strayer J (1983) Effective and Cognitive Components of Children's Empathy. Paper presented at the meeting of the Society for Research and Child Development, Detroit.

Tesch SA (1983) Review of friendship development across the life span. Human Development 26: 226–76.

Thompson RA (1990) Empathy and emotional understanding: the early development of empathy. In N Eisenberg, J Strayer (eds) Empathy and its Development. Cambridge: Cambridge University Press, pp. 119–45.

Tronick EZ, Cohn JF (1989) Infant–mother face to face interaction: age and gender differences in co-ordination and the occurrence of mis-coordination. Child Development 60: 85–92.

Watson JB (1913) Psychology as the behaviourists use it. Psychological Review 20: 158–77.

Winer GA (1982) A review and analysis of children's fearful behaviour in a dental setting. Child Development 53: 1111–33.

Chapter 16
Psychological aspects of adolescence and the development of identities

N.J. BANKS

Key concepts	Key names
Puberty	
Sex-role identity	Bem
Gender-role identity	
Gender constancy	Maccoby and Jacklin
Sex-role stereotypes	
Sexuality	
Oppositional-defiant disorder	
Conduct disorder, conflict	
Personal identity development	Erikson
Identity status positions	Marcia, Berk
Adolescent turmoil, parental conflict	Foster and Robin, Rutter
Ethnic identity development	Banks, Clark and Clark, Helms, Cross

Introduction

This chapter will consider aspects of sexual development that impact on the psychological development of the adolescent. Gender identity, sex role development, adolescent and ethnic identity development issues are also discussed.

Sexual development

Puberty is commonly seen as marking the onset of the stage of 'adolescence'. There are marked changes in height, weight and body proportions in both boys and girls including the enlargement of breasts, penis and testes, and vulva. The sequence of pubertal change may be fairly uniform, although the age of onset and rate of development may vary widely

(Tanner, 1962). Signs of pubertal development appear, in girls of European origin, to occur at an average of about 11 years of age although the range extends from 8 to 13 years. For boys it appears later with a range of 11 to 14 years. The 'completion' of adolescence (age 17 to 19 years) appears socially rather than developmentally determined. Berk (1991) notes that the physical events of puberty and the timing and speed at which they occur have important implications for both social and emotional adjustment. Developmental changes and the adjustment to these are seen to cause more of a focus on 'self' than previously existed. Greif and Ulman (1982) noted that menstruation is not just a sign of physiological development: it is a 'rite of passage' into womanhood – a sign of maturity. However, girls' views about this vary widely – some appear to see it more as 'curse' than 'blessing' and something that has to be endured. The most difficulty was associated with having to prepare for it. For girls who had no warning of their first period the event was seen as quite distressing. Girls who report being unprepared report more severe physical symptoms and less favourable attitudes, and more embarrassment and self-consciousness (Koff et al., 1982). Bell (1980) found that adverse reactions to menstruation could be overcome if parents helped in the girls' preparation. A boy's first ejaculation also marks the coming of maturity although some, without preparation and understanding, may have concerns about whether the experience is 'normal' (Bell, 1980). Some studies have found mixed feelings in boys about their first ejaculation, possibly because they were unprepared (Gaddis and Brooks-Gunn, 1985). Fewer boys told of their first ejaculation than did girls of their first menstruation. It would seem that if young people are prepared early there is more positive adjustment and acceptance of the occurring pubertal changes.

Early maturing boys tend to be more popular whereas this is not always so for early maturing girls who may experience social discomfort. Researchers have found that, in girls of 9 to 11 years of age, breast development correlated with a more positive view of self and greater feelings of peer acceptance and superior psychological adjustment (Brooks-Gunn and Warren, 1988).

Gender and sex-role identity

Sex-role identity refers to a child's personal and private definition of self as 'male' or 'female'. Gender-role identity is related to one's view that one is a 'man' or 'woman', 'masculine' or 'feminine' within a sociocultural role expectation context. Sex-role adoption is the internalization of personality characteristics, preferences and behaviours that mainstream or dominant culture determines as appropriate for one sex or the other (Mussen et al., 1984). The gay and lesbian rights movements have been active in promoting a view that any discrepancy about an individual's definition of self as a sexual being and the opinion of an individual professional may reflect more on the professional's personal bias and world view than an identity 'disorder' of the individual. Psychiatrists are cautioned that the use and application of the term 'gender disorder' may be seen as being more aligned to one's social prejudices and cultural isolation than objective classification. The term 'gender realignment need' may be more in keeping with the social progress of the new millennium.

Many so-called masculine and feminine social qualities are not mutually exclusive. We are seeing something of a social revolution, where 'new men' are expected to participate equally in childcare and women are expected to have professional careers and to work in areas traditionally seen as male dominated. Most research suggests that the development of a gender identity happens between 18 and 36 months of age (O'Brien and Huston, 1985; Bem, 1989). Children acquire a sense of being a 'boy' or a 'girl'. *Gender constancy* refers to the understanding that gender does not change according to the activities a person engages in or the clothes that he or she may wear. This understanding typically occurs at about age five. However, by the time children are three years of age they show quite definite expectations of what they believe is socially expected of males and females (O'Brien and Huston, 1985; Bem, 1981, 1983). By the age of four or five they have a surprising, often rigid, knowledge of *gender-based stereotyped occupational roles* (Martin, 1989). This store of information may be in conflict with the child's actual experience. An anecdote to illustrate this is that the present writer knew of a five-year-old boy who consistently asserted in play that 'ladies are nurses and men are doctors' even though his mother was a doctor. After five years of age, children often adopt the personality characteristics that they believe are associated with masculinity and femininity. This can be most clearly observed during play where character roles are acted out (Huston, 1983). At the age of two or three years, children will also select toys and play-based activities that fit in with their view of 'masculine' and 'feminine'. Girls appear to be more flexible in this play and role selection than boys and this may be related to masculine activities being more socially desirable because of the greater status being afforded to them.

In a review of 1500 societies, Maccoby and Jacklin (1974) found that only four common *sex-role stereotypes* had any degree of accuracy. These related to females having a greater degree of verbal ability than males (displaying itself in adolescence), males having greater visual/spatial ability, males having greater mathematical reasoning ability (showing itself in early adolescence) and males being more physically and verbally aggressive than females. Since this early research, other sex differences have also been found. For example, males tend to be more physically active than females (Eaton and Keates, 1982), more willing to take risks (Ginsburg and Miller, 1982), and more vulnerable to reading disabilities, speech defects, emotional disorders. The reader is referred to Maccoby (1980) for a fuller discussion. The reader is also reminded that individual girls and boys may be more alike than gender group differences predict.

As girls and boys learn about society's expectations of them they also learn about sexuality. *Sexuality* becomes important in Western society during puberty when adolescents become physically (but not emotionally) mature. At this point adolescents integrate aspects of sexual identity into gender identity. They begin to consider how to express their sexuality in relationships. Dreyer (1982) described several changes to adolescent sexual attitudes. Firstly, he found that they tended to believe sex with affection was acceptable. There was a decline in 'double standards' – a lessening of the view of sex being acceptable for men but not women outside of marriage. The third change was confusion about sexual norms and what exactly individuals saw as acceptable with others. Should relationships be seen as long term before sex? Should virginity be maintained? Fenwick and Smith (1993) note that, in early adolescence, the closest relationships tend to be same-sex relationships, which can be intense and exclusive. Friendships with the opposite sex usually mark the beginning of early 'sexual' relationships. Much 'sexual activity' may be make believe or boasting to gain status. Fenwick and Smith note that early 'sex' usually means mutual fondling, with girls having intercourse, on average, later than boys. By the age of 17 half of all British boys and one third of girls claim to have experienced sexual intercourse (Bancroft, 1989). Rates in 1979 for USA males were similar, with 56% having intercourse by age 17 and 77% percent by age 19 (Zelnik and Kanter, 1980).

Adolescent and parent conflict

Conflict can occur as a natural consequence of differing social perspectives and can range from disagreements about makeup and clothes to the other end of the spectrum where temper tantrums and offending behaviour predominate and a communication breakdown exists. At this end of the spectrum the ICD-10 includes the disorder of *oppositional defiant disorder*, which, it states, tends to be observed in children below the age of nine to 10 years of age. Foster and Robin (1989) however, note that the *Diagnostic and Statistical Manual of Mental Disorders* (American Psychiatric Association, 1987) was the first to list a diagnostic category explicitly relevant to parent adolescent conflict: oppositional defiant disorder (p. 493). There appeared, at that time, some difference in the age-related onset. However, the authors went on to say that: 'Because the diagnosis is so new . . . information on its incidence and prevalence in adolescence is unavailable.' Foster and Robin (1989) offer a useful operationally definition of what they term *clinically significant parent–adolescent disorder* as characterized by one or more of the following:

- repeated, unpleasant predominantly verbal disagreements about one or more issues;
- disputes that fail to produce workable agreements, resulting in repeated occurrence of the issues that elicit disputes;
- negative, anger-laden exchanges over problem issues; and
- feelings of dissatisfaction about family relations, the behaviour of others, and/or unresolved issues.

Furthermore, Foster and Robin suggest that non-problematic conflict tends to be of shorter duration, ends in agreement and is not followed by extensive dissatisfaction with family relationships.

One of the tasks of adolescence is striving for autonomy. This may upset previous family patterns of functioning. Robin and Foster (1989) offer a model that aims to predict how conflict is dealt with. They see the outcome of conflict as being dependent on four factors:

- the family's problem solving skills;
- the family's communication patterns;
- the belief system of individuals within the family; and
- how the family interacts on a face-to-face, day-to-day level and how these interactions are structured.

Difficulties in any of these areas are seen to increase the continuation of significant conflict between its members. A further psychiatric classification in the ICD-10, that of *conduct disorder*, is characterized by 'a repetitive and persistent pattern of dissocial, aggressive or defiant conduct'. The defiant behaviour should not be isolated acts but should be 'an enduring pattern of behaviour'. The diagnosis needs to take into account the child's developmental level and what could be expected of a child's behaviour. The ICD-10 gives the examples of temper tantrums being developmentally appropriate for a three year old and violent crime as not being within the capacity of most seven year olds. These behaviours are therefore not relevant diagnostic criteria for those age groups. Herbert (1987) notes that general population surveys show that under half of disorders in adolescence begin before adolescence. Clinic-based surveys suggest adolescent psychiatric disorders begin at early or middle childhood (Rutter, 1977). Robins (1966) found that the parents of many of the anti-social children in his study provided the children with questionable discipline, being unable or unwilling to cope with the presented problems.

Despite the demonstration of *conflict* in clinic-based populations, there appears to be some consensus that *adolescent and parental values are similar*. Allowing for evolving and changing cultural influences, there does appear to be some significant overlap between adolescent and parental values. Hartup (1983) has suggested that parental influence is likely to be seen in the areas of moral and social values and thus *the view of strife and turmoil in adolescence is largely unjustified.* Mussen et al. (1984) argue that, in order to move from adolescence to adulthood, adolescents must become independent from their parents. This may be seen as a culturally embedded viewpoint that may not be considered appropriate outside of the Western world (Lacan, 1977). In complex Western societies that do not have *rites of passage* to act as symbolic markers for the transition from adolescence to adulthood, and where many choices exist, one may expect an *identity crisis* to arise. Marcia (1966, 1980) saw this period as a short-lived time of increased self-consciousness and self-reflection where the adolescent experiments with alternatives before making commitments. It was Erikson's (1968) view that such 'experimentation' did not serve as a commitment or *identity formation* because a truly secure identity resulted from making choices from realistic and unrealistic fantasized 'possibilities' – for example, becoming a rock star versus going on to further education.

Erikson saw *identity development* as a lifelong process. He focused on specific ego development tasks at different stages of a person's life. His eight stages were:

- stage one (infant) – trust versus mistrust;
- stage two (toddler) – autonomy versus shame and doubt;
- stage three (early childhood) – initiative versus guilt;
- stage four (middle childhood) – industry versus inferiority;
- stage five (adolescence) – identity versus role confusion;
- stage six (young adulthood) – intimacy versus isolation;
- stage seven (middle adulthood) – generativity versus stagnation;
- stage eight (older adulthood/middle age) – ego integrity versus despair.

In each stage there was a critical period for the development of a particular ego capability or developmental task that had to be resolved in order to ensure a satisfactory process of development. From the age of six to adolescence, for example, a person had to develop a sense of mastery and competence so as not to feel inferior to others. Erikson saw the major conflict in adolescence as identity formation versus role confusion. An inability to resolve this conflict could result in role confusion or diffusion of identity. However, Rubins (1968) has suggested that an *identity crisis* could occur at any stage and that a *mid-life crisis* may be an identity crisis. Erikson saw some form of identity crisis as a normal and universal part of development. Baumeister (1986), however, suggests that there has been no universality of identity crisis found in the research and some individuals may go through this period while others will not. Furthermore, an identity crisis may be the outcome of cultural, historic and social factors. Therefore, in societies where adolescence is not seen in *psychosocial moratorium* terms, a crisis may not occur. In males, Jordan (1971) found that one factor associated with the occurrence of an identity crisis was the son perceiving his parents as accepting or rejecting. Sons with ambivalent or inconsistent parents were more prone to crisis. Sons with foreclosed identities (identities introjected though parentally imposed values, not chosen or 'achieved' through crisis) tended to be close to their parents, particularly their fathers and saw them as supportive. Disapproving or rejecting parents appeared to create 'diffuse' identities. However, one study has found that crisis was more related to having increased cognitive sophistication and another study found it was related to a developmental advance in cognitive functioning (Leadbeater and Dionne, 1981). Ginsburg and Orlofsky (1981) and Orlofsky (1977) observed that female identity crises may demonstrate more conflict than those of males and that female foreclosures do not demonstrate the same difficulties as male foreclosures (Damon, 1983; Waterman, 1982).

Marcia (1966, 1980) has reconstructed and developed Erikson's theory to form four *identity status positions*, which have been summarized by Berk (1991).

*   Identity achievement. Here individuals have experienced a time of crisis and decision making and now show a secure sense of commitment to a value or belief system.
*   Moratorium. This refers to a temporary delay or pause. Here individuals have postponed commitments while entering an identity crisis, perhaps searching for an appropriate occupational goal or belief system with which to identify.
*   Identity foreclosure. Individuals have committed to belief system positions. They have been able to avoid a period of crisis and have reached a commitment to a parentally determined identity before they have self-sifted choices.
*   Identity diffusion. These individuals are not searching for commitments to define or develop their identity. They typically show lack of direction and purpose.

Berk (1991) has concluded that:

> identity achievement and moratorium are regarded as healthy and adaptive venues to identity formation, whereas foreclosure and diffusion are considered maladaptive . . . in addition identity achieved individuals , more than those in the other three statuses, have moved beyond the preoccupation with an *imaginary audience* that characterises adolescents' entry in to the *formal operational stage*. They are less self-focused and preoccupied with how others regard them and more self assured and other directed than their same age counterparts. (pp. 447–8)

It seems that late adolescence is a particularly important time for identity consolidation (Adams and Fitch, 1982) and Erikson (1968) believed that, for most adolescents, identity formation proceeded in a uniform uneventful way to integrate self and identity in a unifying internal structure.

Powers et al. (1989) have shown that there is only a 2% increase in clinically relevant psychological disturbance from childhood to adolescence, moving the overall rate to close to that existing in the adult population. However, disturbances that do show a rise in adolescence are suicide and depression. Pfeffer (1986) has shown how the suicide rate tripled, with suicide ranking as the most common form of death. The number of boys who kill themselves was up to five times the number of girls. It seems that girls more often make unsuccessful attempts (*parasuicide*). It appears that family discord, marital break-up, bullying, peer relationship disturbance and parental difficulties are common in the lives of those who commit suicide (Curran, 1987; Holden, 1986; Shaffer, 1985). Suicide may be more common in adolescents as they are more able to consider (perhaps inaccurately) how others perceive them and they feel self-conscious about this.

Ethnic identity development

If identity formation is a difficult task for white European adolescents, then it may be particularly difficult for minority cultures living in white societies. There may be conflicts between family *cultural expectations* and those of the wider society. Banks (1992, 1996) has shown how external social pressures within mixed-race families, where one parent is black and the other white, exert disrupting influences which can affect the identity and emotional development of children. As early as 1939 (Clark and Clark, 1939) found that black children appeared to be rejecting *identification* with their own ethnic group. How this research should be interpreted has long been a matter of debate. Milner (1983) showed similar findings. However, during the 1980s these finding were largely reversed. This is seen as being essentially a positive outcome of the black pride movement (Powell, 1982). Although we have discussed *gender constancy* developing at about three years of age, it is not until about eight or nine years of age that *ethnic constancy* appears (Aboud, 1984; Semaj, 1980). This suggests that considerations of 'identity work', except in extreme cases that mimic self-mutilation, may be premature.

Goodman (1952) proposed a three-stage model of *racial attitude development*, which included knowledge, differentiation and emotional links to the learned knowledge base. Stereotypes and discriminatory prejudices were seen as developing from this. It may be questionable whether this knowledge base could be developed independent from associated emotions, as knowledge about 'race' is essentially emotionally charged to begin with and is rarely objective or rational. Aboud and Skerry (1984) offer a more comprehensive view of *racial awareness development* (and consequently racial identity development). They suggest there are essentially four linked areas in development:

- perception of one's own group;
- perceived similarity with one's group;
- perceived similarity/difference with other groups;
- a cognitive response in perceiving others.

The affective or emotional component is largely present in the initial development of own group views but reduces as the cognitive or perceptual components increase. Cross (1978) has also formulated stage models of racial identity development and considers cognitive, affective and behavioural aspects of experience.

What is often overlooked in consideration of ethnic identity development is that white children too, belong to an ethnic group and have ethnic identities. Helms (1990) has developed a model of *white racial identity development*. What is common to all models of racial identity development is that they consider the effect of racism on both white and black people to the exclusion of other types of experience. This becomes an over-focus constraining the development of children exclusively within a racialized context with few other inputs or influences into their developmental world.

Summary

Sex-role identity development and sex-role adoption occur prior to adolescence. Adolescence is a period of rapid physical, social and cognitive change. There are male and female differences both in the rate and effect of the change. Much of the social change is related to cultural expectations and influences and some argue that adolescence as a specific 'stage' in development is a Western concept or 'invention'. Parental conflict during adolescence may not be universal and may be more related to parenting styles, family problem-solving skills and socialization than adolescent change. Identity development does not take place only within adolescence but is seen as being a life-long task, although late adolescence is seen as being a particularly important time. Ethnic identity development is an additional task to master and may bring additional pressures for minority group children and adolescents. There are empirically defined stages of ethnic identity development for both minority group members and white majority group members.

References

Aboud FE (1984) Social and cognitive bases of ethnic identity constancy. Journal of Genetic Psychology 145: 217–19.

Aboud FE, Skerry SA (1984) The development of ethnic attitudes. Journal of Cross Cultural Psychology 15(1): 3–34.

Adams GR, Fitch SA (1982) Ego stage and identity status development: a cross-sequential analysis. Journal of Personality and Social Psychology 43: 574–83.

American Psychiatric Association (1987) Diagnostic and Statistical Manual of Mental Disorders. 3rd ed revised. Wahington DC: ACP.

Bancroft J (1989) Human Sexuality and its Problems. London: Churchill.

Banks N (1992) Some considerations of racial identification and self-esteem when working with mixed ethnicity children and their mothers as social services clients. Social Services Research 3: 32–41.

Banks N (1996) Young, white single mothers with black children in therapy. Clinical Child Psychology and Psychiatry vol. 1, 1: 19–28.

Baumeister RF (1986) Identity: Cultural Change and the Struggle for Self. Oxford: Oxford University Press.

Bell R (1980) Changing Bodies, Changing Lives, A Book for Teens on Sex and Relationships. New York: Random House.

Bem SL (1981) Gender schema theory: a cognitive account of sex-typing. Psychological Review 88: 354–64.

Bem SL (1983) Gender schema theory and its implications for child development: raising children in a gender-schematic society. Signs: Journal of Women in Society and Culture 8: 598–616.

Bem SL (1989) Genital knowledge and gender constancy in pre-school children. Child Development 60: 649–62.

Berk LE (1991) Child Development (2 edn). Boston: Allyn & Bacon.

Brooks-Gunn J, Warren MP (1988) The psychological significance of secondary sexual characteristics in 9–11 year old girls. Child Development 59: 1061–9.

Clark K, Clark M (1939) The development of consciousness of self and the emergence of racial identification in negro pre-school children. Journal of Social Psychology, SSPSI Bulletin 10: 591–9.

Cross WE (1978) The Cross and Thomas models of psychological nigrescence. Journal of Black Psychology 5: 13–19.

Curran DK (1987) Adolescent Suicidal Behaviour. Washington DC: Hemisphere.

Damon W (1983) Social and Personality Development. New York: Norton.

Dreyer PH (1982) Sexuality during adolescence. In BB Wolman (ed.) Handbook of Development Psychology. New York: Wiley.

Eaton WO, Keats GJ (1982) Peer presence, stress and sex differences in the motor activity levels of pre-schoolers. Developmental Psychology 18: 534–40.

Erikson E (1968) Identity, Youth and Crisis. New York: Norton.

Fenwick E, Smith T (1993) Adolescence: A Survival Guide for Parents and Teenagers. London: Dorling Kindersley.

Foster SL, Robin AL (1989) Parent/adolescent conflict. In EJ Mash and RA Barkley (eds) Treatment of Childhood Disorders. New York: Guilford Press.

Gaddis A, Brooks-Gunn J (1985) The male experience of pubital change. Journal of Youth and Adolescence 14: 62.

Ginsburg SD, Orlofsky JL (1981) Ego identity status, ego development and locus of control in college women. Journal of Youth and Adolescence 10: 297–307.

Goodman ME (1952) Race Awareness in Young Children. Cambridge MA: Addison Wesley.

Greif EB, Ulman KJ (1982) The psychological impact of menarche on early adolescent females: a review of the literature. Child Development: 1413–30.

Hartup W (1983) Peer relations. In PH Mussen (ed.) Handbook of Child Psychology, vol. 4. Socialization, Personality and Social Development. New York: Wiley.

Helms JE (ed.) (1990) Black and White Racial Identity: Theory, Research and Practice. Westport CT: Greenwood Press.

Herbert M (1987) Conduct Disorders of Childhood and Adolescence: A Social Learning Perspective. Chichester: Wiley.

Holden C (1986) Youth suicide: new research focuses on a growing social problem. Science 233: 839–41.

Huston AC (1983) Sex Typing. In PH Mussen, EM Heatherington (eds) Handbook of Child Psychology, vol. 4. Socialization, Personality and Social Development (4 edn). New York: Wiley.

Jordan D (1971) Parental Antecedents and Personality Characteristics of Ego-Identity Statuses. Unpublished Doctoral Dissertation, Stage University of New York at Buffalo.

Koff E, Rierdan J, Sheingold K (1982), Memories of menarche: age, preparation and prior knowledge as determinants of initial menstrual experience. Journal of Youth and Adolescence 11: 1–9.

Lacan J (1997) Ecrits: A Selection. London: Tavistock.

Leadbeater BJ, Dionne JP (1981) The adolescent's use of formal operational thinking in solving problems related to identity resolution. Adolescents 16: 111–21.

Maccoby E (1980) Social Development. San Diego: Harcourt Brace-Jovanovich.

Maccoby E, Jacklin EN (1980) Sex differences in aggression: a rejoinder and reprise. Child Development 51: 964–80.

Marcia JE (1966) Development and validation of ego identity status. Journal of Personality and Social Psychology 3: 551–8.

Marcia JE (1980) Identity in adolescence. In J Adelson (ed.) Handbook of Adolescent Psychology. New York: Wiley, pp. 159–87.

Martin CL (1989) Children's use of gender-related information in making social judgements. Developmental Psychology 25: 80–8.

Milner D (1983) Children and Race. Ten Years On. London: Ward Lock Educational.

Mussen PH, Conger JJ, Kagan J, Huston AC (1984) Child Development and Personality. (6 edn). New York: Harper & Rowe.

O'Brien M, Huston AC (1985) Development of sex-type play behaviour in toddlers. Developmental Psychology 21: 866–71.

Orlofsky JL (1977) Identity formation and achievement and fear of success in college men and women. Journal of Youth and Adolescence 7: 49–62.

Pfeffer CR (1986) The Suicidal Child. New York: Guilford Press.

Powell GJ (1982) The impact of television on the self-concept development of minority group children. In GL Barey, C Matchell-Kerman (eds) Television and the Socialization of the Minority Child. New York: Academic Press.

Powers SI, Hauser ST, Kilner LA (1989) Adolescent mental health. American Psychologist 44: 200–8.

Robin AL, Foster SL (1989) Negotiating Parent/Adolescent Conflict: A Behavioural-Family Systems Approach. New York: Guilford Press.

Robins AL (1966) Deviant Children Grown Up. Baltimore: Williams & Wilkins.

Rubins JL (1968) The problems of acute identity crisis in adolescence. American Journal of Psychoanalysis 28: 37–44.

Rutter ML (1977) Prospective studies to investigate behavioural change. In JS Strauss, HM Babigian, M Roth (eds) The origins and Course of Psychopathology. New York: Plenum Press.

Semaj L (1980) The development of racial evaluation and preference: a cognitive approach. Journal of Black Psychology 6: 59–79.

Shaffer D (1985) Depression, mania and suicidal acts. In M Rutter, L Hersov (eds) Child and Adolescent Psychiatry. Modern Approaches. New York: Guilford Press, pp. 698–719.

Tanner JM (1962) Growth in Adolescence (2nd edn). Oxford: Blackwell.

Waterman AS (1982) Identity development from adolescents to adulthood: an extension of theory and review of research. Developmental Psychology 18: 341–58.

Zelnik M, Kantner JF (1980) Sexual activity, contraceptive use and pregnancy among metropolitan area teenagers: 1971–1979. Family Planning Perspectives 12: 230–7.

Chapter 17
Psychological development in adult life

JANET R. WHEATLEY

Key concepts	Key names

Life span development
   organismic
   mechanistic
   psychoanalytic
   lifespan development/contextual/dialectic	

Social learning theory	Bandura
Psychosocial stages	Erikson
Stages and crisis theory of development	Levinson
The family lifecycle	
Mid-life crisis	

Introduction and overview

This chapter examines psychological development during adulthood, spanning the years between adolescence and old age. The period of adult life covers approximately four decades of life from the twenties through to the fifties. It has traditionally been perceived as a stable plateau between the rapid biological, cognitive and social development of childhood and adolescence, and the losses in physical, cognitive and social spheres in later life. Although the extremes of the lifespan, and particularly the early years, have been the focus of much psychological study, the middle years have been relatively neglected. During this period the major changes demanding active adaptation are the individual's and family's life cycle, but there is comparative stability in biological and cognitive functioning.

In the sections that follow, major life events and changes in adult life are reviewed, the main models for conceptualizing human development are introduced, and theories for understanding the process of psychological adaptation in adult life are presented. The impact of a number of particular life challenges and changes is then considered in more detail.

The course of adult life

Three broad categories of life events have been identified as prompting psychological and personal development. These are:

- normative events that are expected to happen within a particular age range;
- idiosyncratic, non-normative life events;
- normative, cohort-related events.

Each of these will be considered in turn.

Age-related normative factors

During the forty or so years of adulthood, prior to old age, there are a number of normative life events that are expected to take place for the majority of the population. The move from childhood into adulthood is marked in modern Western culture, by the ending of formal education, moving away from the parental home and starting to earn one's living. Marriage and parenthood are also regarded as normative in early adulthood. Later in adult life, it would be expected that children will grow up and leave home, that elderly parents may become frail and need care, that the capacity to earn a living will be maintained, that parents will become grandparents, and that a person will eventually retire from work. For women, during middle age, the biological changes of the climacteric – that is the change from the reproductive to the non-reproductive phase of life, including the menopause – take place.

Havighurst (1972) refers to these normative life events as *developmental tasks*, dividing them into those of early adulthood and of middle age as shown below:

Early adulthood
Courting and getting married
Adjusting to being married
Beginning a new family
Rearing children
Developing a career
Taking on civic responsibilities

Middle age
Accepting/adjusting to physiological changes
Reaching/maintaining satisfactory career performance

Assisting teenage children to become responsible, happy adults
Adjusting to ageing parents
Relating in a satisfactory way to one's spouse
Assuming civic responsibilities
Developing leisure-time activities.

It is apparent that such a listing of events relies on societal norms and, as such, it is to some extent both culture bound and tied to a particular era. For example, 50 years ago in Britain, the expectation of marriage prior to child bearing, was stronger than it is now. Some of these expectations have a different emphasis in different cultural groups or may not be relevant. So, for example, moving away from home may not be a signal of adulthood in some societal structures, and bearing children may be of greater significance in, for example, some African cultures than it is in current British culture. The expected course of events has been shown to vary within Western culture to some degree, by gender and social class.

As these are general expectations they do not hold true for everybody in the population. Some individuals will not meet the conventional norms of society. There are those who are gay or who are single. There are those who marry, but are unable to have children or choose not to do so. There are other people who have children but do not get married. There are those who are not willing or able or given the opportunity to make a living. Using Havighurst's perspective, outlined above, one might say that these individuals have failed to successfully negotiate the developmental tasks that society expects of them. Where societal norms are not met, individuals may be put under pressure by family and others to conform and may feel pressure to justify their lifestyle. In the extreme people may be excluded from society because they do not fit with conventional expectations.

Apart from happening or not happening, these events may take place 'on' or 'off' time. Thus a person who goes on studying until his or her late twenties, when they might be expected to be earning a living, is often described, rather disparagingly, as an 'eternal student'. The mother who has her first child at 14 or 41 years of age is looked on, at least in current Western society, as too young or rather old for motherhood. Neugarten (1968) found that people have an internal sense, which she calls the 'social clock', of whether they are on time with regard to their culture's expectations.

These events may also take place, through force of circumstance or individual choice, in an order which is different from that which society expects. Thus a couple who get married when their children are already growing up are seen as unconventional; and a couple who marry and have children before they are financially independent may be looked upon as foolish.

The psychological adaptations and challenges posed by moving through these life events are reviewed further below.

Idiosyncratic or non-normative events

Non-normative life events are those that occur uniquely or only to a minority of people. These include events such as being made redundant, suffering a serious illness, 'coming out' as gay, or winning the lottery. Some non-normative events may occur for a minority of the population of a similar age. For example, divorce, the death of a child, or taking on the role of caregiver for an ageing parent are likely to affect clusters of people at similar life stages. Coping with illness and adjusting to loss are more common in later life than earlier adulthood, and as such they are reviewed in more detail in the chapter on ageing. There is some evidence to suggest that these idiosyncratic events, which are less predictable than age norma-tive events, are more traumatic and it is harder for the individual to adjust to them.

Normative cohort-related events

Many events that influence psychological development are historical and have a unique influence on those alive at the time. The generation born in Britain in the 1950s, growing into young adulthood after the advent of the birth control pill, may have a different moral attitude from those born in the 1970s, who have grown up during a time when AIDS is prevalent. Similarly, for those living in certain parts of Africa or Asia, those born in the 1950s will have grown up while their countries were dominated by a colonial power, whereas those born in the 1970s will have known nothing other than independent rule. These experiences may have influenced self-concept and view of self in relation to others.

Such historical effects, which have cohort-specific influences, need to be recognized when assessing the findings of longitudinal studies, which confound cohort and age effects (this issue is discussed in greater detail in Chapter 18).

Models of lifespan development

A range of models has been used to help understanding of adult human development. The underlying assumptions and emphases of the various models differ with regard to issues such as how much emphasis to lay on the influence of nature and nurture, whether they take a holistic or a reductionist viewpoint, and whether they conceptualize development as occurring in stages or as a continuum.

There are a number of texts that contain chapters giving a summary of models. Hayslip and Panek (1989) divide the main models into organ-ismic, mechanistic, psychoanalytic and lifespan developmental. Rybash et al. (1991) also describe mechanistic and organismic models, including psychoanalytic within the latter category. They call a third approach, which has similar characteristics to the lifespan developmental model, the contextual or dialectic model. These three models are briefly reviewed below. Schaie and Willis (1991) give a more detailed breakdown of 'approaches' rather than 'models', naming seven as follows:

- dialectical;
- psychoanalytic;
- behavioural (labelled by others as mechanistic);
- humanistic (an holistic approach focused on motivation towards self-actualization);
- individual differences (focused on a descriptive measurement of how people differ with respect to personality or intelligence);
- attribution (focused on how people develop schemata by which they understand and respond to events);
- information processing (an approach which uses the analogy of computer functioning to understand cognitive development).

The lifespan developmental perspective

Much of the psychological study of adult life employs a lifespan developmental perspective, which views development as continuing from conception through to death, rather than stopping after the obvious physical, cognitive and social growth periods of early life (Baltes, 1987). The approach sees development as being organized and adaptive change, in response to the gains and losses that occur in every period of life. The psychological development of the individual is seen as involving adaptation to the interplay between internal, biologically driven processes and external social influences to achieve a state of effectiveness and wellbeing. It is therefore sensitive to the impact of context, whether historical or cultural. It recognizes the influences of both continuous, cumulative processes and reaction to specific life events across the years of life, although, as we shall see, some theorists are more inclined to emphasize crises and others focus on continuity. It also allows scope to explain the individual differences that arise from unique combinations of biological and social circumstances.

The organismic model

The organismic model sees genetic forces as determining the way that the individual matures, with genetic programmes lying behind the unfolding of behaviour. The successive stages of growth are therefore seen as largely internally driven, and the influence of context is viewed as less important. According to this approach development would be expected to follow a fairly predictable course; it would not be very susceptible to alteration by the environment and would be similar across cultures and periods of history. Piaget's view of cognitive development proceeding through an orderly series of qualitative stages and Freud's view of the stages of psychosexual development are two well known examples of theories based on this conceptualization of the person as first and foremost an internally driven biological system.

The behavioural model

By contrast, the behavioural model stresses the way the individual develops through learning about the associations between his or her actions and the effects they have on the environment. Thus an action that produces consequences that are reinforcing to the individual is more likely to be repeated (operant conditioning). The individual may also learn from associations between stimuli and responses, with responses becoming conditioned to occur to particular stimuli if these are presented under certain conditions (classical conditioning). In this model the human being is viewed as influenced much more by the environment than in organismic models. This tends to be a reductionist approach, in which it is assumed that we can develop an understanding of the person by breaking down behaviour into its component parts. The focus is more upon the minutiae of reinforcement contingencies than on the broader influences of the social context. This marks a major difference from the lifespan developmental perspective, which is more holistic in its approach. Social learning theory (Bandura, 1977) is one example of a behavioural theory of human development.

Theories of lifespan development

As we have seen in the section above, there is more than one way to look at psychological development during adulthood. This section will consider the most influential theories.

Erikson's theory of psychosocial stages

Erikson was a student of Freud, who accepted the basic theory of early psychosexual development, but who also proposed that development continues across the lifespan, particularly in terms of the developing relationship between the individual and the social system within which he or she lives. From a psychoanalytic point of view, this process is seen largely in terms of ego development. In other words, the development of personality requires the development of an ego that is strong enough to control the basic pleasure-seeking instincts of the id, which keeps the individual properly in touch with reality, and enables him or her to recognize what can be accomplished within the constraints of the superego (conscience) and the environment. Erikson proposed that societies' mores exist to guide the individual along a path that allows the individual and the species to fulfil their genetic potential. The individual is seen as developing in stages, with each stage focused around a particular crisis that stems both from internal, biological drives and cultural and societal expectations. Erikson (1963) puts forward eight such stages, of which three are concerned with the period under consideration here.

In the stage of entering adulthood from adolescence, which is the fifth of Erikson's stages, the main task is for the individual to successfully develop a sense of identity. The *identity crisis* arises as adolescents seek to adjust to and incorporate into their overall sense of identity a changed physical appearance, awakened sexual interest, a sense of difference from parents, new work, and family and societal roles. If this stage is not successfully negotiated there is identity or role confusion. The stage is therefore referred to as that of 'identity versus role confusion'.

The next stage is that of early adulthood, in which the crisis is prompted by the need to establish an intimate relationship. This may be sexual or platonic, but intimacy is viewed as successfully achieved if both partners are committed to the relationship, without one overwhelming the other. If this is not achieved the individual may turn inwards and become isolated. This stage is known as that of 'intimacy versus isolation'.

Having established an intimate relationship, the task of middle adulthood becomes that of *generativity*, which is a concern for future generations. This may be satisfied through bringing up children to become responsible citizens or through contributing productively to society via work, civic or family roles. Where individuals are not able to feel that they are productive, creative or giving, they are likely to have a sense of stagnation. This particular concern is popularly referred to as the *mid-life crisis* and will be examined further below. The stage is known as that of 'generativity versus stagnation'.

Erikson's theory, then, is based on an organismic model of internally driven stages, which are facilitated by the pressures of society. New stages of development are achieved if the crisis that arises at each stage is successfully resolved. The theory has been very influential, partly because it is one of the first to have addressed the whole lifespan and partly because its integrative approach is very attractive. Much of the evidence to support it is drawn from clinical case studies and from biographies, rather than from large-scale research studies.

Levinson's theory of the seasons of a man's life

Daniel Levinson (1978, 1986) also puts forward a stage and crisis theory of the development of the life path. His theory was initially based on in-depth interviews of 10 to 20 hours with 40 middle-aged men. It is therefore based on an analysis of retrospective and speculative accounts of a particular generation of men. Subsequent research, however, has attempted to test out its applicability to women, and it is reported that the ideas hold true, although the life course appears more complex for women (Roberts and Newton, 1987).

Levinson proposed that life can be structured into four eras, these being childhood and adolescence, early, middle, and late adulthood. During each era, the individual creates a 'life structure' by developing a network of relationships and roles. In between each era is a transitional period during which the life structure is reviewed. The doubts or dilemmas raised during such review often cause a period of instability, which must be resolved before the individual moves on.

Thus, the transition between adolescence and adulthood is seen as taking place between the ages of 17 and 22, and is a time when the individual must form an adult identity (cf. Erikson's concept of identity versus role confusion). Early adulthood then lasts until the age of 40 years. During this era the young adult is seen as having to master certain tasks, including pursuing an occupational ambition or 'dream' and raising a family. This is viewed as a productive and demanding era.

Between the ages of 40 and 45 comes the mid-life transition. During this, the individual needs to deal with three tasks. Firstly, he must review what he has achieved so far and perhaps adjust to the reality of not having achieved all he set out to do. Secondly, he must start to move into middle age. Thirdly, he must adjust to four particular issues – growing older, being mortal, accepting the feminine as well as the masculine side of his nature, and needing attachment to as well as separateness from others. This transition links with the notion of mid-life crisis, and leads into middle adulthood, which then continues to the age of 60.

During middle adulthood individuals are in a period when they have the opportunity to make an impact on their families and on society, through family, professional and civic roles (cf. Erikson's notion of generativity). At the ages of 60 to 65 there is a transition into late adulthood.

Consistency and continuity in lifespan development

While stage theories are a seductive way of conceptualizing adult development, the evidence for them, as we have seen, is not extensive. There is evidence to suggest that there is considerable continuity in psychological factors over the adult years. In terms of the major dimensions of personality, it has been found that the degree of extraversion or introversion, and the degree of neuroticism remain stable across adolescence and the adult years. A third dimension, that of 'openness to experience versus rigidity' was found to be less stable. However, overall, it seems that individuals have a certain consistency in their underlying personality traits. The way these are expressed may vary over time – for example, a person may be consistently extravert but may express this through night clubbing in adolescence, through being the life and soul of his children's parties in early adulthood and through visiting friends and relatives in middle age.

Some theorists propose that there is gradual change in psychological functioning during the adult years, rather than change that occurs through a sequence of crises. Vaillant (1977), for example, holds an organismic model, believing that human beings are driven by instinctive needs. In order to meet these needs and resolve conflicts, the individual must develop effective defence mechanisms. Vaillant found evidence that, among a group of highly educated men, there was a shift across the years to more mature forms of defence mechanism. So, projection of feelings or thoughts on to others was more common in earlier adulthood, whereas sublimation, for example, into altruism, was more common in middle age.

Bernice Neugarten, who has researched and written extensively on psychological development in adult and later life employing a lifespan developmental perspective (Neugarten, 1968; Neugarten and Datan, 1973), believes that there is little evidence to support the idea of chronological age having a particular relationship with psychological development during adulthood. She asserts that, particularly in twentieth-century American society, there are so many possibilities for varying life patterns that it is not possible to say that there is a 'right time' for life events. The struggles and crises, for example, of intimacy versus independence or coming to terms with success or failure, are not the exclusive preserve of particular ages, but are revisited on various occasions over the lifespan.

Consideration of particular developmental tasks

Establishing identity

One of the major developmental tasks in establishing oneself as a young adult is to gain a clear sense of who one is. The transition from adolescence to adulthood involves acquiring many new roles within work and family contexts.

The young adult who takes up employment becomes a worker and an independent earner. The nature of people's occupation becomes an aspect of their identity. Being a young farmer, accountant or teacher each contributes, in its own particular way, to self-image. Being a wage earner may, in itself, entail the new role of becoming a budget manager, and being eligible to borrow credit may encourage young people to try out the role of debtor! Within a family context, moving away from home brings about a plethora of new roles. This might involve becoming a tenant, a shopper, a housekeeper and cleaner, a cook, a neighbour and so on. Being away from the parental home allows more freedom to choose a way of living. The young person may struggle with whether to retain aspects of lifestyle and values which they have taken on from their parents. An individual may perhaps continue to be a churchgoer, but also become a late riser; he or she may decide to experiment with drugs, may try out a political affiliation quite different from that of his or her background, or may decide a flashy car has to be part of his or her identity.

For young people moving into adulthood, all these decisions and moves are part of developing a definite and independent identity, distinct from that of their parents. Over a period of time, as new roles are established, so a coherent sense of identity emerges. As we have seen, Erikson views this as the major task of entering adulthood, and for Levinson it is the central feature of the transition into early adulthood. In Erikson's framework, the failure to develop an integrated sense of person results in an identity crisis and a sense of 'role confusion'. Marcia (1967) expands on Erikson's theory to produce a more detailed framework to assess the degree to which identity has been established, with four categories being proposed. The 'identity achiever' has explored the possibilities and has made some firm commitments to values, beliefs and personal goals. Those who have a 'foreclosed' identity have also made some commitment, but have not explored the alternatives. Others are still actively exploring aspects of identity but do not yet have firm commitments to particular goals or values. These people are described as being in a 'moratorium'. Finally, there are those who do not seem to have a sense of identity and who seem to be drifting rather than struggling with the issue. This group is described as having 'identity diffusion'.

The development of identity, however, is not a task that is left behind on entering adulthood, but is one that continues throughout the individual's life. The roles that are established in early adulthood undergo further changes as life progresses, and new roles are taken on. The way a particular individual reacts and adapts to the changes is influenced by the backdrop of temperamental characteristics that they bring to situations, and by the maturation of some of these basic qualities, but it is possible to make some generalizations around the impact that particular role changes and transitions can have on personal identity.

The major areas of role that contribute to development of identity are in the spheres of gender and culture, work and family life. These are easier to consider separately, but of course, they each impact on the other producing a complex matrix overall, contributing to the very different life situations and the rich variety of identities that clinicians are aware of in everyday practice.

Gender roles

The normative expectations of society differ for men and women, with societal norms leading to stereotypes that are taken on by children from a very early age. Studies have shown that by the age of five or six years children already hold distinct views about the characteristics of each gender. In Western society, the male stereotype is focused on the concept of competence. Men are expected to be more aggressive, competitive, active, objective and independent. They are viewed as able to lead and make decisions. The female stereotype is focused on nurturance and warmth. Women are expected to be gentle, empathic and able to express tender feelings. They are also seen as more dependent. Socialization fosters an internalization of these norms, reinforcing behaviour that expresses the stereotype and discouraging behaviour that contradicts it.

Family example has been shown to be influential in modelling behaviour and may have a strong influence on normative and non-normative behaviour. Families may give a young person examples of traditional gender roles, or of variations from the norm. So, for example, studying those generations in which it was not expected for married women to earn a living outside the home, it has been shown that girls whose mothers worked were more likely to develop a career than those whose mothers did not. There has been recent debate in Britain expressing concern about the lack of models for the role of husband and father in households where the son has no father present.

In effect, studies of behaviour show more overlap between genders than distinct differences on many of the stereotypical dimensions mentioned above. There are also considerable numbers of people who do not follow a life path that conforms to the norm. Single men and women are less likely to perform only gender specific roles than those who are married and have a gender-stereotyped division of labour.

Most of the theories of development in adult life have focused on studies of men. As might be expected in a male-dominated society, the process of men's development tends to be viewed as the norm. Thus Erikson's, Levinson's and Vaillant's theories, mentioned above, are all based on male experiences. Any differences that are found between men and women are often described as if female development is a variation upon the normative pattern. This can be difficult to avoid once frameworks for thinking are set up through male-oriented theories. There is emerging evidence to suggest that the path of personal development differs for women in some substantial ways.

In terms of Erikson's stages of development, it has been found that whereas, for men, independence and personal identity may be established before intimacy, for women the two stages are not separately defined. Personal identity is traditionally more closely intertwined with that of their partners and their children. Thus identity and intimacy become parallel and overlapping issues, rather than being separated. Gilligan (1982) describes women as locating their identity and independence within their relationships with others, whereas men subordinate their personal relationships to career demands and personal ambitions. Researchers have found that early adulthood, which is often described as a period of growth and consolidation for men, can be a period of considerable turmoil for women, as they work out how to compromise between personal ambitions, family related desires and societal expectations.

Similarly, in Erikson's stages, generativity follows intimacy, occurring in middle age, but many women report that, for them, generativity was not postponed to this point of life.

The expectations that women should provide care for others can put women at risk from 'role overload' in early adulthood, when career, household and family may all make demands, and in middle adulthood, when adolescents, frail elderly relatives, career and household may all compete for attention. There may also be 'role conflict' when, for example, a woman feels great pressure to succeed in her career as well as successfully bring up her family.

There is some evidence to suggest that when adults deviate from the expected gender roles, this causes psychological discomfort. Longitudinal studies (Livson, 1981) have found that by age 50 those who had followed the gender typical roles as adolescents (girls preparing for family and social roles, and boys for careers) were psychologically healthier than those who had not conformed.

Gender roles change to some degree across the course of adult life, with gender-differentiated behaviour being most extreme in early adulthood when parents have young children. In middle age, men appear to take on more of the traditionally feminine attributes, becoming more tender and more understanding of others, whereas women develop more autonomy. Thus the roles become more androgynous.

Racial identity

Just as gender expectations and stereotypes play a large part in socializing men and women in society, so cultural expectations are also a major influence. Basic aspects of the lifecycle are clearly universal and demand psychological adaptation whatever the cultural context. Thus finding a way of making ends meet, adjusting to marriage and widowhood, and rearing children are developmental tasks for all of us if these events are part of our individual life course. However, as mentioned above, different norms hold true in different places and at different times. Issues of work identity, for example, may be different in a rural, subsistence economy from those in a post-industrial society; family roles may differ between nuclear, extended and polygamous families, posing different psychological issues for the family members.

There are complicating factors that may affect personal identity in a multicultural society, particularly where there is one dominant culture and others are in a minority, or where there has been immigration such that cultural mores are brought from overseas into a differing indigenous culture. Young adults from a minority culture may feel conflicting pressures to conform to the societal norms of the dominant society as well as those of their culture of origin. This may cause identity confusion for young adults. It may also mean that identity is less integrated as expectations may differ more between home and work settings than would be true for the majority of the population. The development of close relationships may be more difficult where a majority have little appreciation of a minority culture, so that a member of a minority group may become more easily isolated.

In some instances, those from a minority culture not only need to adapt to cultural differences but also have to combat the impact of racism. This is the case where the majority culture holds a negative stereotype of members of a minority culture. If the majority culture, for example, holds a stereotype that members of another group are dull, lazy and lacking in ambition, this negative image will affect members of the minority group. The young adult may find him or herself drawn into the prejudiced view, believing that he or she is stupid and unambitious. In this case individuals will be unable to fulfil their potential and develop a satisfactory personal identity unless they are able to see beyond the internalized oppression. Where development of personal identity is strong despite racist stereotypes, the individual will still have the stress of living in a society which projects negative expectations on to them. In Britain, those from immigrant communities are, on average, more likely to experience poor mental health than the indigenous population.

Work identity

The type of job a person does contributes significantly to self-concept. The role in itself has certain expectations attached. So, for example, most of us would hold certain expectations if we were about to meet a psychoanalyst, a hairdresser or a tax collector. These expectations influence the person's own behaviour and that of others toward them. Those who work full time spend so many of their waking hours in the work setting that it has a powerful influence on personal and intellectual development. For example, those who are expected to solve problems on a daily basis retain good skills in flexible thinking; and those who work on their own all day every day may find themselves unable to make conversation.

Although occupation is a major part of self-identity, it appears that, for many people, choice of career path is unplanned. Various theories have been put forward to describe the psychological processes that may be involved in deciding on a career. Rybash et al. (1991) give a summary of three of these, which suggest that selection of an occupation is variously based on fulfilment of self-concept; on a gradual shaping up of decisions through phases of fantasy, tentative thinking and realistic thinking; and on the match between personality and occupational demands. The last of these is perhaps the most well known and will be further elaborated here. This latter theory was put forward by Holland (1985). He proposes that job satisfaction is attained when the personality of the individual fits well with the demands of the job. Where these aspects are not well matched, this leads to job dissatisfaction and consequent career instability as the person searches for a different career. Holland outlined six basic personality types (investigative, realistic, conventional, enterprising, social and artistic) and the work roles that best match them. The investigative person likes to work with ideas and is likely to choose a research or scientific occupation. The realistic individual prefers working with objects and is drawn towards mechanical work. The conventional type is conscientious but not creative and does well in checking roles, such as bookkeeper or receptionist. By contrast, the enterprising person is dominating and persuasive, making a good salesperson. The social person enjoys work with people and is likely to work in human services, and the artistic type likes to work with emotions and may choose a creative, artistic career. These ideas have been found to have some validity, although personality only appears to be one element in career choice. Background, family, opportunity and current context also play a large part.

Following career choice, it has been proposed that the individual's contact with occupation continues through the further stages of career entry and adjustment, maintenance and finally retirement (Rybash et al., 1991). Issues within each of these may lead to further psychological demands and development. Entering an occupation may take a great deal of energy in the initial stages, as the individual is 'socialized' into the role. The person needs to learn to get on with co-workers, respond appropriately to authority, and so on. Levinson, whose theory of development was reviewed above, proposes that among the tasks of early adulthood are those of forming a 'dream' or image of what life, and particularly the preferred occupation, may be like and finding a mentor. As the actual experience does not match the 'dream' in all respects, people need to come to terms with the 'reality shock' of finding out what their chosen career is really like. The existence of a mentor – an older person who can provide guidance – has been found to be helpful to young adults in developing their sense of identity in the workplace.

During the time of adjustment to the realities of working life, Levinson proposes that there is a period during which the person must establish a satisfactory occupational identity and performance. Some people will manage this in a straightforward way, but others may drop out or change direction. For some there may be a period of trying several career directions before settling down to a stable career.

By middle adulthood, many people have achieved considerable advancement in terms of salary, responsibility and status. There is some evidence that different factors contribute to job satisfaction in early adulthood and middle age. Young adults are concerned with salary, job security, relationships with colleagues and managers and possibilities for advancement, whereas older workers are concerned with the degree of autonomy they have and with whether the work is intrinsically satisfying and meaningful. In mid-life those who are satisfied may continue to be settled but for those who are not, there may be a period of reflection and crisis that, for some, results in a radical career change.

The descriptions of development of work identity above, are related to a stereotyped view of a young adult entering a chosen occupation and remaining in continuous employment until retirement age. The research findings quoted tend to be from large-scale studies of employees of large firms. In fact, this pattern is probably not very common. The majority of people change employers a number of times during their working lives. There are also a number of patterns of employment. Continuous employment is the most common pattern for both men and women, but there are also those who have periods in and out of work. These include women who either have a career gap while bringing up children, or who postpone undertaking further education and employment until their children are at school. It also includes those who have difficulty finding employment, experience redundancy, or become disabled and unable to work. The role strain of working while children are small has already been mentioned. For those who are unemployed, or unable to work, there are psychological consequences for self-concept and self-esteem as well as the obvious practical consequences of having too much time and too little income.

Intimacy

The sections above have introduced some of the main findings regarding the development of personal identity in early adulthood and the way identity continues to be forged through role change and development of new roles. The following sections are concerned with two aspects of personal life: development of close relationships and parenting, which also contribute greatly to personal identity.

Intimacy develops in a relationship that involves mutual disclosure and understanding between the two parties. Rogers (1972) analysed the features common in intimate relationships, and found four factors. Firstly, there was a commitment to keep the relationship growing; secondly there was meaningful communication, with each partner feeling that he or she could disclose personal thoughts and feelings and be understood and accepted by the other; thirdly, the goals and needs of the relationship were defined by the two partners, rather than being dictated by society or the families of either partner; and lastly, the identity of both partners was able to grow and develop with neither being stunted or stifled.

As mentioned in the section on Erikson, an intimate relationship is not necessarily one that is sexual or that leads to marriage between the partners. Friendships and sibling relationships may be very close and involve sharing and support. However, within adulthood the marital relationship stands out as one that involves a major commitment, as well as forming the basis of the family context for having and bringing up children.

Finding a mate is generally considered a task of early adult life. Giving commitment to another adult may cause conflict or crisis for the individual. By definition, there needs to be some compromise and some shift in personal values to develop a partnership, but this may feel like a threat to hard won identity and independence. Where the sense of personal identity is not strong one person may have a fear of being overwhelmed or smothered by the other. Where this is the case, the individual's identity may become defined only through the relationship, so that the person loses his or her personal initiative. This can lead to a lack of self-respect. On the other hand, individuals may protect themselves by holding rigidly on to their independent position, leading to a sense of isolation and loneliness.

The process of finding a mate differs across cultures. Some societies have arranged marriages in which the families select, negotiate and agree suitable alliances for their children whereas, in others, the young people take the initiative, with their marriage being, to varying degrees, a matter for approval by the respective families. Where the young people have the choice, the concept of romantic love is often seen as the cornerstone of attraction. Love has received attention from a number of researchers. One of the most well known theories was put forward by Sternberg and Barnes (1988) who propose a triangular theory of love. In this model, a triangle is used as a pictorial representation of love, with three characteristics – intimacy (an emotional factor), passion (a motivational or arousal factor) and decision-commitment (a cognitive factor) – being placed one at each corner. The relative strength of these three components determines the shape of the triangle, making it easy to describe different types of love, and to represent balance or imbalance.

Surveys of marriages demonstrate that as a general rule 'like pairs' are attracted, with the majority of couples being of the same cultural group, social class, and level of education. This is probably multi-determined because there may be psychological reasons why a person would feel better understood by someone of a similar background as well as social reasons why people of a similar cultural group and level of education are more likely to meet in work, religious or social settings.

Marriages last until death or divorce. Similar factors appear to be important to marital satisfaction at any age. One cross-sectional study (Reedy, Birren and Schaie, 1982), looking at young, middle-aged and older adults, found that six factors were ranked in the same order by all three age groups. These, from highest to lowest ranked, were emotional security, respect, communication, shared chores and leisure time, sexual intimacy and loyalty. There are some gender differences in aspects of marriage that are viewed as important, with women valuing intimacy and emotional security and men placing a high premium on loyalty and commitment.

Across the years of married life, again using cross-sectional studies, it has been shown that marital satisfaction is high immediately after marriage, dips when the first child is born, and rises again after the last child leaves home, often to a level higher than that reported by newly-weds. This pattern may simplify a complex picture, partly because it looks at marital satisfaction in isolation from other aspects of life satisfaction, partly because the cross-sectional nature of the studies may mean that those with less happy marriages disappear from samples and partly because the findings may be influenced by cohort effects.

There is some evidence to suggest a number of factors that contribute to happy marriages. Marital satisfaction is higher among those couples who share traditional, conforming views of gender roles; those who treat each other as equals and those who have similar personalities.

Divorce and remarriage

Many less happy marriages end in separation or divorce, although some couples stay together despite the relationship being an unhappy one. Divorce is more common among those who married below the age of 20 years, those where the marriage took place when the woman was pregnant, and those who have a low income. Religious factors, social pressures and young children may be major influences preventing divorce. Although the process of divorce has become easier, and the level of stigma attached to being divorced is much less than it used to be, divorce nevertheless remains a painful, stressful process. It involves loss of roles, causes changes in family and social relationships, and often brings financial and social strain. Adjusting to divorce means adapting to all these changes and at the same time coming to terms with the failure of a relationship that was meant to last for ever. This can have a far-reaching impact on self-esteem and cause severe depression.

Many of those who divorce remarry. People enter remarriages with different expectations, looking for companionship and steady affection. There is some evidence that second marriages are more egalitarian, but that the levels of satisfaction and tension are about the same as in first marriages. A number of second marriages lead to 'blended families' when one or both partners already have their own children, and the couple may go on to have children together. This presents particularly difficult challenges if all involved are to develop trusting relationships with each other.

The family lifecycle

It has been proposed that the family has a lifecycle of its own, which adds up to more than the individual's lifecycles (Duvall, 1971). The family lifecycle is usually seen as starting with the formation of a new marital couple and lasting until the death of both spouses. Arrivals and departures of family members and changes in role are seen as marking different stages in the life of the family, with six to eight stages commonly identified. These might be, for example, married couple with no children; new parents; the family with pre-school children; the family with school children; the family with adolescent children; the family with children leaving home; and the return to a dyad after the children have left home.

Each of these changes involves adjustment for the family and its members. Entering the phase of 'new parents', to take one example, involves emotional bonding of the parents with the new baby; it involves the parents coping with the changes this brings in the relationship between them; it brings new roles and new tasks that must be divided between the adults; and it may involve a renegotiation of roles with the baby's grandparents.

As with many of the issues of adjustment addressed in this chapter, the nature of the life events is, to some extent, culturally dependent, with the majority of the research being focused upon modern Western culture and white, Anglo-Saxon, Protestant (WASP), American norms in particular. In other cultures the normative family lifecycle may have different identifiable stages or phases. So, a polygamous culture or one involving an extended family system may bring different transitions and events. The cultural context may also have an influence on the social resources that facilitate coping with family events. Thus, adjusting to the birth of children may pose different problems for a nuclear family in a suburban setting, than it does for a couple within a multi-generation household in a rural setting.

It should also be remembered that the family lifecycle describes normative events. Non-normative or idiosyncratic life events may bring different family lifecycle patterns, as when there is a blended family, a single parent, a childless couple or a gay couple.

Parenting

The widespread availability of effective birth control has allowed sexual activity to be separated from the production of children and so, for many couples, child bearing may be open to influence from social pressures, rational decision making, and psychological factors as well as biological drives. Effective contraception, combined with lower infant mortality, has led to a trend in industrialized countries, across the first half of the twentieth century, towards smaller families.

Social influences towards having children remain strong, with socialization preparing both girls and boys for the idea that they will become mothers and fathers when they grow up. During childhood and adolescence children learn a great deal through the role models of their parents and through portrayals in the media about what is expected of parents. The majority of young adults expect to become parents and to find the experience a fulfilling one. However, this is an area that has been strongly influenced by cohort related events for recent generations. Not only has birth control made a difference, but, alongside this, the feminist movement has led to changing expectations of and for women. Many, particularly those who have the opportunity to benefit from education, and those who face financial need, expect to have a career of their own and a life that stretches beyond the horizon of the family. This has led to many couples postponing having children and to a greater number of mothers of young children working outside the home.

Psychological factors also play a part in the decision to have children. Children may be seen as a way of meeting a need to love or be loved, and have been described by Erikson (1963) as fulfilling the drive towards 'generativity'.

Studies show that parents find the experience of having and rearing children both satisfying and stressful. The satisfactions are described as a sense of fulfilment and a sense of being needed. Parents describe feelings of joy, pride and maturity. For many women there is a strong link between their sense of self-esteem and their performance as parent, although this does not appear to be the case for men. The strains of parenthood lie within the role strain and financial strain that may come from the extra work and costs involved. There is also an impact upon the marital relationship as the parents have less time to spend together and their roles become more separate. Women still take on the majority of childcare tasks, and may, at times, feel oppressed by the routine and undervalued by their families. Where parents have received poor parenting themselves, it may be difficult for them to know how to succeed in bringing up their own children and this may prove particularly stressful.

The balance of satisfactions and strains are influenced by the context, including factors such as when the children are born in relation to the age and life stage of the parents, the age and sex of the children, and the financial and wider family situation of the parents.

Mid-life crisis

It is a widely held belief that many people face a mid-life crisis on entering middle age. The possible basis of this for men has been reviewed above in the section on Erikson's psychosocial stages of development, in which the crisis arises from the conflict between generativity and stagnation, and in the section on Levinson's approach to the seasons of man, which proposes that the mid-life transition may be a time of crisis. For women, mid-life crisis has been suggested as being linked to the need to adjust to the physical signs of ageing, in a society that places so much emphasis on youthful aspects of beauty, as well as to the menopause, which prompts women to think about their reproductive opportunities being over. It has also been proposed that adjusting to the *empty nest* is especially difficult for women. Middle age may also be a time, prompted by children growing up as well as by parents ageing, when the individual first really takes on board the fact that they are mortal and that time is finite.

The evidence for the existence of a mid-life crisis is equivocal. Some American studies (for example, Levinson, 1978), particularly those of men, have found that the majority report a period of turmoil on entering middle age. However, others have not found this to be the case. Vaillant (1977) suggests that changes of occupation, divorce and depression are no more or less common in middle age than any other period of adult life.

Studies of women show that the physical effects of the menopause (including nausea, hot flushes and headaches) may be both a trouble and a worry to some women. However, there is no other noticeable increase in emotional disturbance during middle adulthood. The end of the risk of pregnancy may be a welcome relief for some women. For those women whose personal identity has been closely bound up with that of their children, it may be hard to adapt to life without them at home. Neugarten (1968), however, found that most women did not view the menopause or the 'empty nest' as traumatic. Where self-concept did show a major change in mid-life, it was not linked to these life events. In fact, many studies show an increase in life satisfaction and marital happiness after children have left home. The post-parental period may allow parents to fulfil goals that were put on one side while children were growing up and permit them to once again pursue joint interests and develop a renewed intimacy.

Summary and conclusions

This chapter has looked at psychological adjustment during adulthood, identifying the major influences as social rather than cognitive or biological. Such social events were classified as falling into the three categories of normative, cohort-related and idiosyncratic life events. Organismic, behavioural and lifespan developmental models were described as the main frameworks for understanding development in adulthood. They are distinguished by their differing emphases on internal drives and external learning, and reductionist and holistic perspectives. Some of the major theories were introduced, including the stage approaches of Erikson's psychosocial theory and Levinson's theory of the seasons of man. Approaches that put more emphasis on continuity, such as Neugarten's lifespan developmental approach and that of Vaillant were also briefly reviewed.

We examined particular aspects of development in adult life, including the development of identity, with particular reference to gender issues, 'racial' identity and work roles, the development of intimate relationships with reference to marriage, and aspects of the family lifecycle, including parenting and the mid-life crisis. The frame of reference for much of the work in this area of social psychology lies within Western and particularly American culture, so care needs to be taken when applying the ideas to particular individuals. However, research indicates that, far from being a sterile period, adulthood is a rich and fascinating time of life.

References

Baltes PB (1987) Theoretical propositions of lifespan developmental psychology: on the dynamics between growth and decline. Developmental Psychology 23: 611–26.

Bandura A (1977) Social Learning Theory. Englewood Cliffs NJ: Prentice-Hall.

Duvall E (1971) Family Development (4 edn). Philadelphia: Lippincott.

Erikson E (1963) Childhood and Society (2 edn). New York: Norton.

Gilligan C (1982) In a Different Voice: Psychological Theory and Women's Development. Cambridge MA: Harvard University Press.

Havighurst RJ (1972) Developmental Tasks and Education (3 edn). New York: McKay.

Hayslip B, Panek P (1989) Adult Development and Aging. New York: Harper & Row.

Holland JL (1985) Making Vocational Choices: A Theory of Vocational Personalities and Work Environments (2 edn). Englewood Cliffs, NJ: Prentice-Hall.

Levinson DJ (1978) The Seasons of a Man's Life. New York: Knopf.

Levinson, DJ (1986) A conception of adult development. American Psychologist 41: 3–13.

Livson FB (1981) Paths to psychological health in the middle years: sex differences. In D Eichorn, J Clausen, N Haan, M Honzik and P Mussen (eds) Present and Past in Middle Life. New York: Academic Press.

Marcia JE (1967) Ego identity status: relationships to change in self-esteem, 'general adjustment' and authoritarianism. Journal of Personality 35: 118–33.

Neugarten BL (1968) Personality in Middle and Late Life (2 edn). New York: Atherton Press.

Neugarten BL, Datan N (1973) Sociological perspectives on the life cycle. In PB Baltes, KW Schaie (eds) Lifespan Developmental Psychology. New York: Academic Press.

Reedy MN, Birren JE, Schaie KW (1982) Age and sex differences in satisfying love relationships across the lifespan. Human Development 24: 52–66.

Roberts P, Newton PM (1987) Levinsonian studies of women's adult development. Psychology and Aging 2: 154–63.

Rogers C (1972) The Coming Partners: Marriage and its Alternatives. New York: Dell.

Rybash JM, Roodin PA, Santrock JW (1991) Adult Development and Aging (2 edn). New York: William C Brown Publishers.

Schaie KW, Willis SL (1991) Adult Development and Aging (3 edn). New York: HarperCollins.

Sternberg RJ, Barnes ML (eds) (1988) The Psychology of Love. New Haven: Yale University Press.

Vaillant G (1977) Adaptation to Life. Boston: Little, Brown.

Chapter 18
Normal ageing

JANET R. WHEATLEY

Key concepts	Key names
Chronological vs functional vs biological vs social age	
Cross-sectional design	
Longitudinal design	
Cross-sequential design	
Impairment vs disability vs handicap	
Fluid and crystallized intelligence	Cattell
Memory	
Complex reaction time	
Terminal drop	
'Post-formal' cognitive functioning	Knight
Developmental tasks	Havighurst, Erikson
Integrity vs despair	
Disengagement theory	Cumming and Henry
Activity theory	
Interiority	
Life review	
Psychoticism, neuroticism, introversion–extraversion	Eysenck
Caregiving	
primary strain	
secondary role strain	
secondary intrapsychic strain	Pearlin et al.
Coping style	
Stages of bereavement	Parkes
Grief work	Worden
Stages of facing dying	Kubler-Ross
Seven propositions of ageing	Baltes and Baltes
Maturity, specific challenge model	Knight

Introduction and overview

Ageing refers to the process of becoming old, with the study of human ageing usually concentrating on the later years of life. This chapter is concerned with psychological aspects of the process of becoming older, from about the sixth decade through to the end of life. It examines normal ageing and its impact on physical, cognitive, emotional and social aspects of functioning.

The chapter begins with definitions of old age, and a consideration of some of the methodological concerns of importance in collecting and understanding information. It then reviews physical, social and cognitive changes in later life and the challenges that these present for older people in terms of psychological adjustment.

Theories of psychological development and adjustment in old age are then introduced, before moving on to describe what is known about emotional adaptation and coping in later life. The chapter ends with two models that attempt to provide integrated frameworks for understanding the psychology of later life.

Definitions of old age

In discussing the psychology of later life it is necessary to have a definition of the period of life encompassed. This might seem obvious but it is not as straightforward as it first appears. *Chronological age* (how old a person is) is commonly used to define an age band of older adults. However, the number of years lived only tells us about a person's psychology in so far as aspects of ageing correlate exactly with the passage of time. In fact, there is wide variation among functions and among people in their susceptibility and their response to age-related changes.

The start of the period of 'later life' is not immutable, but ages between 50 and 70 years are looked upon as signalling the start of old age in most societies. In British society generally, 60–65 years is looked upon as the threshold of old age. The reason for this is possibly related to societal norms (retirement age and pensionable age) and to an age at which degenerative changes of ageing become noticeable.

This age band of approximately 65 years to 100 years or more is clearly a very broad one, including a range of 30–40 years and more than one generation. It is quite possible in an old age mental health service to have patients in their 80s being supported by an adult children in their 60s. The life stage is sometimes sub-divided into young-old (60s), middle-old (70s) and old-old (80+ years), or young-old (65 to 75 or 80), old-old (75-80 to 90) and very old (90+).

An alternative way of defining age is to use *functional age* – to assign a person a functional age depending on their performance in relation to age-graded norms. Thus, a person might have a chronological age of 70 (be 70 years old) but have a functional age of 50 for reaction time and of 60 for speed of information processing. This type of definition therefore allows a separation of the degree of ageing of different functions, and tells us more precisely about the nature of the individual's performance.

The related term of *biological age* may be used to relate individual function to age-based norms of physiological functions and, similarly, *social age* may be used to refer to societal norms of how people should behave at particular ages. Thus it might be expected, in British culture, that most people would retire from paid employment in their 60s, or that most people over 30 years would have lost interest in going to nightclubs. It is then possible to describe an individual as 'on or off time' with regard to the various expectations of society.

Methodology

Studies of the psychology of human ageing try to understand the impact of ageing using one of three contrasting methods. The relative qualities of these influence the nature of the research-based evidence obtained. A thorough description of the impact of ageing on any psychological variable should include a statement on the type of methodology that has produced the conclusions.

The most common research design is *cross-sectional*. These studies compare different age groups on a particular variable, such as intelligence. They can be conducted at a single point in time, making them practical and speedy to carry out. The disadvantage of cross-sectional studies is that they confound the influences of age and cohort. So, using the example of intelligence, we can cite cross-sectional evidence from studies in the 1950s showing that intelligence declines steadily from the mid-20s onwards. However, further consideration tells us that there may be reasons other than age that contribute to this finding. Those in the older age groups were born in earlier years and therefore had less education and probably poorer health and material living conditions than the younger generations. These factors would be expected to have an adverse influence on the performance of older generations.

The second major type of research design is a *longitudinal* one. In this case a cohort of participants is tested on successive occasions as they grow older. This allows us to isolate the impact of ageing for this particular group. Such studies have the drawback of taking many years to carry out, but also have two further disadvantages. Firstly, the fittest and most well-motivated participants are more likely to stay in for successive sessions than the less fit, and less motivated, so that such studies may not retain a normative sample. Secondly, longitudinal studies reflect the characteristics of a particular generation. So, for example, the generation that was young in the economic depression of the 1930s and then lived through the Second World War may, as a consequence, hold certain beliefs and attitudes. Similarly, the post-war baby boomers, growing up after the advent of the Welfare State and in an era of stability may, in their turn, be influenced by this context. Thus, while it is important to understand the influences on each cohort, findings cannot necessarily be generalized to those born in a different time or culture.

A third research design provides a combination of cross-sectional and longitudinal aspects, yielding results that allow the disentangling of ageing from generation effects. This design involves establishing a panel of participants of different age groups, as in a cross-sectional design, and then following each over time. This is known as a *cross-sequential design*. The Seattle Longitudinal Study of adult cognitive functioning is one of the most well known and thorough studies of this type. The study began in 1956 with 500 participants aged from 22 to 70, grouped into seven-year age bands. These participants were followed up on five occasions between then and 1984, with further participants also being recruited in successive waves. This major study has produced a sophisticated understanding of the influence of ageing on intelligence (see below).

Challenges of later life

In moving into old age the individual is likely to face many life events and challenges, all of which demand psychological adjustment. Some of these are physical in nature and others are social. Our interest in them here is primarily concerned with how they affect psychological wellbeing. The major changes will be briefly considered below, and the subsequent section will examine frameworks for understanding the nature of the psychological tasks these changes pose.

Physical aspects of ageing

As people grow older their bodies suffer from a number of age-related changes. This section will give a brief account of how ageing affects the senses and the nervous system; and will survey levels of disease and illness with a view to examining their effect on the individual.

Vision

In terms of vision, older people tend to have poorer accommodation, often resulting in long sightedness; there is a loss of acuity (ability to see detail); speed of adjustment to changes in luminescence is slowed; there is a change in colour perception, with colours at the blue end of the spectrum becoming more difficult to distinguish.

The practical consequences are that older people often need glasses to read and brighter light to see clearly. Moving from light to darkness or vice versa may become difficult so, for example, going to the bathroom at night in an unfamiliar environment or night driving may prove hazardous. Subtle colour schemes may cause confusion about, for example, whether there is a step when a carpet changes to lino.

The consequences may, in turn, have a significant influence on lifestyle as older adults adapt their pattern of life to manage within the confines of age-related changes. Thus, an elderly driver, conscious of finding glare difficult to cope with in the dark, may no longer go to visit friends or attend meetings on winter evenings. Bookwork or sewing may be carried out in the daylight in a seat by the window rather than at the fireside in the evenings. This type of accommodation is often gradual and would not usually be experienced as upsetting.

A significant minority of over 75s, estimated as 16% (Crandall 1980), are blind or partially sighted due to cataracts, glaucoma or macular degeneration. This may cause more drastic changes in a person's life and consequently has greater implications for psychological adjustment.

Hearing

There is some deterioration in hearing from about the age of 40 years, but sharper deterioration occurs after the age of 60 years. Approximately 75% of 75 to 79 year olds have some degree of hearing difficulty, and it has been found that by the age of 80 years, 25% of speech is not heard. Much of the deterioration is in the perception of high frequency sounds but pitch discrimination also becomes less sensitive and it becomes harder to pick out meaningful sounds such as speech from any masking background noise. In addition, about 10% of over 65s suffer from tinnitus.

Problems with hearing may have the consequence of interfering with interaction and relationships. Elderly people may withdraw from conversation rather than face the embarrassment of misperceiving what is said, or may be perceived by others as being deliberately awkward rather than disabled. This may cause hearing-impaired people to become socially isolated, and may play a part in causing depression for some. For the person with paranoid tendencies, what cannot be accurately heard may be misinterpreted as hostile.

Other senses

Studies of taste indicate that there is little change with ageing, though the palate may become more sensitive to bitter taste. The sense of smell appears to be only minimally affected in well, elderly people. Touch becomes a little less sensitive in old age but, possibly more significantly, there is some evidence that pain thresholds are higher.

Nervous system

There is a loss of neurons in the central nervous system with age, and there is decreased efficiency in those remaining. The brain becomes about 10% to 15% lighter during normal ageing, and there are changes in electrical and probably neurochemical activity. Sleep becomes lighter and more broken and basic reaction times are, on average, slower.

It is a common belief that loss of brain cells inevitably causes cognitive problems for older people. However, the relationship between the brain and cognitive functioning is complex and cognitive decline is not inevitable. This area is discussed further below.

Disease and illness

Older people are more likely to suffer from acute and chronic illness than younger people. Data from the General Household Survey (GHS, 1993), which is conducted by the Office of Population Censuses and Surveys, indicates that at any one time 15% to 18% of over 65s are suffering from an acute condition, whereas the rate for other adult age groups is below 15%. The rate of accidents, injuries and poisoning is particularly high for older women, with falls, broken bones and medication toxicity all playing a part.

Over 60% of the over 65s have a chronic condition, with arthritis being the most common, affecting approximately 20% of people, followed by heart disease, hypertension and back trouble.

Widowed people and those from less favourable socioeconomic conditions are more likely to have a long-term limiting illness.

In discussing the impact of illness, a distinction may be drawn between *impairment* (damage), *disability* (functional limitation resulting from impairment), and *handicap* (limited capacity to function due to an interaction between disability and the environment). Many of those with a degree of impairment suffer no disability unless tested to the limits of competence. Where impairment starts to cause disability, many older adults may change their routine – for example by substituting a less strenuous sport for one that arthritic knees cannot manage. It is possible for a small degree of disability to cause handicap. Surveys have shown that problems in bending and stretching cause old people to have trouble with such varied tasks as cutting their own toenails and changing their curtains. Where disease cannot be cured, handicap can often be reduced through a prosthetic environment.

The fear that impairment will lead to dependency is a major worry of older people. For those who do become very disabled or dependent on others, this has a considerable impact on the self and on relationships with others. One of the aims of modern medicine is not so much to lengthen life but to reduce or compress morbidity, disability and handicap so that a good quality of life may continue to be enjoyed into very old age. Coping with chronic illness will be reviewed further below. Sidell (1995) provides an excellent overview of health in old age examined from a psychosocial perspective.

In Western society, death has become a feature of old age. In 1987, 79% of all UK deaths occurred over the age of 65 years. Coming to terms with mortality has therefore become a task of middle age or later life.

Social aspects of ageing

For many people in British society, the status of being 'old' in the eyes of the state comes abruptly with their sixtieth or sixty-fifth birthday when they retire from work, and become entitled to an old-age pension. This change, as is the case for many transitions, has a number of aspects, each of which demands adjustment. There is a loss of routine and structure to the day and the week, as well as the loss of work-related activity. Individuals have to construct for themselves alternative purposes for getting up in the morning and new ways of using their time. There is also an impact on the rest of the household. In the case of current older generations, it was often the case that the husband worked and the wife looked after the house. On retirement, the husband may feel at a loose end, but the wife still has all her usual chores to do and may find that her husband is always 'under her feet'. If the husband tries to help, he may not do things to the wife's standards and therefore runs the risk of criticism; or he may give the wife the impression that he is trying to take over. For most couples this is a period of adjustment. It often results in a shift to a greater degree of sharing of household tasks, and as gender roles become less distinct there is said to be more androgeny. There are also financial aspects to retirement, as income is reduced, limiting lifestyle possibilities for many.

In addition to these practical aspects, retirement may mean a change in status, particularly for those whose identity has been closely linked to their job, either because it carried a high status, commanding respect from others, or because the status of being the 'breadwinner' carried kudos of its own. The individual may need to adjust to this change in self-image and may suffer a temporary lowering of self-esteem.

Retirement is possibly the major social adjustment task of the 'young-old'. For those who have good health and adequate material provision, the period following retirement can be a period of high life satisfaction. Within this period, individuals may pursue ambitions or interests that were held in check during years of employment. For those with grandchildren there may be a period where they are able to help working sons and daughters with childcare. Others turn to voluntary work as a way of feeling useful and contributing to society. It has been suggested that, in many ways, the concerns of this period have more in common with middle age than with the older old.

In the seventh, eighth and ninth decades, those who survive are likely to lose many of their contemporaries through bereavement. This may lead to a smaller social circle, a loss of deep-rooted friendships and a sense of isolation and loneliness. It is also a constant reminder of mortality.

A substantial minority of older people provide care for a frail, elderly spouse. This is a role that often carries physical and emotional demands and can be stressful, resulting in psychological or physical morbidity for a proportion of caregivers.

Many older people will have to adjust to the death of a spouse. This is a major loss that often demands a lengthy period of grieving and readjustment (discussed further below).

Cognitive aspects of ageing

Lay views

The lay person's concept of the impact of age on intelligence has two contrasting aspects. On the one hand we associate old age with wisdom, usually picturing a sage as a wise old man with a flowing white beard. On the other hand, one of the myths of ageing is that it leads to an inevitable decline in cognitive functioning. Shakespeare is often used as a source of quotations demonstrating this, for example, in *As You Like It* where the state of old age is described as 'sans eyes, sans teeth, sans everything'. As we will see, research bears out both these views to some extent, showing that although there is extreme decline for some, there is maintenance and possibly growth of intellectual function for the majority of well, elderly people.

General intelligence

The majority of psychological studies of cognitive functioning in adult life have used a psychometric approach, in which standardized intelligence tests or tests of 'primary mental abilities' are administered to those of various ages. The most common test used is the Wechsler Adult Intelligence Scale (WAIS) or its predecessors (Wechsler-Bellevue) or successor (WAIS-R or WAIS-III). The WAIS contains 11 subtests, of which six (information, comprehension, vocabulary, arithmetic, similarities and digit span) are grouped together to yield a verbal intelligence quotient (IQ) and five (digit symbol, picture completion, block design, picture arrangement and object assembly) are grouped to give a performance IQ. It was developed in the United States of America but also has British norms.

The early cross-sectional studies of age differences in performance on intelligence tests supported the pessimistic lay view that cognitive functioning shows a decline from age 25–35 onwards. As reviewed under the heading of methodology above, there is reason to believe that these studies fail to separate the influence of differences between the generations from the impact of ageing, thus over-estimating the decline that occurs due to age.

Longitudinal studies, by contrast, show a picture in which IQ continues to increase into the fifth decade of life and to be maintained at least into the sixties. This more promising picture is too optimistic because most of the studies tested those with higher educational levels, and therefore the results cannot be generalized to the whole population.

Specific abilities

There have been attempts to distinguish between those functions that 'hold up' with age and those that 'don't hold'. In general, the cross-sectional studies show a differential decline on the WAIS between performance and verbal intelligence, with verbal intelligence peaking later and declining less slowly than performance intelligence. In making sense of this R.B. Cattell (1971) and Horn (1982) proposed that the difference was due to a contrast between *fluid* and *crystallized* intelligence. Fluid intelligence is described as the ability to solve novel problems quickly and accurately. It is often viewed as being an innate capacity. Crystallized intelligence, on the other hand, involves recollecting and using information acquired through education and experience. Older people show more decline in abilities that rely on fluid intelligence, whereas crystallized abilities are maintained or continue to grow and develop into later life. In clinical situations, functions that hold up well in the face of ageing, such as reading or vocabulary, are often used to give an index of pre-morbid functioning.

One of the most thorough studies of the various mental abilities across adult life is the cross-sequential study known as the Seattle Longitudinal Study, referred to above (Schaie, 1990). The major factors studied were verbal meaning, inductive reasoning, spatial orientation, numerical ability and word fluency.

The results show that, on average, these abilities are maintained through to 60 years, with the exception of word fluency, which shows a decline. Following the age of 60 years there is a significant average decline in every ability for every seven-year period. However, this average decline is accounted for by a small number of individuals who show a marked fall in performance, whereas the majority continue to maintain their abilities. So, for example, 1.1% of the sample showed a decline in all five abilities between the ages of 67 and 74 years, and 2.3% between 74 and 81 years. Over 80% maintained or improved on three or more of the five abilities between the ages of 67 and 74 years and over 75% between 74 and 81 years.

In terms of cohorts, there is evidence that inductive reasoning, spatial abilities and verbal meaning have improved across the generations from the 1889 birth cohort through to the 1959 birth cohort, though in the latter two areas this improvement has now levelled off. Numerical ability initially improved but has shown a steady decline since the 1924 cohort, and verbal fluency has shown little change.

Memory

The effect of age on memory deserves special attention because it is commonly believed that memory fails with age, and memory is clearly affected in the minority of older adults who have a dementia. The picture from research in this area is fairly complex but has been summed up by Bromley (1990) in the following succinct sentence: 'A useful practical assumption is that all learning and memory functions are impaired by ageing to a lesser or greater degree, but that steps can be taken to minimize these effects'. Memory is not a unitary entity; there are different types (verbal, visual, spatial or semantic and episodic), different time spans (sensory, short-term (primary), long-term (secondary), and remote) and different processes (registration, encoding, retention and retrieval) involved.

Older people show little difference from younger adults in sensory memory – very short-term memory for sensory images. Short-term memory is usually tested by span (for example digit span or word span). The example often used to demonstrate short-term memory is that of remembering a telephone number from the directory long enough to dial it. If the number is too long it cannot be remembered without writing it down, as the short-term memory store is limited. If the number has to be remembered beyond a few seconds it must be rehearsed or it is forgotten. Short-term memory shows little ageing effect, although older people are less likely to spontaneously 'chunk' a string of digits or words, so they may not use their memory span as effectively as younger adults. If any additional demand is made upon short term memory, for example by asking the participant to manipulate information or by including some distraction, then performance is poorer among those over about 60 years of age. A number of explanations have been suggested for this, including the possibility that there is a decrease in the capacity of working memory.

When attention is examined, older adults are found to have well-preserved sustained attention, commonly examined through a vigilance task. However, large age decrements are found in selective attention (i.e. the ability to maintain attention in the face of distraction) and divided attention.

The largest changes related to age are found in long-term memory. Long-term memory processes are invoked whenever material needs to be retained for a longer length of time than is possible in short-term memory – any time longer than about a minute. Older adults appear to encode information less effectively than younger adults. Whereas younger adults spontaneously organize material to be remembered, for example grouping words into categories, older adults do not. The depth of processing also appears to be shallower among older adults, who are more likely to try to commit material to memory through simple repetition rather than, for example, examining the meaning of the material and its connection with previous knowledge. In addition to less effective encoding, retrieval is also poorer among older adults, who have difficulty recalling information, but perform better on recognition tests.

Remote memory – memory for 'public' events of past years – is hard to test in a valid manner, but it shows no obvious decline with age.

There is considerable evidence to show that older people can improve the effectiveness of their short-term and long-term encoding when they are given instruction and practice in using strategies for organizing information.

While we usually think of memory as relating to past events, prospective memory or remembering what needs to be done in the future, is of great practical importance for day to day functioning. Evidence suggests that prospective memory is well preserved in later life. Those older people who do best appear to rely on external rather than internal cues to help them to remember.

Finally, in this section, we will look at semantic and episodic memory. Semantic memory refers to memory for facts and information. This is an integral part of crystallized intelligence, so it is no surprise to find that semantic memory is well preserved in later life. Episodic or autobiographical memory is hard to research. However, it has been shown that older adults are actually slower to produce reminiscences, and that these are often less detailed in their content. Events from early childhood have often been recalled and recounted many times and such 'memories' have been shown to change and develop over time.

Speed

About half of the age difference in cognitive functioning in tests of fluid intelligence has been shown to be due to older people being at a disadvantage in timed tests. The slowing of performance may be partly a result of peripheral factors, because conditions such as poor eyesight and arthritis may have an impact. It is also influenced by a basic slowing in reaction times. Ageing has consistently been found to affect the speed with which a person responds to a stimulus (simple reaction time). *Complex reaction time* is also slower, with the degree of slowing increasing proportionately with the complexity of the choice. Practice reduces the amount of lag but still does not produce a performance as fast as that of younger people.

Physical health

It is hard to disentangle the impact of ageing per se from the impact of poor health. Cardiovascular disease, for example, affects more people in older age groups, and has been shown to be related to reduced cerebral blood flow, which in turn is related to poorer cognitive function. Physical exercise, which increases cerebral blood flow, has been shown to improve reaction time in older adults. It is important, therefore, that we recognize factors that correlate with age and that offer a more satisfactory explanation of cognitive decline than age itself.

A further issue is related to the increased incidence of brain pathology in older adults, with cognitive functioning being drastically affected in the

5% of over 65s who suffer from dementias. However, the relationship between brain pathology and intellectual functioning is not clear cut. Minor or moderate atrophy, for example, does not necessarily affect cognitive competence and the changes due to ageing do not appear to be part of a continuum with the severe decline due to dementia.

Terminal drop

The Seattle Longitudinal Study was able to show that decline in intelligence tended to be step-wise and sudden rather than gradual. There is evidence to suggest that this type of critical drop is associated with increased mortality in the young-elderly.

Concept of intelligence

In discussing the impact of ageing on intelligence it should be noted that the concept itself is centred in the ideas of educational success and occupational selection. Thus it is focused on development in the early part of life. Tests often stress the type of information and skills that are emphasized during formal education. The relevance for the older population of this particular way of measuring intelligence may be questioned. Older people may be at a disadvantage in these tests because it is longer since they received their formal education. In addition, particular non-cognitive factors, such as motivation, may influence their performance because they perceive the tests as silly or irrelevant. Some psychologists have questioned the pertinence of the juvenile base of intelligence in adult life. Schaie (1977/8) proposes a model of adult cognitive development containing five stages. Whereas the stress in childhood and adolescence is on acquisition of knowledge, in later life he proposes that it is on re-integration of knowledge related to interests, attitudes and values held. Knight (1986) proposes that, as part of maturity of cognitive function, many older adults achieve a stage of *'post-formal' cognitive functioning*. This is seen as being a level beyond Piaget's final stage of formal operations and is characterized by an ability to see and weigh both sides of an argument simultaneously, as well as to take the moral dimension of decision making into account.

The psychological tasks of later life

This review of physical and social life events shows how much human beings have to adapt to in later life at a time when their cognitive resources may not allow the flexibility to adapt easily to novel situations. Until fairly recently, this area was ignored by developmental psychologists who viewed childhood and adolescence as the times of life when development set the path for the future, with subsequent decades being stable and fairly sterile.

However, in recent decades the picture has begun to change, so that there is an interest in 'lifespan development', which includes adult years as well as childhood, and old-age psychologists have generated frameworks for understanding the developmental challenges of later life.

Baltes and Baltes (1990) propose that successful ageing needs to be judged by a range of indicators, including length of life, state of biological and mental health, cognitive efficacy, social competence and productivity, personal control and life satisfaction. In this model there are factors that tap the physiological and social changes of ageing, and also the degree of adaptation to them, measured through life satisfaction and personal control. Individual status can be judged against these indicators according to what is normative for the age group.

Others have more explicitly picked out the areas that demand psychological adjustment, including Havighurst (1972) who listed six *developmental tasks* to which the individual must adapt in later life. Many of the life events discussed above are encompassed within them. The six tasks are:

* adjusting to decreased physical health and strength;
* adjusting to retirement and reduced income;
* adjusting to death of spouse;
* establishing an explicit association with one's age group;
* adopting and adapting social roles in a flexible way;
* establishing satisfactory physical living arrangements.

Erik Erikson (1963, 1982) proposed that eight stages of development can be identified across the lifespan, with each stage being identified by a conflict that must be resolved for satisfactory adjustment to be achieved. The final conflict identified, which occurs in old age, is prompted by awareness of life being finite and the end drawing near, and is that of *integrity versus despair.* The attempt to resolve this conflict involves a process of life review and coming to terms with the life that has been lived. Individuals who blame themselves for lack of fulfilment or who realize that they no longer have time to make amends for past errors may fall prey to despair. However, most individuals will come to accept the achievements, and failings of their life, with this process bringing about 'ego integrity'.

Peck (1968) developed Erikson's theory, proposing that there are three conflicts to be resolved in later life. These are ego-differentiation versus work-role preoccupation (referring to adjusting to the loss of work status), body transcendence versus body preoccupation (referring to adjusting to bodily and physiological ageing) and ego transcendence versus ego preoccupation (adjusting to mortality).

The remainder of this chapter will present what we know about how old people do develop and adapt.

Emotional adaptation in later life

Disengagement or activity

It has been variously proposed that it is most appropriate and helpful to wellbeing for older people to disengage from life, or to continue with a high level of activity. Disengagement may be described as a withdrawal from roles and responsibilities that were previously held. The proponents of disengagement theory (Cumming and Henry, 1961) proposed that disengagement occurs as a universal phenomenon in old age, and consists of an internally driven, intrapsychic process in which individuals voluntarily withdraw from their investment in the wider world. This allows more time for life review and contemplation prior to the end of life.

Disengagement theory, however, can be criticized in a number of ways. The disengagement of many older people is not of their volition but is imposed by circumstances. So, for example, retirement from work removes roles of responsibility, children leaving home or grandchildren living in a geographically distant location automatically reduces the involvement in roles of parent and grandparent. Physical limitations, such as impaired mobility, vision or hearing may reduce the possibilities for outings and interaction with others, against the wishes of the ageing person. Taken to the extreme this view can present an unattractive image of passive, inactive older adults patiently waiting for death. Psychological studies have tended to show that it is only a minority of people who are content with disengagement, particularly where this is imposed rather than sought.

The 'activity theory' of ageing provides a completely alternative perspective to disengagement theory – that in order to have a high level of life satisfaction it is important for individuals to maintain active involvement with life. This might involve finding alternative activities following retirement or if hobbies are ruled out by physical or mental limitations, and making alternative friendships if close friends are lost through bereavement. This view carries some validity, as engagement with activity has been consistently found to be associated with wellbeing. However, if crudely applied it can also lead to unattractive outcomes, if professional workers or well-meaning relatives make an assumption that any activity is better than none, even if it is meaningless or does not appeal to the person in question. The stereotype of old people's clubs or ward activities involving bingo and singalongs does not appeal to all! Choice and control are important factors that influence whether or not activity contributes to quality of life.

The Kansas City Longitudinal Studies looked at levels of activity and their connection with life satisfaction among people in their seventies (Neugarten et al., 1968). From their studies they drew up eight categories reflecting the various combinations that emerged between level of activity and level of life satisfaction. They were able to label these to show eight different types of personality, within three categories, as shown in Figure 18.1:

Category	Personality type	Level of activity	Level of life satisfaction
Integrated	Reorganizers	High	High
	Focused	Medium	High
	Disengaged	Low	High
Armoured/ defended	Holding on	High	Moderate
	Constricted	Moderate	Moderate
Passive/ dependent	Succourance seeking	Moderate	Moderate
	Apathetic	Low	Moderate
Unintegrated	Disorganized	Low	Low

Figure 18.1: Kansas City Longitudinal Studies, eight personality types.

Their findings indicate that high levels of life satisfaction can be found among people who are highly active, substituting new activities after retirement (reorganizers); those who are moderately active, with one or two main hobbies (focused) and among people who are disengaged, having chosen to give up roles and responsibilities, though the latter were a small minority. The 'armoured/defended' types have tried to adapt to ageing by either desperately clinging on to their middle-aged lifestyle (holding on) or by withdrawing so as not to be confronted with failure, yet continually dwelling on what they had lost (constricted). Their life satisfaction is only moderate, possibly indicating that high levels of activity, without adaptation, or premature disengagement through defensiveness may both lead to reduced levels of wellbeing. Those described as 'passive/dependent' also attain a moderate degree of life satisfaction, though this seems to depend on reliance on others. In the 'succourance seekers' this appears to be a strategy adopted in later life, whereas those who are 'apathetic' have perhaps never been very actively engaged. The unintegrated personality type described a small percentage of people who were having difficulty functioning in the community, possibly due to early dementia.

So this is an example of a study that demonstrates that the relationships between activity and life satisfaction are complex. The individual needs to have the flexibility to adapt to changes of ageing, and although disengagement may suit some, purposeful activity is often more satisfying.

The role of life review

Despite the mixed findings regarding disengagement, a number of studies of personality in later life have shown that older people may spend more time on reflection, becoming more inward looking with age – they are described as having greater *interiority*. This fits with Erikson's view of the major developmental task of later life, and connects with studies of the part that reminiscence plays in the lives of older people.

Coleman (1986) in a longitudinal study of reminiscence, found that he could divide the older people he interviewed into four groups. Firstly, there were those well-adjusted, satisfied individuals who enjoyed talking about pleasant memories of the past. These people are perhaps close to the stereotype of the elderly person who likes to tell stories. Their repetition of the past may serve to reinforce personal identity and self-esteem. Secondly, there was a group that was also well adjusted but that spent little time looking back at the past. These were mainly very old people and it is possible that they had come to terms with their past lives, achieving the state of ego-integrity described by Erikson. Thirdly, there were a number of people who spent time mulling over troubled memories of difficult events in the past. These people appeared to be trying to resolve problems and may benefit from therapy that includes life review. Finally, there was a small group of people who avoided thinking about the past because it was too painful.

Thus, as with activity, there is no simple result to say that reminiscence is a good or bad thing for older people. However, age does appear to bring more reflection, with its nature and function depending on the nature of the memories and the current context of the individual.

Other personality changes

The body of research on personality in old age shows that, for the most part, there is continuity, with traits established in early adulthood persisting into old age. Age brings a time when long-established reactions and ways of problem solving may no longer be appropriate because of changes in circumstances, but personality is more likely to be adapted rather than radically changed.

Some general trends have, however, been found in addition to that of greater interiority mentioned above. Eysenck (1987) using his well-known framework of the three traits of *psychoticism* (P – the degree to which a person is emotionally cold), *neuroticism* (N) and *introversion-extraversion* (E) found that older men showed a large decline in P, bringing their scores down to a similar level to women, who also showed some decline with age. Men and women tended to be more introvert at greater ages, but this decline was greater in men, who began at higher levels of extraversion, crossed over with women in middle age and, on average, were more introverted than women in later life. Both men and women showed some decline in neuroticism.

It is tempting to see this as a psychogenic process. However, it is easy to overestimate the concrete nature of personality traits. Although people may be consistent enough in their responses across a number of settings to be described as having certain personality traits, nevertheless it is also the case that individual responses vary according to context. It is therefore possible that the general changes in personality measures with age reflect a typical response to some of the social changes that take place in later life.

Coping style

There has been an increasing amount of work in recent years on coping style, seeking to establish whether particular ways of coping are more adaptive than others (for example, Lazarus and Folkman, 1984). Coping styles have been divided into active and passive. Active or problem solving coping styles are those which try to address the stressor and make it less stressful, by changing the environment to prevent it occurring, or by changing the way it is viewed to find it less distressing. Passive or emotion-focused coping styles do not address the root of the problem, but address the emotions that result from it. This could be, for example, by voicing distress to others or by drinking to lessen tension. It has been found, across many situations, such as coping with stroke and illness, that problem-focused coping tends to be associated with better adaptation than emotion-focused coping.

Many older people, however, may face situations that are not easy to alter. In some circumstances they may be left with little alternative than to accept events that occur. A cross-sequential research study carried out in Germany (Brandtstädter and Baltes-Götz, 1990) demonstrated that, during middle age and later life, events were perceived as being less within the control of the individual than in younger age groups, and the lack of perceived control was more likely to be correlated with feelings of depression or resignation. To adapt to this, older people appeared to adopt a more accommodative (accepting) and less assimilative (problem-focused) coping style. The accommodative style may actually be more helpful for those who have to adapt to inevitable events than active coping, which may feel like banging one's head against a brick wall and therefore causes frustration.

Coping with specific events

The sections above indicate that, in order to achieve satisfactory development in later life, the individual needs to adapt to the various life events and changes that so often occur. The process of adjustment may be facilitated, for many individuals, through:

• flexibly adapting level and type of activities to compensate for social and physical changes;

- adopting active coping styles where change is possible;
- accommodating to events where they are inevitable;
- looking back to resolve and accept what life has brought.

These elements may be applied to many of the events of ageing, such as the onset of disability and coping with loss. However, there has been more specific work on the impact of some of the major events of later life and this will be briefly reviewed below.

Disability

There has been a considerable amount of research in this field particularly over the past two decades, with some focused on particular diseases such as stroke, Parkinson's disease or arthritis. In reviewing the literature, Sidell (1995) proposes that a number of common issues emerge as being the major psychological consequences of illness. These are:

- coping with the loss of self – the impact on one's self-concept;
- disrupted biographies – in other words, the fact that personal and family life are interrupted;
- the problem of finding meaning – working out the answer to 'why me?'
- dealing with uncertainty and unpredictability;
- and the sense of isolation that may come about because of disrupted relationships.

Work on the best ways of coping with illness fits with the description in the section on coping above. Sidell (1995) reports, for example, on a study by Williams (1990), investigating how older Scottish people viewed coping with disability. He found three active strategies, all of which led to positive adaptation. These were carrying on as normal, using determination to struggle against illness, and adjusting activities to the restrictions of illness. There were two passive and accepting strategies. One was viewing illness as a loss to be endured and the other was looking on illness as a release from effort. These produced more negative emotions, but where acceptance played a large part, bitterness was avoided. These findings connect well with the studies of personality types and ageing, as well as with the work on activity and disengagement.

Social support is a further important factor in helping people to cope with chronic illness. It may be difficult to maintain because the illness itself may change the dynamics of relationships. However, there are suggestions that having an intimate, confiding relationship enhances health and wellbeing, and that social support may act as a buffer against the effects of stress by giving individuals social resources to draw upon to help them to cope.

Caregiving

Where an older person becomes disabled and needs to rely on another for care, then if the person is married this nearly always falls to the spouse, whether this is a husband or wife. Research in this area has burgeoned since the 1980s and there have been many studies showing that providing care for a frail, elderly relative is stressful, with psychological morbidity occurring in approximately a third of caregivers. One model by Pearlin et al. (1990) suggests that the degree of wellbeing of the carer depends on the amount of *primary strain* (that caused by providing care), *secondary role strain* (the knock-on effects of caregiving on other roles), and *secondary intrapsychic strain* (impact on self-esteem, sense of control and mastery) taking into account also the influence of context (nature of relationship, previous history) and coping resources (internal and external). Those who cope with least damage to wellbeing would be expected to be those who have effective ways of reducing the strain, perhaps through the adoption of an active coping style in a setting where there is good social support.

Bereavement and loss

As seen in the sections on changes in biological, social and cognitive spheres during ageing, there can be many losses in later life, including bereavement, loss of job, income, health and home. Studies of various losses have shown a typical pattern of emotional reaction, which is perhaps best illustrated through an account of Murray Parkes' (1972) definition of phases in the reaction of women to the death of their spouses. He described an initial phase of numbness, in which the individual is unable to take in the loss and feelings are dominated by shock and disbelief and accompanied by physiological arousal. This may be followed by a period of yearning, during which the person longs for the deceased to return, and remembers the deceased with painful intensity. Bereaved people may have vivid dreams or hallucinations of the deceased, and may find themselves searching for them. Emotions in this phase are of intense sadness. A third phase is that of disorganization and despair, during which the bereaved person is coming to terms with the fact that the deceased person will not return. There may be feelings of anger towards the dead person for abandoning them or towards professionals for not saving them. There may be feelings of guilt as the survivor turns over what they could have done to save the deceased, or regrets words said or not said during their lifetime. Finally, there is a phase of reorganization, during which the emotions of attachment become less intense and the deceased can be remembered with less pain and more pleasure. The bereaved person is able to pick up the threads of life again and may be able to develop trusting and close relationships with others.

The process of recovery from a major bereavement may take one to two years, although it is hard to generalize. Not all individuals will move neatly through the phases highlighted by Parkes; they may go to-and-fro between various stages, or miss phases out altogether. This type of model should not therefore be rigidly applied as a yardstick for 'normal' grieving. Nevertheless, *stage and phase* frameworks for bereavement provide a useful description and show that many unusual experiences can be part of a normal reaction to loss.

Worden (1991) describes the process of grieving from the active perspective of 'grief work' and describes the bereaved person as having to complete four tasks in their adaptation to loss. Firstly, they must acknowledge that the loss is real; secondly they must go through the pain of separation; thirdly they must learn to live without the deceased and lastly they need to be able to reinvest in new relationships.

Facing death

As stated above, death in modern Western society has become an event of old age. Coming to terms with mortality is something that all elderly people face. Research shows that by the time they reach old age, many people have become familiar and comfortable with the idea of life ending. However, people fear dependency, pain and loss of dignity during the process of dying. Much of the work in this area has examined how people cope when faced with a diagnosis of terminal illness such as cancer. Through her extensive work with dying people, Kübler-Ross (1969) proposed that those who are facing death move through five stages of reaction, not too unlike those experienced by the bereaved. This similarity is not surprising if one conceptualizes dying as facing major loss. The stages she described were denial, anger, bargaining, depression and acceptance.

Bringing it all together

This chapter has reviewed the main findings in the psychology of later life. It has looked at a definition of old age, and at the methodological issues that must be borne in mind when investigating ageing. It has then reviewed the main biological, social and cognitive changes, before moving on to look at some of the theoretical frameworks for understanding psychological reaction and development in later life, as the individual adjusts to these life changes. The chapter then reviews what is known about emotional adjustment and coping in later life. From this review it is apparent that old age is a challenging time, but not a time when quality of life and adjustment are inevitably poor. This chapter will conclude with two models that attempt to draw all these threads together.

Baltes and Baltes (1990) put forward seven propositions to summarize the nature of human ageing from a psychological point of view. All these can be recognized from the text above. The seven propositions are:

* there are major differences between normal, optimal and pathological ageing;
* there is much heterogeneity (variability) in ageing;
* there is much latent reserve;
* there is an ageing loss near limits of reserve;
* crystallized intelligence and technology can offset age-related decline in fluid intelligence;
* with ageing the balance between gains and losses becomes less positive;
* the self remains resilient in old age.

Examining this position, the authors propose a model of 'selective optimization with compensation'. The process describes an element of selection – that is, flexibly adapting and focusing interests and activities to fit with the limitations imposed by changes. Secondly, it adds a process of optimization – that is, engaging in a way of life that makes the most of possible capacities, through taking care of physical and mental health. Thirdly, the process of compensation refers to the need to compensate when impairment leads to disability, through technological means (such as a hearing aid) or psychological means (such as learning better encoding strategies). This model is put forward as a strategy that would lead to successful ageing.

Alternatively, Bob Knight (1986), one of the major contributors to thinking about therapy in later life, puts forward the contextual, cohort-based, maturity, specific challenge model. Although this is quite a mouthful, it embodies the major findings of the psychology of later life. Firstly, it recognizes the importance of two background factors – context – both political, economic and cultural – and cohort – reminding us that every generation has experiences of its own that shape its particular response to ageing. Then it brings in the wisdom of experience that ageing can bring by highlighting maturity. This refers to the various ways in which experience can overcome adversity and limitations. Finally, the specific challenge is a reference to the many life events that impinge on later life, encouraging us to identify, for any one individual, which specific challenge is facing that person at a particular time.

These two models provide convenient ways of summarizing the psychology of later life, giving frameworks that are both realistic and optimistic in their view of the potential we all hold to cope with the challenges of later life.

References

Baltes PB, Baltes MM (1990) Successful perspectives on successful aging: the model of selective optimization with compensation. In PB Baltes, MM Baltes (eds) (1990) Successful Aging: Perspectives from the Behavioural Sciences. Cambridge: Cambridge University Press.

Brandtstädter J, Baltes-Götz B (1990) Personal control over development and quality of life perspectives in adulthood. In PB Baltes, MM Baltes (eds) (1990) Successful Aging: Perspectives from the Behavioural Sciences. Cambridge: Cambridge University Press.

Bromley DB (1990) Behavioural Gerontology: Central Issues in the Psychology of Ageing. Chichester: John Wiley & Sons.

Cattell RB (1971) Abilities: Their Structure, Growth and Action. Boston: Houghton Mifflin.

Coleman PG (1986) Ageing and Reminiscence Processes: Social and Clinical Implications. Chichester: John Wiley & Sons.

Crandall RC (1980) Gerontology. A Behavioral Science Approach. Reading MA: Addison-Wesley.

Cumming E and Henry W (1961) Growing Old: The Process of Disengagement. New York: Basic Books.

Erikson EH (1963) Childhood and Society (2 edn). New York: Norton.

Erikson EH (1982) The Life Cycle Completed: A Review. New York: Norton.

Eysenck HJ (1987) Personality and ageing: an exploratory analysis. Journal of Social Behaviour and Personality 3: 11–21.

General Household Survey (1993) London: Office of Population Censuses and Surveys.

Havighurst RJ (1972) Developmental Tasks and Education (3 edn). New York: McKay.

Horn JL (1982) The theory of fluid and crystallized intelligence in relation to concepts of cognitive psychology and aging in adulthood. In FM Craik and S Trehub (eds) Aging and Cognitive Processes. New York: Plenum.

Knight B (1986) Psychotherapy with Older Adults. Beverly Hills CA: Sage.

Kübler-Ross E (1969) On Death and Dying. New York: Macmillan.

Lazarus J, Folkman S (1984) Stress, Appraisal and Coping. New York: Springer.

Neugarten BL, Havighurst RJ, Tobin SS (1968) Personality and patterns of aging. In BL Neugarten (ed.) Middle Age and Aging. Chicago: University of Chicago Press.

Parkes CM (1972) Bereavement: Studies of Grief in Adult Life (2 edn). New York: International Universities Press.

Pearlin LI, Mullan JT, Semple MA, Skoff MM (1990) Caregiving and the stress process: an overview of concepts and their measures. Gerontologist 30: 583–94.

Peck RC (1968) Psychological developments in the second half of life. In BL Neugarten (ed.) Middle Age and Aging: A Reader in Social Psychology. Chicago: University of Chicago Press.

Schaie KW (1977/1978) Toward a stage theory of adult cognitive development. Aging and Human Development 8: 129–38.

Schaie KW (1990) The optimization of cognitive functioning in old age: predictions based on cohort-sequential and longitudinal data. In PB Baltes and MM Baltes (eds) Successful Aging: Perspectives from the Behavioral Sciences. Cambridge: Cambridge University Press.

Sidell M (1995) Health in Old Age: Myth Mystery and Management. Buckingham: Open University Press.

Williams R (1990) The Protestant Legacy: Attitudes to Death and Illness Among Older
    Aberdonians. Oxford: Oxford University Press.
Worden JW (1991) Grief Counselling and Grief Therapy: A Handbook for the Mental
    Health Practitioner. New York: Springer.

Part Three:
Social Psychology

Chapter 19
Social psychology

GUY CUMBERBATCH and PAUL HUMPHREYS

Key concepts	Key names
Attitude measurement	
equally appearing intervals	Thurstone
summated ratings	Likert
semantic differential	Osgood
attitude–behaviour difference	La Pierre
Cognitive consistency	
balance theory	Heider
cognitive dissonance	Festinger
Persuasive communication	
message learning approach	Hovland
cognitive response approach	Greenwald
elaboration-likelihood model	Petty and Cacciopo
heuristic–systematic model	Eagle and Chaiken
Self	
the self	James
self recognition	Lewis and Brooks-Gunn
naive psychologists	Heider
correspondence theory	Jones and Davis
covariation model	Kelley
Leadership	
social power	Raven
contingency theory	Fiedler
path–goal model	House
attributional model	Pfeffer
obedience	Milgram
conformity	Sherif, Asch
de-individuation	Zimbardo

(contd)

(contd)

Key concepts	Key names
Crowd and mob	
contagion theory	Le Bon
emergent norm theory	Reicher
Discrimination	
stereotypes	Lippman
prejudice	Elliot
Aggression	
frustration	Dollard
catharsis	Freud
ethology	Darwin, Lorenz
social learning	Bandura
media violence – sleeper effect	Heusman
coercive behaviour	Patterson
Altruism	
bystander apathy	Latane and Darley
social exchange theory	Thibaut and Kelley
reciprocity	Gouldner
selfish gene	Dawkins

This chapter covers some key areas in social psychology. According to a classic definition by Allport (1985), social psychology represents 'an attempt to understand and explain how the thought, feeling and behavior of individuals are influenced by the actual, imagined or implied presence of others' (Allport, 1985: 3). As such it embraces a wide number of issues to be found in psychology but will always include some idea of other people even if this is so broadly conceived as to include cultural influences on the individual such as through the mass media.

Attitudes

Since Thurstone (1928) published his seminal paper 'Attitudes can be measured', the study of attitudes has become a cornerstone of social psychology (Eagly and Chaiken, 1993) and indeed a very big business supported by numerous organizations that routinely survey public opinion and beliefs. The study of attitudes in some shape or form pervades decision making by governments and commerce and, with the increasing accountability required in the public sector, it is an important facet of the health professions. Arguably, some of the central issues that psychiatrists face in their work are essentially to do with the attitudes of people who present with deviant behaviour. This section can only touch the surface of some aspects worth considering.

First of all, what do we mean by 'attitude'? The concept of social attitude seems to have been first introduced by Thomas and Znaniecki (1918) to explain the striking behavioural differences between Polish farmers in Poland and Polish immigrant farmers in the USA. However the concept of attitude goes back a long way in art to describe the arrangement or pose of figures that has frozen the behaviour captured by the artist. This meaning continues today in dictionary definitions that include the technical term 'attitude of an aircraft', which refers to the direction in which it intends to go. Thus the idea of attitude has long been linked with the idea of behavioural consequences.

Although a rich concept like attitude cannot be simply summarized, perhaps the classic definition is that by Gordon Allport (1935) who described it thus: 'An attitude is a mental and neural state of readiness, organized through experience, exerting a directive or dynamic influence upon the individual's response to all objects and situations with which it is related' (Allport, 1935: 198).

A further classic account of attitudes by Secord and Backman (1964) synthesized the various interpretations offered by researchers. They suggested that most approaches to the study of attitudes included three components:

- a cognitive component: what someone believes about the attitude object;
- an affective component: what someone feels about the attitude object;
- a behavioural component: how someone will behave towards the attitude object.

They suggested that behaviour will be a function of both the cognitive and affective elements.

This idea is useful in suggesting that beliefs are somewhat narrower than attitudes in that they are centrally about the cognitive part of attitudes such as knowledge and information (however distorted these cognitions may be). Values are more about liking and preferring as in the affective component. Allport defined a value as 'a belief upon which a man acts by preference'. Various other related terms such as 'ideology' (a stronger form of belief) can be seen to emphasize different aspects of the attitude concept. Today there is a general agreement with Eagle and Chaiken (1993) that the core feature of attitudes is that they are essentially evaluative: 'Attitude is a psychological tendency that is expressed by evaluating a particular entity with some degree of favor or disfavor' (Eagle and Chaiken, 1993: 1).

Measuring attitudes

Although Thurstone (1928) is often credited with inventing attitude measurement, various quite elaborate techniques were developed during the 1920s. Thurstone himself devised a number of ways of measuring attitudes, perhaps the most famous of which is the *method of equally appearing intervals*. The method is quite time consuming but in essence it is simple enough. The researcher draws up a large pool of around 100 attitude statements that vary in terms of how positive or negative they are towards the attitude object. Examples from Thurstone's own research on attitudes to the church include: 'I believe the church is the greatest institution in America today' (a very positive statement) and 'I think the church is a hindrance to religion for it still depends upon magic, superstition and myth' (a very negative statement).

A group of judges then classifies each attitude statement about the attitude object by sorting them into 11 piles from 1 = very positive to 11 = very negative. Statements on which judges disagree are discarded as unreliable measures and the final pool of statements is selected to represent each of the scale points. It is this final pool that makes up the attitude scale where respondents have simply to indicate the statements with which they agree. The attitude score of each respondent is then calculated by adding up all the 'agree' statement scores using the mean (average) rank position that the original judges gave to the statements.

Today the most popular method is the so-called *Likert scale* or *summated ratings scale* (after Likert, 1932). Here the judging stage of the Thurstone technique is abandoned and a pool of attitude statements is offered to respondents to rate how much they agree or disagree with each attitude statement. The rating scales are typically from 1 to 7 with the extremes being strongly disagree and strongly agree, but there are numerous variations such as using an even number of response categories to avoid a midpoint and thus forcing respondents to decide one way or another. In practice, too, the number of response categories can be reduced to 3 or 4 or even stretched well beyond 7 when each scale number would not receive a description, and merely the end points labelled as a bipolar scale. An example would be:

'I think this book chapter is really interesting.'
Strongly agree – 1 – 2 – 3 – 4 – 5 – 6 – 7 – Strongly disagree.

We might hope that readers would pick 1 (or possibly even 2).

Apart from the greater simplicity of Likert scales, they are more convenient when researchers wish to explore attitudes to a range of attitude objects. Thurstone-type techniques were developed to explore attitudes to only one attitude object (originally the Catholic Church). The weakness of Likert scales is that strictly speaking statistically they are not scales since the difference between a scale 2 and a scale 4 is not the same as between 4 and 6, which is the problem that Thurstone's methods attempted to overcome.

Perhaps one of the most intriguing and subtle methods used to measure attitudes is Osgood's *semantic differential* (see, for example, Osgood, Suci and Tannenbaum, 1957). Osgood contributed two books on the subject of meaning: one on the meaning of meaning, the second on the measurement of meaning. He argued that words we use have two meanings. One is the semantic or *denotative meaning*, which will be found in a dictionary. The second is the *connotative meaning*, which is how someone feels about the word. These connotative dimensions can be tapped by asking respondents to rate the words using adjective pairs called *bipolar adjective scales*, such as

Good – 1 – 2 – 3 – 4 – 5 – 6 – 7 – Bad.

In measuring attitudes, researchers usually focus on evaluative connotative meanings such as how good/bad, desirable/undesirable, pleasant/ unpleasant the word is. However, Osgood shows how when words are rated using a variety of descriptors, the results point to three connotative components: an *evaluative component* (for example, good/bad), a *potency component* (for example, powerful/weak) and an *activity component* (for example, fast/slow). The technique can be dramatically illustrated by asking a respondent to rate, using a series of bipolar scales, first of all 'poison' and then 'honey' – they tend to have very different connotative meanings. Of course individuals will vary in the connotative meanings attached to significant others such as 'my father' and this has helped the development of the technique in clinical settings. Indeed, Osgood first demonstrated the value of the tool with the famous case of multiple personality studied by Thigpen and Cleckley (1957). Osgood concluded that the 'three faces of Eve' reported by Thigpen and Cleckley were, in fact, quite unstable and predicted later personality changes that eventually appeared. In this field, Osgood's books are essential reading.

At first sight the development of attitudes must seem to depend on experience, but the distinction between attitude formation and change is not easily made. Attitudes tend to develop as part of larger attitude constellations over time and are reinforced by the social groups to which individuals belong. Thus, by and large, attitudes tend to be resistant to change as we will see later in examining attitude change and as we can begin to understand by exploring the idea of cognitive consistency.

Cognitive consistency

One of the earliest and still influential proponents of the view that cognitive consistency is a strong human motivation was Heider (1958) whose balance theory has origins in gestalt psychology. He argued that people seek harmony in their values, attitudes and beliefs. More than this, people tend to evaluate things that are related in similar ways and prefer relationships that fit well together. He emphasized the 'sentiment relationship', which people seem to show to objects in their social worlds. Thus, when a friend (whom we like) does something we do not like, we have a balance problem that we can resolve in numerous ways. A commonly observed phenomenon would be to disbelieve or distort what the friend actually did.

This idea was also developed by Abelson in his model of *symbolic psycho-logic* (for example, Abelson et al., 1968). They explored more widely how people deal with imbalance to include the important notion that people can even deny that two inconsistent categories are related. Thus liking ice cream and wanting to slim could lead to a denial that ice cream was part of the part of the category of weight gaining foods.

In the research literature more attention has been given to the varying consequences of attitude imbalance rather than the less puzzling phenomena of attitude consistency. In this field, theories of cognitive dissonance dominate.

Cognitive dissonance

Festinger (1957) pioneered *cognitive dissonance theory*, demonstrating, through a series of elegant experiments, some surprising consequences of the psychological discomfort that cognitive imbalance can cause. The classic experiment is that of Festinger and Carlsmith (1959) where participants were required to perform exceptionally tedious motor tasks for an hour. They were paid either $1 or $20 for their efforts. On leaving they were asked if they would tell the next participant (actually a confederate of the researcher) waiting outside that the experiment was 'very enjoyable' or 'fun'. Later Festinger and Carlsmith in apparently unrelated research were able to measure the attitude of the original participants in the experiment. Those who had been paid $1 to participate and lie about how interesting it was, rated the experiment as more interesting than those who had been paid $20. Festinger concluded that this shows that the cognitive dissonance caused by lying was resolved by the $20 dollar group by reasoning that it was financially worth it, but the $1 group could only justify their lie by persuading themselves that the experiment was interesting. As the authors conclude, it may sometimes be easier to buy people's beliefs with $1 rather than $20. There has been a considerable research literature stimulated by cognitive dissonance theory but the basic idea can be traced back at least to Aesop who, in his fables, describes a fox that, after repeated attempts to gather some sweet-looking grapes just out of reach, turns away concluding that they were probably sour anyway! Denigrating what we cannot achieve is certainly one way of achieving cognitive consistency.

Persuasive communication

The above sections have introduced some ideas relevant to understanding attitude change and the problems faced in persuasive communication.

Certainly we may expect that merely urging people to change is not likely to be effective and yet this is still the approach taken in many health education messages.

A major development in persuasive communication research took place in North America during World War Two for various reasons. On the one hand, German propaganda orchestrated by Goebbels was manifestly impressive. On the other, the United States quickly discovered that few Americans were enthusiastic about laying down their lives for a distant war. Thus Carl Hovland at Yale University was commissioned to orchestrate a large research programme for the war effort, supported by a number of prominent social psychologists. Their various studies (for example, Hovland et al., 1949) entered the public arena mainly in the post war era, for obvious reasons. Hovland concluded that the distinction between effective and ineffective communications can be understood in terms of what he called the *message learning approach*. Here attitude change is dependent on three factors: on people paying attention to the message, on people comprehending the message and people accepting the message. The Yale team carried out an evaluation programme of various 'propaganda' in terms of who says what to whom, by what means and with what received meaning. They identified four factors as important: *source factors* (notably the credibility of the communicator); *message factors* (notably that the message was comprehended); *receiver factors* (where intelligence and education can increase message learning but reduce yielding to the message); *channel factors* (face-to-face communications were more effective than mediated ones).

Further understanding of individual differences in susceptibility to persuasive communications was offered by Greenwald (1968) who suggested a *cognitive response approach* where recipients are seen as more active processors of information, relating the messages to their own beliefs and feelings. He used a *thought-listing technique* where recipients list all their thoughts and ideas about a topic, which independent judges then rate in terms of how positive and consistent they are with the persuasive communication.

Petty and Cacciopo (1986) use the term *elaboration* to refer to the extent to which a recipient thinks about issue-relevant arguments in a message. This *elaboration-likelihood model* emphasizes that such thinking provides a *central route to persuasion* that is likely to be enduring. However, even when unable or unwilling to comprehend a message, recipients can still be influenced to a lesser extent by the attractiveness or credibility of the communicator (the *peripheral route to persuasion*).

A very similar approach was offered by Eagle and Chaiken (1993) in their *heuristic–systematic model*. As above, the idea is that people may scrutinize arguments engaging in systematic processing (for example, I understand and believe what my doctor tells me), or accept the message according to peripheral aspects, which they called heuristic processing (for example 'doctors are good people, therefore I believe what my doctor says'). However they also draw attention to the motives people may have in information processing. People may have an *accuracy motivation* for unbiased processing. However they may also have a *defence motivation* to confirm the validity of their own position or even an *impression motivation* to express attitudes which are socially acceptable.

The above models perhaps begin to challenge notions that persuasive communication is usually effective. We may remember too that Festinger's model of cognitive dissonance predicts that people would tend to avoid communications with which they disagree (a somewhat controversial issue in the research literature). However it is clearly the case that the journey from persuasive communication to influencing attitudes and changing behaviour may well be a long one.

Attitudes and behaviour

Although we might expect some consistency between attitudes and behaviour, this is quite controversial. The classic study that cast some doubt on the attitude–behaviour relationship was that by LaPierre (1934). At a time of anti-Chinese sentiment in the United States, LaPierre travelled the country for two years with two Chinese friends. He was somewhat surprised at the level of courtesy they received in hotels and restaurants. In fact out of 250 establishments visited they were refused service only once – in a small autocamp. This experience inspired a novel experiment where LaPierre wrote to all the hotels and restaurants in the regions that they had visited asking if they would accept 'members of the Chinese race as guests in your establishment?' Fewer than 1% replied 'yes' (92% said 'no' and 7% were undecided). Moreover one half of the replies were from establishments that they had actually visited and where they had received such courtesy. Of course, discrimination by letter is obviously easier than in a face-to-face situation, the Chinese couple were middle class and did not conform to the prevalent pigtail stereotype of Chinese people, those who replied were the managers and not the staff who served LaPierre, and so on.

In a review of 42 studies examining how well attitudes predict behaviour, Wicker (1969) concluded that 'it is considerably more likely that attitudes will be unrelated or only slightly related to overt behaviours than that attitudes will be closely related to actions'. However this view may be unduly pessimistic if the attitudes measured are not ones relevant to actual behaviour and even less so if the behaviour is not voluntary.

Fishbein and Ajzen (1975) pioneered a new approach to the attitude–behaviour controversy in their *theory of reasoned action*. They suggested that our attitudes as evaluative feelings are only part of the equation. *Subjective norms* about what people who are important to us think will also be important. Finally, attitudes and subjective norms will combine to influence our *behavioural intentions*. A later development of the theory was to include some measure of *perceived behavioural control* – how much a person feels capable of achieving the behavioural intentions (Ajzen, 1991). Known as the *theory of planned behaviour*, this approach has been used successfully in predicting a range of real-life behaviours, including safe and unsafe sexual practices in the age of AIDS.

It seems clear that the attitude–behaviour controversy was fuelled as much as anything by a failure to achieve specificity matching between the specific predicted behaviours and the attitudes, which tended to be measured quite generally (Ajzen and Fishbein, 1977; Fazio, 1995). Moreover, Festinger and Carlsmith's 1957 study of cognitive dissonance demonstrated that the behaviour that people engage in may determine their attitudes. This may well have stimulated the idea that attitudes can arise from observing our own behaviours – a view developed by Bem (1972) as self-perception theory.

Functions of attitudes

Attitudes tend to be fairly resistant to change and one reason for this is to be found in the various functions that they seem to serve for people. Katz (1960) suggested that they serve four main functions:

- an ego defensive function, protecting our self-concept;
- a value-expressive function, providing a sense of self-expression and personal integrity;
- an instrumental function, providing us with social approval from important others;
- a knowledge function, summarizing the world for us.

Thus any understanding of attitudes needs to be informed by an understanding of what they mean to individuals in a social world where the 'self' is an important concept. This concept is explored in the following section.

The self

Definitions of the self

Throughout history, philosophers and poets have written of the 'self' to describe the stable inner core of our nature. It has been taken to represent our perception of our personal identity, our uniqueness and our consistency, our beliefs and all that makes us the people that we are. However the concept is, as we shall see a little later, more complex than this, with both stable and variable components. The term is also most often used as a prefix (for example, self-esteem, self-image, self-presentation) and thus takes on a number of different forms and meanings.

The concept of the self was introduced into psychology by the first great American psychologist, William James. In his pioneering book *Principles of Psychology* (1890) – still in print over a century after it was first published – James argued that the self has two components, the 'I' and the 'Me'. He regarded the 'I' as the inner self or the perceiving self – our sense of our awareness and existence. The 'Me', on the other hand, may be regarded as our social selves – the many different faces that we display or allow others to see. An analogy would be the 'I' as an actor, the 'Me' as the parts (s)he plays (Gross, Humphreys and Petkova, 1997).

We do, of course, have many 'Me's. James wrote: 'A man has as many social selves as there are individuals who recognize him and carry an image of him in their minds' (James, 1890: 294).

He believed these social selves (or 'Me's) could be placed into the following categories: the spiritual self, the material self, the social self and the bodily self.

One of the most widely published contemporary social psychologists is Michael Argyle, Emeritus Reader in Social Psychology at Oxford University. He contended (1994) that there are four dimensions of the self:

- The self-image. This contains 'some enduring aspects and others which vary with the situation and the role being played'. It contains a 'core' (for example, body image, sex, age, identity) and the roles played by the individual in a characteristic, individualized manner.

- Self-esteem. This is how a person judges himself or herself: either absolutely or relatively (compared with others). It is the value we place upon ourselves. Needless to say, the outcome of the evaluation will be different on different occasions in our lives (for example when we feel we are loved by someone, when we are depressed) and it will depend heavily upon with whom we are comparing ourselves, upon specific situations, and upon role relationships.

- The ego-ideal. This is what we would ideally like to be and is often what we aspire to. Psychologists are often interested in the gap between the perceived self (self-image) and the ideal self (ego ideal).

- Integration of the self. This is concerned with the consistency of the different elements of the self.

- Argyle adds: 'This consistency may take various forms, depending on whether the self-image is based on the attributes of some person, on a set of ethical or ideological rules of conduct, or on an occupation or social-class role' (Argyle, 1994: 86).

Acquisition of the self

How do we acquire our sense of personal identity? This is a question of some considerable significance. As Miell (1990) puts it:

> to achieve a sense of self, one of the first things we need to be able to do is to perceive ourselves as having a stable, permanent identity. This begins with recognizing our own physical appearance – perceiving a stable physical identity – but this is not a straightforward process for a young child. (Miell, 1990: 32)

An ingenious series of experiments was carried by Lewis and Brooks-Gunn (1979) investigating this issue. They observed how children aged between 9 and 24 months of age acted when they were in front of a mirror and recorded the number of times the children engaged in mirror-directed behaviours (for example touching the mirror), self-directed behaviours (such as pointing to their own bodies), and imitation. These behaviours acted as a baseline for a later study: 'the red nose condition'.

In this experiment, mothers discreetly marked the infants' noses red (by wiping their faces with a cloth that had rouge on it). Lewis and Brooks-Gunn reasoned that if the children had developed a sense of self-recognition and personal identity, they would try to touch or wipe the red spot from their noses but, if they had not, then they would try to do this on the mirror. The results showed that for the children aged between 9 and 12 months less than 5% touched their noses compared with around 40% who touched the mirror (the remainder did neither). By 15 to 18 months the percentage touching the mirror had barely changed but now over 20% touched their noses. Finally, by 21 to 24 months more children (approximately 70%) were touching their noses than were touching the mirror (approximately 60%).

Miell summarizes:

> The observation of some self-directed behaviour across the age-range suggests that infants as young as 9 months show some, slight self recognition, with a steady development from this age in their ability to recognize their own images in detail. (Miell, 1990: 38)

So what is it that enables the children to recognize themselves? In a final study, Lewis and Brooks-Gunn separated out two important factors: physical appearance and movement. They gave 96 infants aged between 9 and 24 months three video presentations:

- a live image of themselves (physical image and movements the same as themselves);
- a video of themselves recorded a week earlier (physical image the same; movements different);
- a video of another child (both physical image and movements different).

The results showed that, even at 9 months, the infants were more interested in the live images of themselves than the other videos (measured by time spent looking, positive attitude and so forth) but it was not until 15 months that they displayed a preference for the week-old video of themselves rather than that of the other child. This suggests that it is not until this age that the child is able to consistently identify itself by physical appearance.

It is thus clear that the growth of the self is a fairly slow and complex developmental process.

Interpersonal issues

In the previous section we considered how we build up a stable and persisting sense of individuality, our self-concept. For many people, unfortunately, their self-perception lacks veracity and any real sense of reality. For example, it is well documented (Dobson et al., 1981) that anorexics perceive themselves as being fat and overweight even when they are practically skeletal. In this section we will begin by examining the insights that psychological research has given us into the way we perceive others, and will briefly examine some of the ways in which people suffering from various mental illnesses/disorders also make errors in their perceptions of others.

Person perception

The term *person perception* has been used within psychology to differentiate it from general perception (or more specifically, object perception). Person perception has several significant differences from object perception resulting from factors such as those offered by Gross (1996):

- people behave but objects do not;
- people interact with other people but we do not interact in the same way with objects nor they with each other;
- people perceive and experience but objects cannot.

To draw appropriate attention to the interaction emphasized above we will use the term *interpersonal* rather than person perception. This acknowledges the dynamic and interactional nature of the processes involved.

Cook (1971) defined *interpersonal perception* as: 'the study of the way people react and respond to others, in thought, feeling and action' (Cook, 1971: 2).

This draws our attention to different levels of activity. It informs us that interpersonal perception is cognitive, affective, behavioural and social. Cook identifies two general categories of psychological models or theories of interpersonal perception: *intuition theories* and *inference theories*. He argues that the former are categorized by an adherence to the following propositions:

- Perception is innate. As far back as 1764 Thomas Reid claimed 'Nature is so constituted that certain empirical facts are signs of certain metaphysical facts and *human nature is so constituted as to be able to be able to interpret these signs intuitively*' (our emphasis) (Reid, 1764: 33).
- Perception is global. In other words we perceive people as whole entities rather than making judgements about particular aspects of them (such as their honesty or intelligence). Spranger (1928) said that we understand people by 'an act of intuition encompassing their personality as a whole'.
- Perception is immediate or direct. This contends that there are no mediation or intervening activities between 'reception' and 'response'.

This model concords with the lay belief that some people are 'just better' judges of others than some other people. It is viewed almost as a gift that some of us are blessed with, and that others (sometimes almost totally) lack. Cook, however, clearly demonstrates that there is very little empirical evidence indeed to support the intuition theories.

The *inference theories*, on the other hand, have been well supported by research evidence. These theories state that, when perceiving others, we make use of knowledge we already hold about people and then apply this to a specific person. Cook summarizes it thus:

> The first proposition states a general principle about people. The second notes that the person under consideration has particular attributes and the third draws the inference that he has a further attribute. (Cook, 1971: 13)

Thus, for example, if I believe that most psychiatrists are intelligent people, and I meet Person A who is a psychiatrist, I judge that she or he will be intelligent. A good deal of the above deals with stranger perception. Let us now briefly consider two examples of human relationships where we build familiarity, intimacy and dependency: affiliation and friendship.

Affiliation

Cardwell (1996) says:

> Affiliation refers to the tendency for people to seek the company of others. It is also seen as a motivational variable in that people differ in their need to affiliate. People may affiliate for a number of possible reasons:
>
> - to avoid loneliness that may exist in the absence of a social network of friends and relatives.
> - to reduce anxiety, either because others provide a source of information that might reduce our anxiety, or because others provide emotional support.

- to gain attention, where people seek the company of others so that they might be the centre of attention. (Cardwell, 1996: 5).

The importance of affiliation is further emphasized by Hogg and Vaughan (1995) who say: 'The need to affiliate underlies the way in which we form interpersonal relationships. Most people need to be with and to interact with others' (Hogg and Vaughan, 1995: 400).

This is empirically supported by a study carried out by Trevarthen (1980), which demonstrated that infants as young as two months showed a desire to interact with their mothers, even via closed-circuit television! Psychologists such as Schaffer and Bowlby have shown how children seem to develop strategies such as crying, smiling and holding on to clothing to increase the likelihood of people they like staying in close proximity to them. Bowlby (1969) went on to argue that a denial of affiliative access can result in a failure to be able to form warm and secure attachment bonds.

Friendship

Argyle (1994) says:

> Friends can be defined as those people whom we like and trust, and whose company we enjoy . . . They don't just come in pairs, though; they form networks, with cliques and chains, which can be more or less dense, in terms of the proportion of possible links taken up. (Argyle, 1994: 62)

He argues that we derive three main sources of satisfaction from our friendships:

- Common interests (doing things together, talking about things that we believe to be interesting or important, sharing common beliefs and values).
- Social and emotional support. For example, friends are supposed to help each other out and support each other in social situations.
- Instrumental rewards (for example, 'getting strokes', being appreciated, having someone who values and appreciates us).

Insofar as psychologists have studied friendship as a motivational need in humans, it is thus possible to see it as a development out of early affiliation processes and desires. In passing we should note that, although friendship is accorded a high importance and salience in Western cultures, this is not always true of non-Western societies where kin and family are often seen as more significant and influential (Moghaddam et al., 1993).

People as 'scientists': naive psychology

Heider (1958) was the first psychologist to argue that all people are basically psychologists (albeit naive ones). Just as psychologists try to make sense of the human world and understand what makes us think, feel and behave as we do, so does everyone else! Nisbett and Ross (1980) put it thus:

> We are all psychologists. In attempting to understand other people and ourselves, we are informal scientists who construct our own intuitive theories of human behaviour. In doing so, we face the same basic tasks as the formal scientist. (Nisbett and Ross, 1980: 94)

Around the concepts of naive psychology and the layperson as a psychologist, Heider developed one of the most fruitful and stimulating ideas in social psychology. His insights into social perception stimulated a research field usually described as *attribution theory*.

Attribution theory

Studies of how people explain human behaviour and more generally make causal attributions about their world developed rapidly in the 1970s. The important point is that, in this role as naive psychologist, the lay person is busily engaged in trying to understand causation. That is to say, we not only observe things that happen around us – we endeavour to understand what caused it to happen. For example, do we explain a person's behaviour with reference to something 'within' them (for example their value systems, their motivations – an internal attribution)? Or do we explain it by something 'outside' them (for example a response to the behaviour of another person or some physical feature of their surrounding environment – an external attribution)? As Clarke (1996) puts it: 'An attribution is the process by which people use available information to make inferences about the causes of a particular behaviour' (Clarke, 1966: 9).

Imagine the following scene. In a crowded university lecture theatre, halfway through a psychology lecture being given by a visiting professor, a young student suddenly stands bolt upright and walks 'stormily' out of the hall. Attribution theory would predict that those observing the action would try to understand what caused her to do this by determining whether it is something to do with her ('she's easily offended', 'she's always doing something like that') – a *dispositional* attribution – or something to do with the visiting professor ('that was such a sexist and offensive thing to say', 'she clearly doesn't know that we just don't say those sort of things over here') or something to do with the immediate environment ('the person sitting by the side of her obviously has vulgar habits') – a *situational* attribution.

The two principal attribution theories, both based on Heider's pioneering work, are *correspondent inference theory* (Jones and Davis, 1965) and the *covariation model* (Kelley, 1967).

Covariation was a term introduced by Heider in his original formulation of attribution theory. The concept goes back to John Stuart Mill's outline of methods of induction, which provides the basis of scientific logic. One method of induction described by Mill to infer causality is the method of difference or covariation. Kelley developed this idea to suggest that perceivers need three kinds of information to make causal attributions. These can be illustrated:

- Consensus. For example 'does everyone says my dog Tasso smells foul?'
- Consistency. For example 'do they always say that Tasso smells?'
- Distinctiveness. 'Do they say other dogs smell?'

The answers to these questions were 'Yes', 'Yes' and 'No'. This allowed me to conclude that Tasso really was a smelly dog.

According to Jones and Davis the goal of the attribution process is to infer whether the observed behaviour corresponds to some underlying stable quality of the actor. The authors suggest that three factors are important in our attributions:

- Choice: was the behaviour freely chosen or coerced?
- Expectedness: is the behaviour typical or part of a social role that is expected?
- Effect: does the behaviour achieve many desirable outcomes or only one? If only one outcome is achieved it is easier for us to infer motive.

Attribution error

It is hardly surprising that people often reveal biases in their attributions. We tend to attribute our successes to our own ability and our failures to external factors. A commonly observed example is where teachers will claim credit for a student's academic success but will attribute a student's poor performance to the student's laziness. A common bias is to underestimate the role of situational factors in explaining the behaviour of others and exaggerate the importance of dispositional factors. This bias has often been described as the *'fundamental attribution error'* but the term 'error' is somewhat strong to refer to a judgement that is not actually wrong but merely biased.

Social behaviour and mental health

There is considerable evidence (Argyle, 1994) that many people suffering from mental health difficulties have severely impaired social skills. Social psychologists have demonstrated that the majority of us have no difficulty in deciding, for example, how close we should stand to the person we are interacting with (Hall, 1966), where we are allowed to touch specific others (Jourard, 1966) and how much eye-contact is appropriate (Argyle and Ingham, 1972). However, many patients seem unable to make and/or enact such judgements.

Argyle (1994) gives the following list of 'social failures' found in many patients:

- Non-verbal communication. Low levels of gaze and smiling; flat, tense or negative tone of voice.
- Conversation. Little initiation; cannot sustain conversation.
- Perception and judgement. Failure to perceive or interpret the behaviour of others correctly; inability to solve interpersonal problems.
- Social relationships. Inability to form or sustain relations with friends, family or others, through low rewardingness or other skill failures.
- Self-image. Low self-esteem; egocentricity, inability to take an interest in other people, empathize with them or see their point of view.
- Social competence. Low rewardingness and assertiveness; performance disrupted by anxiety or fear of negative evaluation; ineffective in social situations.

What is not currently known is the direction of causality: do people suffer from mental illnesses such as anxiety disorders or depression because (at least partially) of severely inadequate social skills? (Others might find it difficult and unrewarding to interact with them.) Or are the social failures a result of the mental disorder (or even a part of the particular disorder)? Almost certainly there is interaction between the factors, so that one exacerbates the others.

Unless we are of the opinion that what Argyle terms 'social failure' is completely unresponsive to experience and learning (for example is determined wholly genetically or by anatomical abnormality), and few psychologists are, then it should be possible to alleviate some of the difficulties by exposure or social skills training. Social skills training would typically include coaching in reading and displaying appropriate non-verbal communication skills, learning how to present oneself, taking the role of the other, analysing the requirements of situations that the patient finds difficulty in handling, and developing conversational skills (such as good listening and turn taking). The needs of individual patients will, of course, vary.

Does this training work? The answer is, it really does depend upon the specific type of mental disorder we are dealing with. It tends to be less successful with disorders that used to be termed 'psychoses' – especially where the aetiology is genetic – than with those previously termed 'neuroses'. (Both terms were dropped from the DSM (IV) and ICD (10). For more detail the reader is referred to Hollin and Trower (1986).)

Leadership and social power

Leadership has been one of the perennial research areas in social psychology. There has been a proliferation of theories and a good deal of research into what makes some of us socially influential to the point where others are drawn to do as we say or to follow our example. Perhaps this is because psychology has long been interested in individual differences between people, and this clearly stands out as a massive individual difference when one compares leaders who have influenced and often inspired whole generations of peoples (such as Jesus, Martin Luther King, Margaret Thatcher) with lonely isolated people whom the world seems to sadly pass by. Perhaps another reason psychologists have studied leadership is that most psychology is carried out in the West (particularly North America) – cultures predominantly characterized by an ethos of individualism as opposed to collectivism (Moghaddam et al., 1993). Arguably such research is funded to a political end because so much of it has been carried out on leadership in industry (Pennington, 1999) – for example what makes a good chief executive? what motivates a workforce? We will leave readers to draw their conclusions about this.

The ethnocentricity mentioned might well be taken to explain one of the most influential of the early studies of leadership, conducted by Lewin, Lippitt and White in 1939. They carried out a field experiment in which three different types of adult leadership style supervised groups of 10-year-old boys attending an after-school model-making club:

- autocratic, where the boys were told what to make and whom to work with;
- democratic, where the leaders discussed activities with the boys;
- *laissez-faire* where the boys were left to their own devices and the leader only intervened when asked to do so.

Clarke and Meldrum (1996) summarize the outcome thus:

> The results showed that boys in the democratic group were more satisfied, organised, independent and efficient than those in the other two groups. In the autocratic group they were more submissive and were aggressive toward each other when things went wrong, although the quality of work was equivalent to that in the democratic group. When the autocratic leader left the room, arguments broke out and work stopped. In the laissez-faire group very little work was completed whether the leader was present or not. By switching the styles of leadership . . . Lewin et al. were able to establish that it was indeed the style of leadership that was causing the different outcomes and not the personality of the boys or the leaders. (Clarke and Meldrum, 1996: 57)

Although this would seem to clearly indicate that one style of leadership is clearly preferable (for the followers) and more efficient, we should be mindful of generalizing to other situations. In particular we should note, as mentioned above, that North America is characterized by individualism and the country is an electoral democracy. The outcome may merely be mirroring the preferences of the culture in which the study was carried out.

Later studies, such as those by Bales (1953), have often concentrated on two different leadership concerns or emphases: task-centred leadership (getting the job done efficiently) and emotion-centred leadership (achieving a good working atmosphere and ensuring that the group is a pleasant and supportive experience). We will return to this when we consider what has been (at least according to Smither, 1988) the most influential contemporary leadership theory: Fiedler's *contingency theory*. But let us pause to define our terms.

What is leadership?

Leadership is usually understood as a process through which one individual in a group (its leader) influences other group members towards the attainment of specific goals (Yukl, 1989).

Notice that no mention is made of the size of the group (it could be a two-person group [a dyad] or a whole nation) or the longevity or nature of the influence. What is inescapable, however, is the notion of *social influence* or *social power*.

Raven (1993) argued that there are six types of social power. These are outlined in Figure 19.1. The reader may be interested in considering whether the forms of social power given in Figure 19.1 are generally located in the person (agentic) or are situational. For example, one psychiatrist may have *legitimate power* over another simply because of senior 'rank'. Referent power is more likely to be agentic.

Type of social power	Description
Reward	The leader has the capacity/resources to reward certain actions
Coercive	The leader is able to administer or threaten punishments for 'unacceptable' behaviours
Expert	The follower will allow him or herself to be influenced because they perceive the leader to have expertise
Legitimate	The leader has a position of formal authority
Referent	The follower identifies with the leader and consequently grants him or her influence
Informational	Information is used to influence or change the behaviour of a follower

Figure 19.1: Raven's six types of social power.

Theories of leadership

Smither (1988) contends that there are four models of leadership, each of which is characterized by many theories. These are as follows:

- *The personological model.* This holds that there are specific qualities or attributes in people that ensure they become leaders. The best known of these theories is the 'great man theory', or trait theory, which argues that some people are literally born to greatness and their special characteristics set them apart from their peers. The major problem is that there is precious little empirical evidence to support this notion (Pennington, 1999) and, at a common sense level, if one compares some 'great leaders' (for example Lenin, Hitler and Gandhi) it is immediately apparent that they shared very little in common (Gross, 1996).

- *The behavioural model.* This model contends that it is what leaders do that is important. The most important and influential theory, mentioned above, is Fiedler's *contingency theory* (Fiedler, 1967). Picking up upon the task/person orientations already noted, Fiedler developed a measuring technique based around people thinking of their least-preferred co-worker (LPC) (this does not necessarily tie the approach to a work situation – it could be used in a school or college for example). The person has to judge this LPC on a number of criteria (for example, tense/open/insincere/kind and the overall score determines the person's leadership style. Those who rate their LPC relatively highly are person oriented, those who rate them poorly are task oriented. The key for Fiedler, who believed that these leadership styles are largely fixed in any given individual, was finding the right match in style between leader and group. However, we should note in passing that research has shown rather low test/retest reliability between LPC scores from the same individual on different occasions (Rice, 1978), which strikes at the very heart of Fiedler's arguments.

- *The cognitive model.* These theories consider what leaders do to be relatively unimportant – it is what followers (actual or potential) make of them that is significant (beliefs and attitudes are the governing factors). Many of these theories focus upon how leaders can gain power by convincing followers that they can satisfy their needs and wishes (for example, House's *path–goal model*, 1971) but Bass (1981) extended the debate through his theory of *transformational leadership* in which he argued that highly effective leaders do more than this – they are able to actually change these wants and needs (usually to ones that they are able to deliver). A classic example in recent times was Margaret Thatcher's successful conversion of very many working-class families from home renters to home owners and in turning Britain into a nation of shareholders, both of which encouraged conservative values.

- *The social model.* Moscovici (1965) said 'If asked to name the most important invention of modern times, I should have no hesitation in saying it was the individual by which I take him to mean the freestanding, autonomous empowered individual' (Moscovici, 1965: 13). For example, Staub (1991) showed just how Hitler met the needs of a nation in crisis and the leadership he was given for providing this. In talk of leadership we should not fail to notice the importance of followership: at the risk of stating the obvious, one cannot have one without the other. Pfeffer (1977) put forward an *attributional theory of leadership*, which argues that in trying to make sense of events around us we try to attribute causation – put crudely, we try to decide who is responsible for the event we have just witnessed (such as a general election success – was it the new Prime Minister, the other politicians, a spin doctor or maybe situational factors?). Pfeffer argues that we are biased to explain leadership success of any kind (even Richard Branson's entrepreneurial achievements) in terms of dispositional characteristics of the person himself (or herself) and largely ignore the contributions of others and situational or circumstantial factors (such as being in the right place at the right time or just luck).

Obedience

Another way of looking at how one individual influences another is through obedience, literally doing as we are told or what we think we are expected to do. One of the all-time classic studies in social psychology was carried out in this field by Milgram (1963). The following synoptic account is based on Humphreys (1994).

The study, carried out at the highly prestigious Yale University, was concerned with the size of electric shock that a person would give another in the context of a study on the effects of punishment on learning efficiency. The participants were volunteers who had responded to a newspaper advertisement. Each was paid $4.50 in advance of taking part. They were tested one at a time and the experiment began with them being introduced to their 'partner' for the study (actually a stooge playing the part). A rigged draw took place, which assigned the genuine participant the role of teacher and the other that of learner. The 'learner' was strapped into a chair with electrodes attached to his wrist (the teacher was given a short, but painful shock as 'illustration'). The teacher was then taken to an adjacent room and seated in front of an impressive-looking (at least for the early 1960s) shock generator with a row of flick-down switches. Under each switch was an indication of the voltage, increasing in 15 V units from 15 V to 450 V. The teacher was told that every time the learner made an incorrect response on a paired-associate task he was to be given a shock and that the teacher should move up one switch (15 volts) every time.

In fact the learner received no shocks but the predetermined responses from the actor were extremely convincing. If the teacher indicated that he would not continue, the following 'prods' were given by the experimenter:

- 'Please continue'. 'Please go on'.
- 'The experiment requires you continue'.
- 'It is absolutely essential that you continue'.
- 'You have no other choice, you must go on'.

Approximately halfway through the escalation of shocks, the learner – who had previously warned them of a heart condition – suddenly became completely silent after violent screaming following the preceding shocks. The teacher was told to treat no response as an incorrect one and continue to increase the shocks.

What did Milgram find? In advance of the study he had asked staff and students to predict how many of the original 40 volunteers would continue administering the shock to the end (450 V). The student mean prediction was 1.2%; for staff it was 0.1%. The actual figure was 65% of participants giving apparently lethal levels of electric shock.

Conformity: the influence of the group

We are not only influenced by other individuals – we are often influenced by being a member of a group. This was demonstrated in a classic study by Sherif (1935), taking advantage of a visual illusion known as the autokinetic effect (a phenomenon where a stationary small beam of light viewed in total darkness appears to move). Sherif originally tested people individually, telling them that he was going to move the light and their task was judge the distance involved. After some initial variation, individuals tended to settle upon consistent answers. However the answers differed considerably between individuals. The light was not actually moving at all. Sherif then tested the people in small groups (usually three) and found that, after initial differences of opinion, the group members converged on a group norm but, once again, there was considerable variation between the different groups. Furthermore, when later tested individually again the members retained the group norm.

Asch (1952) believed that this conformity may have been due to the ambiguity of the stimulus and so tested participants in groups when on some trials all the other members (who were stooges) gave the same, wrong answer to a simple line comparison task (requiring them to state which line out of three given was the same length as the reference one). Despite the apparent simplicity and clarity of the task, participants gave the same (factually) wrong answer as the stooge group on one-third of the trials. Moreover three-quarters of participants conformed at some stage to the group influence, showing just how powerful this can be on a lone individual.

What happens in the group?

One possibility is that, as we saw in the Sherif study, group members may converge on a way of viewing a problem. Much work was carried out in the 1960s on ways in which groups tended to straightjacket the thinking of individuals (for example, Kretch, Crutchfield and Ballachey, 1962). Cardwell (1996) explores this further:

Groupthink is the name given to the tendency for certain types of groups to reach decisions that are extreme and which tend to be unwise or unrealistic. If the group is a highly cohesive collection of individuals with similar views on the subject under discussion, and they are cut off from alternative opinion, they are more likely to reach this highly polarized form of decision. Group members may ignore or discount information that is inconsistent with their chosen decision and express strong disapproval against any group member who might disagree. The eventual decision then appears to be endorsed by all. The social and political consequences of groupthink may be far reaching, and history has many examples of major blunders that have been the results of decisions made in this way. (Cardwell, 1966: 110)

Zimbardo (1969) wrote about the choice of independence or group-influenced behaviour following his participation (as one of the experimenters) in a field study named the Stanford University Prison Study. Students had volunteered to be either prisoners or guards in an unscripted mock-enactment of prison life. The allocation of role was randomly determined. The prisoners were 'arrested' by the local police who had agreed to do this to enhance authenticity and were taken to a local gaol that had been hired. Zimbardo and his colleagues settled back to observe what developed as the students adopted their roles. The results were so dramatic that the study had to be terminated before half of the predetermined time had elapsed. Guards had become so immersed in their role that they were putting 'prisoners' into solitary confinement, denying them blankets and bedding, even making them clean out lavatory basins with their bare hands.

Zimbardo explained this through *de-individuation*. The individual, hidden behind the uniform and the role, loses all sense of individual morality and responsibility. This notion of lack of rationality has an early psychological history in the writings of Le Bon (1895) on crowd and mob behaviour.

Crowd and mob behaviour

Le Bon proclaimed that 'Isolated a man may be a cultured individual; in a crowd he is a barbarian' and further that 'crowd behaviour [is an] irrational and uncritical response to the psychological temptations of the crowd situation' (Le Bon, 1895: 3).

He believed that there are several so-called *situational determinants* that operate when a crowd or mob assemble, these being:

* suggestibility: for Le Bon the 'conscious personality' disappears and the 'racial unconscious' takes over;
* social contagion: (see contagion theory, below);
* impersonality: in riots, attacked groups (such as groups of football supporters) lose their individual identity and simply become 'the enemy';

- anonymity: Le Bon believed that individuals lose themselves in a crowd and lose their own set of personal responsibility (see de-individuation, above).

McIlveen (1998) argues that three main psychological theories of collective behaviour (such as that characteristic of crowds and mobs) are *contagion theory*, *convergence theory* and *emergent norm theory*.

Contagion theory

The earliest exponent of this theory was Le Bon (1879/1895) – rationality is lost and it is as though the individual 'catches' the mood of the group, almost like an illness or disease. Empirical investigation of contagion has provided mixed outcomes. For example, Gergen et al. (1973) have shown that more prosocial and affiliative behaviours can occur when individuals 'lose' their personal identities in large groupings.

Convergence theory

This theory states that in a large grouping there can be a 'meeting of minds' as crowds facilitate a homogenization of beliefs and behaviours. Remember Sherif's study on conformity discussed above.

Emergent norm theory

As McIlveen puts it:

> One weakness of contagion theory is that it does not explain why a crowd takes one course of action rather than another. According to emergent norm theorists, contagion theorists are guilty of exaggerating the irrational and purposeless components of crowd behaviour. (McIlveen, 1998: 14)

Two studies that support this notion of the rational crowd are those by Marsh, Harre and Rosser (1978) and Reicher (1984). In the former, participant observation studies of football gangs suggested that their behaviour was far from mindless and 'randomly aggressive'. Behaviours appeared to be carefully orchestrated with clearly demarcated rules of acceptability and unacceptability. Moreover the football gangs were themselves characterized by adherence to a clear hierarchy of internal status and power. Reicher's study of the so-called 'race riots' which occurred in the St Paul's district of Bristol in 1980 once again showed a group acting with arguably some clarity of purpose. Riots broke out following what was perceived as further intolerable racial harassment of the black community by the police. However, as McIlveen once again neatly puts it:

> [the crowd] damaged only marked and suspected unmarked police cars, and did minimal damage to property. They also confined their behaviour to the St Paul's district and prevented any other forms of violence from taking place.

> For Reicher, the crowd saw the police's presence as illegitimate. The community members . . . behaved in a way they perceived as being legitimate given the police's presence. (McIlveen, 1998: 14)

Oscar Wilde once said that the intelligence of a crowd is not its average but its lowest common denominator. Perhaps, for once, he was wrong.

Intergroup behaviour

Sadly, if perhaps understandably, much of the work on the social psychology of intergroup behaviour has focused upon 'the dark side' of this aspect of human life. We will begin with the area that has probably been researched as much as, if not more than, any of these.

Prejudice and intergroup hostility

Prejudice literally means to pre-judge others – to form a judgement about someone without knowing all there is to know about them or without knowing everything about the situation in which we are making the judgement. Defined in this way all our judgements would be classified as prejudice. However, in psychology (and general understanding for that matter) this is clearly not what we mean. Cardwell (1996) identifies some of the main features in the following definition:

> As used within psychology [this term] means to 'prejudge' somebody on the basis of their membership of a particular category or group . . . Prejudices are specifically those prejudgements which are resistant to reversal when exposed to contradictory knowledge. Prejudice involves more than just having preconceived ideas about another person or group – it involves forming an evaluation of them . . . Prejudice can be either positive or negative, but . . . it is normally taken to mean a negative . . . attitude towards that person or group. Prejudice is usually maintained through stereotyping, the belief that all members of a particular group share the same characteristics. (Cardwell, 1996: 181)

Given this emphasis upon stereotyping, let us examine this process a little further.

Stereotypes represent the cognitive component of prejudice. The term was introduced to psychology by Lippman in 1922 who defined stereotypes as 'pictures in the head'. More recently, 1969, Taguiri described stereotyping as 'the general inclination to place a person in categories according to some easily and quickly identifiable characteristic such as age, sex, ethnic membership, nationality or occupation and then to attribute to him [sic] qualities believed to be typical to members of that category' (Taguiri, 1969: 326).

Gross (1996) argues that stereotyping involves the following reasoning:

- we assign someone to a particular group;
- we bring into play the belief that all members of the group share certain attributes (the stereotype itself); and

- we infer that this particular individual must possess these characteristics.

This is consistent with what Cook (1971) terms *implicit personality theory*, indicating that it is consistent with much of we do when judging others. What is particularly worrying is that stereotypes have been found to operate, even when the individual has had no personal contact with the groups that he or she may be asked to judge.

Gross (1996) notes that most of the 'concern' about stereotyping has been expressed in North America where everyone:

> is first and foremost American regardless of the country they might have come from or their ethnic or cultural origins. By contrast, European social psychologists, notably Tajfel, have been brought up in contexts where it was normal to categorize people into groups, where they expected society to be culturally diverse and where people were proud of their cultural identity. (Gross, 1996: 401)

This is reflected in the words of Brislin (1993):

> Stereotypes should not be viewed as a sign of abnormality. Rather, they reflect people's need to organize, remember, and retrieve information that might be useful to them as they attempt to achieve their goals and to meet life's demands. (Brislin, 1993: 104)

Discrimination?

Discrimination refers to the behavioural, as opposed to the cognitive aspects of 'pre-judging'. It may come about because of enactment of prejudicial beliefs such as the mass killing witnessed in Rwanda or the denial of certain job opportunities because of particular impairments such as visual or auditory ones that would not impede job performance. It may be the result of group pressure whereby fear of rejection by other group members is sufficient to cause an individual to display discrimination against a member of the outgroup. It may even be because of what psychologists call the 'just world hypothesis' – a belief that people get what they deserve in life (thus black people are given a hard time because they 'refuse to integrate').

Making prejudice, and making it go away again

We will look shortly at prejudice and discrimination in the real world, but let us first consider a most informative study carried out by a practising teacher, Jane Elliot, who wanted to demonstrate the ease with which prejudice can be created. One day she informed members of her class that blue-eyed children were inferior, and by the end of the day blue-eyed children were performing poorly at their work and were describing themselves as 'stupid' and 'bad'. At the same time the brown-eyed children had become vicious and discriminatory. A fight broke out because the insult of 'blue eyes' was thrown at one of the children.

The next day she informed the children that she had made a mistake and that it was brown-eyed children who were inferior. Within a matter of a few hours the situation had completed reversed. The next day Elliot told the children just what had happened.

Significantly, the children benefited greatly from this 'there but for the Grace of God go I' experience. When followed up 10 years later these children were more tolerant of group differences and strongly opposed to discrimination.

Attempts to reduce real-world prejudice and discrimination have proved to very largely unsuccessful (Coolican, 1997). Prejudice and discrimination are not always based on hatred and intolerance: *social identity* has also been shown to play a significant part. Tajfel's work beginning in the early 1970s on so-called minimal groups showed that even the most meagre and meaningless of ascription of participants into different groups (such as 'A' and 'B') caused them to act differently to each other (for example, regarding how rewards were to be distributed between the groups). Tajfel and Turner (1986) developed *social identity theory* which, coming out of minimal-group work, contends that people seek to enhance both their individual and their social identities. One of the ways that we do this is to denigrate the 'outgroup', viewing them as being in social competition with our own group(s). The competition may not be real – it rarely is. The social perceptions of in/outgroup boundaries and conflict over a scarce or significant resource are all that is required.

More recently, Pettigrew and Meertens (1995) have argued that we have moved from blatant to subtle prejudice. Blatant prejudice has become politically and socially unacceptable and, as a result, has transformed. Pettigrew and Meertens contend that whereas blatant prejudice was characterized by:

- perceived threat and rejection of the outgroup;
- opposition to close contact with the outgroup,

subtle prejudice (frequently identified by the opening remark of 'I'm not prejudiced but . . .') is characterized by:

- the defence of traditional values; and
- the exaggeration of cultural values; and
- the denial of positive emotions to 'others'.

To see racism as residing in prejudiced others, however, may be too comfortable. We should learn a lesson from history. According to Gross, Humphreys and Petkova (1997: 63):

> A classic demonstration of racism within psychiatry are the two diagnostic categories proposed by the American writer Cartwright in 1851. At this time of slavery, the diagnostic categories were meant to apply exclusively to black people:

(a) *Dysesthesia Aethiopis* was a disease which afflicted all 'free Negroes' without a white person to direct and take care of them, 'the natural offspring of Negro liberty – the liberty to be idle . . . wallow in filth . . . indulge in improper food and drinks'. Symptoms included breaking, wasting and destroying everything they handle, tearing or burning their clothing, stealing from others to replace what they have destroyed, and apparent insensitivity to pain;

(b) *Drapetomania* was, quite simply, the disease that caused slaves to run away.

Aggression

The particular form of social behaviour known as aggression has long interested psychologists. Indeed it has often been used to illustrate the nature versus nurture debate and as a way of introducing different levels of explanation in social psychology (for example, see Lippa, 1994). Most theoretical perspectives in psychology have some contribution to understanding aggression.

Definitions

A good working definition is that offered by Baron and Richardson (1994): 'Aggression is any form of behavior directed toward the goal of harming or injuring another living being who is motivated to avoid such treatment' (Baron and Richardson, 1994: 3).

This goes beyond a behavioural definition of an act of hurting/harming to include the intention to do so (thus excluding accidents or medical treatment, which might hurt). It also emphasizes the intention of the other person involved (thus excluding sado-masochist indulgences).

A major distinction is that between instrumental and hostile aggression. *Instrumental aggression* is aggression where the goal is not aggression but the achievement of something else (as in a street robbery). *Hostile aggression* has hurting/harming as the goal and is assumed to involve emotions such as anger and thus is sometimes referred to as *affective aggression.* To these we may add other distinctions such as predatory aggression, territorial aggression, maternal aggression, and so on. However, as an adjective, aggression often enjoys a less anti-social meaning (as in aggressive marketing) and in this context it is interesting to note the increasing use of the stronger term *violence* in discussions of 'aggression' (as in television violence).

Measurement

Measures of aggression vary considerably but principally involve attitude surveys and self-reported behaviour in field studies. Laboratory experiments have tended to rely either on the electric shock simulation equipment made popular by Milgram or on verbal reports.

Frustration

Perhaps the earliest attempt to achieve a unified theory of aggression was provided by Dollard and his colleagues in their *frustration-aggression hypothesis*. Dollard et al. (1939) attempted to synthesize the concepts of contemporary learning theory with Freudian notions. They suggested that *frustration* (defined as anything that blocks attaining a goal) always leads to an aggressive drive, which has the same strong functional status as an instinct. Once aggression has occurred, drive reduction takes place in a similar way to the satisfaction of other drives such as appetite. Dollard described this drive reduction as *catharsis* – the term Breuer and Freud (1895) had used. Finally they suggested that aggression may be *displaced* from the target to a safer one – as when the boss humiliates his clerk who shouts at his wife who yells at her son who kicks the dog who bites the postman.

Their book, which remains one of the most influential in the field, produced some convincing research evidence for the thesis. Miller (1941) showed children attractive toys. Half of the group was allowed to play with them immediately and the other half told to 'look but don't touch'. This frustrated group, when eventually allowed to play with the toys, did so more aggressively – often smashing the toys. Hovland and Sears (1940) showed that lynching of African Americans in the South increased when the price of cotton fell. They attributed this to economic frustration in white Southerners.

The main criticism must be that frustration does not always lead to aggression as Dollard insisted. However, it is more likely when the person believes that the hindrance was unfair or deliberate (Averill, 1982). The idea of catharsis has received little empirical support over the years, with rather more studies concurring with Darwin's (1872) observation 'He who gives way to violent gestures will increase his rage'. Thus Buss (1966) and Geen (1990) both concluded that people who are given the opportunity to aggress against someone who has frustrated them often become more aggressive and not less.

Ethological approaches

Ethology may be defined as the study of human behaviour from a naturalistic and evolutionary perspective. Beginning with Darwin in the last century, the field developed rapidly in the period after the Second World War, largely due to Konrad Lorenz whose research career began in the 1930s. His book *On Aggression* (1966) is probably the best-known and comprehensive ethological account of aggression, which he defined as 'the fighting instinct in beast and man which is directed against members of the same species'. Thus like Freud, Lorenz believed aggression to be instinctive, noting the particular stimuli which would elicit aggressive responses in different species from jackdaws to sticklebacks. Lorenz describes the *ritualization* of aggressive behaviour in most species, where antagonists may show threats and indicate defeat through *appeasement behaviour* without actually engaging in combat. Dogs and wolves will end a fight with the loser exposing its throat and jugular vein as an appeasement to the victor. This ritual nature of animal aggression controls behaviour to prevent animals destroying one another. However in humans Lorenz argues that such controls are weak. It is not so much that appeasement behaviour (for example begging for mercy) is not effective. It is more that the technology of aggression (such as guns and bombs) distances protagonists from one another so that appeasement rituals cannot be effective.

The pessimistic view of Lorenz that humans are naturally aggressive warriors has become tempered by a growing appreciation of cultural differences where hunter-gatherer behaviour is more evident than aggression. Here behaviour is essentially adaptive to the world and rarely shows the stereotyped patterns that so impressed Lorenz in the animal kingdom. The notion of instinct has also developed with the new sociobiology, which sees aggression as a potential rather than an inevitable aspect of human behaviour (Archer, 1992).

Arousal

In the face of rather limited support for the frustration-aggression hypothesis, Berkowitz (1969, 1989) attempted a major reformulation of the role of frustration. He suggested that if frustration did lead to aggression this was because it caused negative affect and that many other factors could also produce this, such as high temperatures and pain. More than this, physiological arousal and a bad mood does not necessarily result in aggression. This will depend on aggressive cues triggering aggressive behaviour. These cues may include anything associated with violence or unpleasantness. For example in one experiment, participants were allowed to aggress (deliver electric shocks) in the presence of either badminton rackets and shuttlecocks or a shotgun and a revolver. In the weapons condition, participants gave more electric shocks. As Berkowitz (1968) concludes: 'Guns not only permit violence, they can stimulate it as well. The finger pulls the trigger, but the trigger may also be pulling the finger' (Berkowitz, 1968: 22).

A closely related idea of *excitation transfer* was proposed by Zillman (1978, 1991). In this model, the physiological arousal caused by one stimulus can be transferred to a second stimulus. In one experiment, participants were either insulted or treated neutrally by the experimenter. Half of the groups then either engaged in strenuous physical exercise on a stationary bicycle or did not. Finally all participants were allowed to give electric shocks to the experimenter. The angered group who had engaged in the exercise gave the most shocks. This, Zillman concludes, demonstrates that the physical exercise 'energized' aggression in the group who had been angered. Similar effects were achieved with a wide variety of arousing stimuli such as loud noise, vigorous music, sexual scenes and violent movies (Zillman, 1991).

Operant learning

The pioneering work of Dollard et al. on frustration-aggression attempted to integrate contemporary approaches based on learning theory with older Freudian concepts. A central idea in learning theory was that reinforcement helped establish behaviour patterns. Any behaviour that is rewarded or reinforced in some way should be more likely to occur in the future. However research on *operant conditioning* revealed that the manner of the reinforcement was quite subtle, as shown by Walters and Brown (1963). In this experiment they rewarded children for hitting a doll. Half were rewarded each time they acted aggressively, the other half were rewarded only periodically. Both groups increased in aggressive behaviour. However when rewards were withdrawn, the group that had received irregular reinforcement continued to act aggressively for longer than the group that was continuously reinforced.

We may suspect that in the real world aggressive behaviour would receive irregular reinforcement, which may explain why it remains so persistent and stable over long periods of time within individuals. Some insights to this are provided by the Oregon Social Learning Center (Patterson, 1982; Patterson et al., 1984), which attempted to map the patterns of actions and reactions in families to determine factors encouraging aggressive behaviour. Not surprisingly, aggressive acts are quite common – as when one child hits another in order to stop annoying behaviour such as being teased. What is interesting is that roughly four times out of ten such aggressive behaviour is successful and thus could be said to receive *negative reinforcement* (the removal of a noxious stimulus).

Social learning theory

The Oregon Social Learning Center examined the development of aggressive behaviour in a comprehensive fashion. However *social learning theory* has a specific association with Albert Bandura (1973, 1986) and is more commonly referred to as *observational learning* or *modelling*.

In his pioneering research in the early 1960s Bandura began by studying imitation in young children. He wondered whether a teacher who was particularly nurturant would be more likely to be imitated than one who was less so. While this appeared to be the case with most behaviours modelled, Bandura noted that an 'aggressive' act performed by the models was imitated with equal enthusiasm regardless of the teacher. In the next experiment Bandura introduced a new toy – a Bobo doll, which is a child-size inflated clown with a weighted base which when struck will quickly bounce back up again. Five year olds were exposed to one of two conditions:

- either to an adult who played quietly with some Tinker toys
- or to an adult who after playing with the Tinker toys for a minute went up to the Bobo doll and began to kick it, punch it, hit it with a mallet while yelling 'sock him on the nose', 'knock him down', and 'kick him'.

After being exposed to the strange antics of the models, children were then frustrated. This was achieved by taking the children to another room, which contained some wonderful toys that they were invited to admire before being told they could not play with them because they were being 'saved for the other children'. Finally children were then led to a third room containing both Tinker toys and the Bobo doll where they were left to play. The children who had been exposed to the non-aggressive model played quietly, but those exposed to the aggressive model attacked the Bobo doll, imitating the model's behaviour and vocalizations.

Bandura believed that children can observe and learn aggression in many ways but the main sources are the family, the child's subculture and the mass media. In a series of experiments he replicated the earlier studies but used films of models behaving aggressively to conclude that film-mediated models were almost as effective as real life models in eliciting imitative behaviour.

Television

Bandura's experiments using film-mediated models stimulated a series of studies that replicated and extended his findings that children can readily learn from observing others. However part of the success in these studies is due to the novelty of the toys used. For example Kniveton and Stephenson (1973) found that children who were not familiar with the Bobo doll imitated five times more often than children who had previous exposure to it. An additional consideration must be that more naturalistic field studies of the effects of film and television have found that a wide variety of material can lead to an increase in aggressive behaviour. Such material includes *Sesame Street* and *Mr Roger's Neighborhood* – programmes designed to encourage prosocial behaviour in children (Gadow and Sprafkin, 1993).

It may be, as Zillman (1991) has argued, that the essential ingredient of film and television that encourages aggressive behaviour in the short term at least is the arousing property of the content rather than the violence as such. Thus any fast-paced programme might arouse children sufficiently to elicit a higher level of aggressive play.

This may be the explanation for many early laboratory studies of the effects of film-mediated violence on adolescents. For example Berkowitz in a number of studies compared the effects of a violent film (*Champion*) with a control film about canal boats to conclude that those who had been anger aroused were more likely to behave aggressively after seeing an aggressive film. Zillman and Johnson (1973) compared a violent film (*The Wild Bunch*), with a neutral film (*Marco Polo's Travels*) and with a no-film condition. Physiological measurement indicated that the neutral film depressed arousal compared with the no-film condition. Interestingly, when participants were allowed to aggress (by giving electric shocks) there was no difference between the violent film and the no-film condition, both of which produced more aggression than the neutral film.

As Howitt and Cumberbatch (1975) and Freedman (1984) have argued, the artificiality of laboratory studies of film aggression is a weakness and participants may guess what the experimenter expects or even desires. Such problems are less obtrusive in the various longitudinal studies that have been conducted. For example, Huesman and Eron (1986) orchestrated a cross-national comparison of the effects of television on aggression where children in six countries were followed up over a number of years. The researchers claim a Rip Van Winkle (or 'sleeper') effect whereby preferences for violent television programmes predicted later aggression. However the results were not significant in Holland, nor in Australia, nor in an Israeli kibbutz, nor for boys in America. In Poland, the authors note that the effects are small and 'must be treated cautiously'. Overall the results seem far less compelling than the authors claim (Cumberbatch and Howitt, 1989).

Contrary to expectations, Hagell and Newburn (1994) found that delinquents reported far less interest in film or television than a control group, had more difficulty nominating anyone on television they would like to be like, and named similar programmes as their favourites (popular soaps).

The issue of media violence is clearly a controversial one where understandable concerns about crime and violence in society make the mass media a too-easy scapegoat (Cumberbatch, 1994, 1995).

Family and social influences

A number of studies have tracked children over long periods of time in an attempt to predict the development of aggression. In reviewing the considerable literature, Smith (1995) notes that aggression has been found to be quite stable over the life course at least from the age of eight and is related to criminal offending later in life. However childhood aggression seems to predict both violent and non-violent offending, thus suggesting a possibly more general problem of anti-social attitudes and behaviour.

There is a consistent body of evidence (for example, Maccoby and Jacklin, 1980) showing pronounced gender differences in aggression and in offending behaviour. For example the Epidemiological Catchment Area Study (Robins et al., 1991) showed a lifetime prevalence of anti-social personality of 4.5% for males and only 0.8% for females. Similar gender differences are reported for offending behaviour across many cultures but here the gap has narrowed where for example the ratio was 11:1 male: female in 1957 reducing to 5:1 in 1977 since when it has remained quite stable.

Twin studies suggest a weak genetic contribution to offending behaviour (DiLalla and Gottesman, 1989). However Rowe (1983) using self-reported anti-social behaviour concluded a heritability factor of 70%. This may well be relevant to the developing child's socialization experiences whereby adolescent aggressive children will select deviant peers who will reinforce their aggression (Loeber and Hay, 1994).

As suggested earlier, Patterson (1982) has long maintained that family research has identified the effects of parental and family processes in the development of aggression. Risk factors include high levels of coercive behaviour, harsh and inconsistent discipline, weak supervision and an absence of positive parenting. Moreover, because of the limited opportunity to acquire prosocial skills, the child begins to assume coercive behaviour to be normative. As always, the evidence remains controversial regarding causal factors in the aetiology of aggression. We may agree on risk factors but how these operate in the dynamic of a child's socialization is less clear. One thing is clear – interventions need to begin at a very early age.

Helping behaviour

One striking feature of psychology is that it has tended to focus on the darker side of human nature and behaviour with the brighter aspects of life such as humour and laughter, music and love relatively neglected. And so it was with altruism, kindness and helping behaviour until recently.

Augustus Comte (1798–1857) provided a useful conceptual distinction between two forms of helping behaviour: egoistic helping and altruistic helping. The former is where someone wants something in return, the latter is only to increase another's welfare as given in the parable of the Good Samaritan who was 'moved by pity' (Luke, 10: 30–35). In practice the distinction may be less clear, as we shall see. Thus many writers prefer to categorize all altruism and helping research under a general heading of prosocial behaviour, which is defined as voluntary behaviour carried out to benefit another person (Bar-Tal, 1976).

Although research in this field did not begin with the murder of Kitty Genovese, she is one of the most frequently cited examples in reviews. As the *New York Times* reported (27 March 1964):

For more than half an hour 38 respectable, law abiding citizens in Queens watched a killer stalk and stab a women in three separate attacks in Kew Gardens. Twice the sound of their voices and the sudden glow of their bedroom lights interrupted him and frightened him off. Each time he returned, sought her out and stabbed her again. Not one person telephoned the police during the assault; one witness called after the woman was dead . . .

Two psychologists, Latane and Darley had arranged to meet over dinner and they discussed their own reactions to the case. By the time they had finished dinner they had begun to map out a research programme into the phenomenon of bystander behaviour. Their influential book: *The Unresponsive Bystander: Why Doesn't He Help?* (1970) captures one major conclusion. Latane and Darley's research involved staging various fake emergencies to investigate bystander behaviour. They concluded that there are a number of factors that will determine helping behaviour:

* Perception. People must notice the event – not all bystanders will.
* Definition. People must define the event as an emergency. In the case of Kitty Genovese, for example, one interviewee said 'we thought it was a lovers' quarrel'.
* Responsibility. Do people believe that they personally should do something? Perhaps not if there seem to be 37 other bystanders, some of whom might be better qualified to interpret the event and help. Latane and Darley speak of the *diffusion of responsibility*.
* Decision. People must decide what type of help is appropriate.
* Implementation/intervention costs. There are time and risk costs to helping. People need to evaluate the costs and rewards of helping before implementing a decision to help.
* Perhaps the most complex element in all of the above is the final one: 'shall I, shan't I?' Here the framework of social exchange theory is relevant.

Social exchange theory

Attempts to understand interpersonal relations have drawn on many metaphors. Social exchange theory draws heavily on economics combined with elements of learning theory (Thibaut and Kelley, 1959; Homans, 1974). The perspective has been simply put by Rubin (1973): 'We must face up to the fact that our attitudes to other people are determined to a large extent by our assessments of the rewards they hold for us' (Rubin, 1973: 39).

Thus, Homans (1974) speaks of the 'profits' in relationships that are a function of the rewards minus the costs. Blau (1964) describes social relations as 'expensive' in time, energy, commitment and so forth, and adds that we may hope to get more than we put in. It should be stressed that this pessimistic approach does not necessarily attempt to model how we rationalize relationships but rather attempts to explain patterns in those relationships.

In this model we may consider to what extent prosocial behaviour may be disguised by self interest. Clary and Snyder (1991) explored the reasons why people volunteer for tasks such as befriending those with AIDS. They identified six motivations:

- Knowledge: to understand people better and learn people skills.
- Career: to improve job prospects especially through 'contacts'.
- Social adjustment: to be part of a group and obtain social approval.
- Ego defence: to reduce guilt or escape from personal worries.
- Esteem enhancement: to build confidence and raise self-worth.
- Value expression: to support humanitarian values and demonstrate a concern for others.

Note that only the last of these approaches the idea of selfless altruism.

Altruism from empathy

Here it is worth remembering Abraham Lincoln's discourse on the issue of helping behaviour. After arguing that selfishness prompts all good deeds, he stopped the stagecoach he was travelling on to rescue some piglets that were in danger of drowning before their distressed mother. He explained his 'selfish' act thus: 'I should have had no peace of mind all day had I gone and left that suffering old sow worrying over those pigs. I did it to get peace of mind' (cited by Batson, 1991).

However empathy seems to be a natural 'instinctive' reaction to suffering. Hoffman (1981) notes that day-old infants cry more when they hear another baby cry and can stimulate a chorus of crying in a nursery.

Moreover helping is not the only 'selfish' solution: although the Good Samaritan helped, others who did not help quickly withdrew themselves from the scene.

Social norms

The evident variation in helping behaviour across cultures suggests that simple social exchange models are inadequate. Perhaps a basic and probably universal moral code is that of *reciprocity*: we should return help to those who have helped us (Gouldner, 1960). However, beyond this there are *norms of social responsibility* that different cultures develop (Berkowitz, 1972). This seems to have been the point in the Good Samaritan parable when Jesus asks: 'If you love those who love you, what right have you to claim credit?. . . I say to you love your enemies' (Matthew 5: 46, 44).

Pandora's box

As Montagu (1976) and Wrightman (1979) have argued, our view of 'human nature' is somewhat coloured by a large collection of pessimistic but influential writers. Darwin, in observing that man 'still bears the indelible stamp of his lowly origins', captured the idea of Tennyson's *In Memoriam* of 'nature, red in tooth and claw' where survival of the fittest would seem likely to drive out altruism. Like Konrad Lorenz, we remain fascinated by the violence of animals. Today we enjoy this in wild life documentaries and in crime programmes. However the reality is that such behaviour remains rare compared with the preponderance of cooperative, nurturing, helping behaviour in most animals.

The growing realization of this at first presented a paradox for evolutionary psychologists and ethologists. Why should an animal behave to benefit others when it may be replaced by others that act only to benefit themselves? Sociobiologists such as Dawkins (1976) provided one explanation – that natural selection operates at a genetic level and not that of the individual. However a more economical explanation might be that being selfish and anti-social is actually rather hard work, with quite uncertain outcomes. Basically, it is a lot easier to live being nice rather than being nasty. Now, doesn't that make treating anti-social personalities a little easier?

References

Abelson RP, Aronson E, McGuire WJ, Newcombe TM, Rosenberg MJ and Tannenbaum P (eds) (1968) Theories of Cognitive Consistency: A Source Book. Chicago IL: Rand-McNally.

Ajzen I (1991) The theory of planned behavior. Organizational Behavior and Human Decision Processes 50: 179–211.

Ajzen I and Fishbein M (1977) Attitude–behavior relations: a theoretical analysis and review of empirical research. Psychological Bulletin 84: 888–918.

Allport GW (1935) Attitudes. In C. Murchison (ed.) A Handbook of Social Psychology. Worcester MA: Clark University Press.

Allport GW (1985) The historical background to social psychology. In G Lindzey, E Aronson (eds) The Handbook of Social Psychology. New York: Random House.

Archer J (1992) Ethology and Human Development. London: Harvester Wheatsheaf.

Argyle M (1994) The Psychology of Interpersonal Behaviour. Harmondsworth: Penguin.

Argyle M, Ingham R (1972) Gaze, mutual gaze and distance. Semiotica 6: 32–49.

Asch SE (1952) Social Psychology. Englewood Cliffs NJ: Prentice-Hall.

Averill JR (1982) Anger and Aggression. New York: Springer-Verlag.

Bales R (1953) The equilibrium problem in small groups. In T Parsons, RF Bales, EA Shils (eds) Working Papers in the Theory of Action. Glencoe: Free Press.

Bandura A (1973) Aggression: A Social Learning Analysis. Englewood Cliffs NJ: Prentice-Hall.

Bandura A (1986) Social Foundations of Thought and Action: A Social Cognitive Theory. Englewood Cliffs NJ: Prentice-Hall.

Baron RA, Richardson DR (1994) Human Aggression. New York: Plenum Press.

Bar-Tal D (1976) Prosocial Behavior: Theory and Research. Washington DC: Hemisphere.

Bass BM (1981) Stogdill's Handbook of Leadership. New York: Free Press.

Batson CD (1991) The Altruism Question: Toward a Social Psychology Answer. Hillsdale NJ: Erlbaum.

Bem DJ (1972) Self perception theory. In L Berkowitz (ed.) Advances in Experimental Social Psychology 6. New York: Oxford University Press, pp. 1–62.

Berkowitz L (1968) Impulse, aggression and the gun. Psychology Today 2(4): 18–22.

Berkowitz L (1969) The frustration-aggression hypothesis revisited. In L Berkowitz (ed.) Roots of Aggression. New York: Artherton Press.

Berkotwitz L (1972) Social norms, feelings and other factors affecting helping and altruism. In L Berkowitz (ed.) Advances in Experimental Social Psychology 6. New York: Oxford University Press, pp. 63–108.

Berkowitz L (1989) Frustration-aggression hypothesis: examination and reformulation. Psychological Bulletin 106: 59–73.

Blau PM (1964) Exchange and Power in Social Life. New York: John Wiley & Sons.

Bowlby J (1969) Attachment and Loss (vol 1: Attachment). Harmondsworth: Penguin.

Breuer J, Freud S (1895/1982) Studies in Hysteria. New York: Basic Books.

Brislin R (1993) Understanding Culture's Influence on Behaviour. Orlando: Harcourt Brace Jovanovich.

Buss AH (1966) Instrumentality of aggression, feedback and frustration as determinants of physical aggression. Journal of Personality and Social Psychology 3: 153–62.

Cardwell MC (1996) The Complete A–Z of Psychology. London: Hodder & Stoughton.

Clarke D (1996) Social cognition. In MC Cardwell, L Clark, C Meldrum (eds) Psychology for A-level. London: Collins.

Clarke D, Meldrum C (1996) Social influence. In MC Cardwell, L Clark, C Meldrum (eds) Psychology for A-level. London: Collins Educational.

Clary EG, Snyder M (1991) A functional analysis of altruism and prosocial behavior. In MS Clark (ed.) Prosocial Behavior. Newbury Park: Sage.

Cook M (1971) Interpersonal Perception. Harmondsworth: Penguin.

Coolican H (1998) Thinking about prejudice. Psychology Review 4(2): 26–9.

Cumberbatch G (1994) Legislating mythology: video violence and children. Journal of Mental Health 3: 485–94.

Cumberbatch G (1995) Media Violence: Research Evidence and Policy Implications. Strasbourg: Council of Europe.

Cumberbatch G, Howitt D (1989) A Measure of Uncertainty: The Effects of the Mass Media. London and Paris: John Libbey.

Darwin C (1872) The Expression of Emotions in Man and Animals. London: John Murray.

Dawkins R (1976) The Selfish Gene. Oxford: Oxford University Press.

DiLalla LF, Gottsman II (1989) Heterogeneity of causes for delinquency and criminality: lifespan perspectives. Development and Psychopathology 1: 339–49.

Dobson CB, Hardy S, Heyes S, Humphreys A, Humphreys P (1981) Understanding Psychology. London: Weidenfeld and Nicolson.

Dollard J, Doob LW, Miller NE, Mourer OH, Sears RH (1939) Frustration and Aggression. New Haven CT: Yale University Press.

Eagle AH, Chaiken S (1993) The Psychology of Attitudes. Fort Worth TX: Harcourt Brace Jovanovich.

Fazio RH (1995) Attitudes as object-evaluation associations. In RE Petty, JA Krosnick (eds) Attitude Strength: Antecedents and Consequences. Hillsdale NJ: Erlbaum.

Festinger L (1957) A Theory of Cognitive Dissonance. Stanford CA: Stanford University Press.

Festinger L and Carlsmith JM (1959) Cognitive consequences of forced compliance. Journal of Abnormal and Social Psychology 47: 203–10.

Fiedler FE (1967) A Theory of Leadership Effectiveness. New York: McGraw-Hill.

Fishbein M, Ajzen I (1975) Beliefs Attitudes Intention and Behaviour: An Introduction to Theory and Research. Reading MA: Addison-Wesley.

Freedman JL (1984) Effects of television violence on aggression. Psychological Bulletin 96 (2): 227–46.

Gadow KD, Sprafkin J (1993) Television violence and children with emotional and behavioral disorders. Journal of Emotional and Behavioral Disorders 1(1): 54–63.

Geen RG (1990) Human Aggression. Milton Keynes: Open University Press.

Gergen KJ, Gergen MM, Barton W (1973) Deviance in the dark. Psychology Today 7: 129–30.

Gouldner AW (1960) The norm of reciprocity: a preliminary statement. American Psychological Review 25: 161–78.

Greenwald AG (1968) Cognitive learning cognitive response to persuasion and attitude change. In AG Greenwald, TC Brock, TM Ostrom (eds) Psychological Foundations of Attitudes. New York: Academic Press.

Gross RD (1996) Psychology: The Science of Mind and Behaviour. London: Hodder & Stoughton.

Gross RD, Humphreys PW, Petkova B (1997) Challenges in Psychology. London: Hodder & Stoughton.

Hagell A, Newburn T (1994) Young Offenders and the Media. London: Batisford.

Hall ET (1966) The Hidden Dimension. New York: Doubleday.

Heider F (1958) The Psychology of Interpersonal Relations. New York: John Wiley & Sons.

Hoffman ML (1981) The development of empathy. In P Rushton and RM Sorrentino (eds) Altruism and Helping Behavior. Hillsdale NJ: Erlbaum.

Hogg MA, Vaughan GM (1995) Social Psychology: An Introduction. Hemel Hempstead: Prentice-Hall/Harvester Wheatsheaf.

Hollin CR, Trower P (eds) (1986) Handbook of Social Skills Training. Oxford: Pergamon Press.

Homans GC (1974) Social Behaviour. New York: Harcourt Brace Jovanovich.

House RJ (1971) A path–goal model of leader effectiveness. Administrative Science Quarterly 16: 321–38.

Hovland CI, Sears RR (1940) Minor studies in aggesssion VI: correlation of lynchings with economic indicators. Journal of Psychology 9: 301–10.

Hovland C, Lumsdaine AA, Sheffield FD (1949) Experiments in Mass Communications. Princeton NJ: Princeton University Press.

Howitt D, Cumberbatch G (1975) Mass Media Violence and Society. London: Elek.

Huesman LR, Eron LD (1986) Television and the Aggressive Child: A Cross National Survey. Hillsdale NJ: Erlbaum.

Humphreys PW (1994) Obedience after Milgram. Psychology Review 1(1): 2–5.

James W (1890) Principles of Psychology. New York: Holt.

Jones EE, Davis EE (1965) From acts to dispositions: the attribution process in person perception. In L Berkowitz (ed.) Advances in Experimental Social Psychology 2. New York: Academic Press.

Jourard SM (1966) An exploratory study of body-accessibility. British Journal of Social and Clinical Psychology 5: 221–31.

Katz D (1960) The functional approach to the study of attitudes. Public Opinion Quarterly 24: 163–204.

Kelley HH (1967) Attribution Theory in Social Psychology. In D Levine (ed.) Nebraska Symposium on Motivation 15. Lincoln: Nebraska University Press.

Kniveton BH, Stephenson GM (1973) The effect of pre-experience on imitation of an aggressive film model. British Journal of Social and Clinical Psychology 9: 31–6.

Kretch D, Crutchfield RS, Ballachey EL (1962) The Individual in Society. New York: McGraw-Hill.

LaPierre RT (1934) Attitudes – vs – action. Social Forces 13: 230–7.

Latane B, Darley JM (1970) The Unresponsive Bystander: Why Doesn't He Help? New York: Appleton Century Crofts.

Le Bon G (1895) The Crowd: A Study of the Popular Mind. London: Fisher Unwin.

Lewin K, Lippitt R, White R (1939) Patterns of aggressive behaviour in experimentally created social climates. Journal of Social Psychology 10: 271–99.

Lewis M, Brooks-Gunn J (1979) Social cognition and the acquisition of self attitudes. American Sociological Review 19: 68–76.

Likert R (1932) A technique for the measurement of attitudes. Archives of Psychology 140: 1–55.

Lippa RA (1994) Introduction to Social Psychology. Pacific Grove CA: Brooks-Cole.

Lippman W (1922) Public Opinion. New York: Harcourt.

Loeber R, Hay DF (1994) Developmental approaches to aggression and conduct problems. In M Rutter and DH Hay (eds) Development Through Life: A Handbook for Clinicians. Oxford: Blackwell Scientific.

Lorenz K (1966) On Aggression. New York: Harcourt Brace and World.

Maccoby EE, Jacklin CN (1980) Sex differences in aggression: a rejoinder and reprise. Child Development 51: 964–80.

McIlveen R (1998) Collective behaviour. Psychology Review 4(4): 12–15.

Marsh P, Harre R, Rosser E (1978) The Rules of Disorder. London: Routledge & Kegan Paul.

Miell D (1990) The self and the social world. In I Roth (ed.) Introduction to Psychology. Hove: LEA and Open University Press.

Milgram S (1963) Behavioral study of obedience. Journal of Abnormal and Social Psychology 67: 391–8.

Miller NE (1941) The frustration-aggression hypothesis. Psychology Review 48: 337–42.

Moghaddam FM, Taylor DM, Wright SC (1993) Social Psychology in Cross-Cultural Perspective. New York: WH Freeman.

Montagu A (1976) The Nature of Human Aggression. New York: Oxford University Press.

Moscovici S (1965) The Age of the Crowd: A Historical Treatise on Mass Psychology. Cambridge: Cambridge University Press.

Nisbett RE, Ross L (1980) Human Inference: Strategies and Shortcomings of Social Judgement. Englewood Cliffs NJ: Prentice-Hall.

Osgood CE, Suci CJ, Tannenbaum PH (1957) The Measurement of Meaning. Urbana IL: University of Illinois Press.

Patterson GR (1982) Coercive Family Process. Eugene OR: Castallia Press.

Patterson GR, Dishion TJ, Bank L (1984) Family interactions: a process model of deviancy training. Aggressive Behavior 10: 253–67.

Pennington D (1999) Psychology Review 5(4) (In press).

Pettigrew TF, Meertens RW (1995) Subtle and blatant prejudice in Western Europe. European Journal of Social Psychology 25: 57–75.

Petty RE, Cacciopo JT (1986) Communication and Persuasion: Central and Peripheral Routes to Attitude Change. New York: Springer-Verlag.

Pfeffer J (1977) The ambiguity of leadership. Academy of Management Review 2: 104–12.

Raven BH (1993) The bases of power: origins and recent developments. Journal of Social Issues 49: 227–51.

Reicher SD (1984) St Pauls: a study in the limits of crowd behaviour. In J Murphy, M John, H Brown (eds) Dialogues and Debates in Social Psychology. London: LEA.

Reid T (1764) Inquiry into the human mind and the principles of common sense. In The Works of Thomas Reid. Edinburgh: McLachlan & Stewart.

Rice RW (1978) Construct validity of the esteem for least preferred co-worker (LPC) scale. Psychological Bulletin 85: 1199–237.

Robins LN, Tipp J, Przybeck T (1991) Antisocial personality. In LN Robins, DA Regier (eds) Psyciatric Disorders in America: The Epidemiological Catchment Area Study. New York: Tree Press.

Rowe DC (1983) Biometrical genetic models of self-reported delinquent behavior: a twin study. Behavior Genetics 13: 473–89.

Rubin Z (1973) Liking and Loving. New York: Holt, Rinehart & Winston.

Secord PF, Backman CW (1964) Social Psychology. New York: McGraw-Hill.

Sherif M (1935) A study of social factors in perception. Archives of Psychology 27.

Smith DJ (1995) Youth crime and conduct disorders: trends patterns and causal explanations. In M Rutter, DJ Smith (eds) Psychosocial Disorders in Young People: Time Trends and their Causes. Chichester: Wiley.

Smither RD (1988) The Psychology of Work and Human Performance. New York: Harper & Row.

Spranger E (1928) Types of Men. Tübingen: Niemeyer.

Staub E (1991) The Roots of Evil: The Origins of Genocide and other Group Violence. Cambridge MA: Cambridge University Press.

Taguiri R (1969) Perception. In G Lindzey, E Aronson (eds) Handbook of Psychology (Vol 2). Reading MA: Addison-Wesley.

Tajfel H, Turner JC (1986) The social identity theory of group behavior. In S Worchel, W Austin (eds) Psychology of Intergroup Relations. Chicago: Nelson Hall.

Thibaut JW, Kelley HH (1959) The Social Psychology of Groups. New York: Wiley.

Thigpen CH, Cleckley H (1957) The Three Faces of Eve. New York: McGraw-Hill.

Thomas WI, Znaniecki F (1918) The Polish Peasant in Europe and America. Boston MA: Badger.

Thurstone LL (1928) Attitudes can be measured. American Journal of Sociology 33: 529–44.

Trevarthen C (1980) The foundations of intersubjectivity: development of interpersonal and cooperative understanding in infants. In DR Olson (ed.) The Social Foundations of Language and Thought. New York: Norton.

Walters RH, Brown M (1963) Studies of the reinforcement of aggression. Child Development 34: 563–71.

Wicker AW (1969) Attitudes – vs – actions: the relationship between verbal and overt behavioral responses to attitude objects. Journal of Social Issues 25(4): 41–78.

Wrightman LS (1974) Assumptions about Human Nature: A Social Psychological Approach. Monterey CA: Brooks-Cole.

Yukl GA (1989) Leadership in Organisations. Englewood Cliffs NJ: Prentice-Hall.

Zillman D (1978) Attribution and Misattribution of Excitatory Reactions. In J Harvey, W Ickes, RF Kidd (eds) New Directions in Attribution Research 2: Hillsdale NJ: Erlbaum, pp. 335–68.

Zillman D (1991) Television viewing and physiological arousal. In J Bryant, D Zillman (eds) Responding to the Screen: Reception and Reaction Processes Hillsdale NJ: Erlbaum.

Zillman D, Johnson R (1973) Motivated aggressiveness perpetrated by exposure to aggressive films and reduced by non-aggressive films. Journal of Research in Personality 7: 261–76.

Zimbardo PG (1969) The human choice: individuation reason and order versus impulse and chaos. In WJ Arnold, D Levine (eds) Nebraska Symposium on Motivation. Lincoln: University of Nebraska Press.

Index